Brain Tumors: A Practical Guide to Diagnosis and Treatment

Brain Tumors: A Practical Guide to Diagnosis and Treatment

Editor: Maxton Johnson

MURPHY & MOORE
www.murphy-moorepublishing.com

www.murphy-moorepublishing.com

MURPHY & MOORE

Cataloging-in-Publication Data

Brain tumors : a practical guide to diagnosis and treatment / edited by Maxton Johnson.
p. cm.
Includes bibliographical references and index.
ISBN 978-1-63987-083-7
1. Brain--Tumors. 2. Brain--Tumors--Diagnosis. 3. Brain--Tumors--Treatment. I. Johnson, Maxton.
RD663 .B73 2022
616.994 810 59--dc23

Murphy & Moore Publishing,
1 Rockefeller Plaza,
New York City, NY 10020, USA

ISBN 978-1-63987-083-7 (Hardback)

Contents

Preface

The collection of abnormal cells in the brain is termed as a brain tumor. It causes pressure to develop within the skull, which in turn causes damage to the brain. Brain tumors can be classified as primary or secondary tumors. The primary tumors can be either cancerous or non-cancerous. The primary tumor originates in the brain while secondary tumors spread to the brain from another organ. The secondary tumors are always cancerous in nature. Some of the common symptoms of brain tumors are headaches, confusion, clumsiness and memory loss. They can be diagnosed through physical exam and imaging tests such as CT scan of the head. Tumors are generally treated through surgery. This book includes some of the vital pieces of work being conducted across the world, on various topics related to the diagnosis and treatment of brain tumors. It presents researches and studies performed by experts across the globe. The extensive content of this book provides the readers with a thorough understanding of the subject.

After months of intensive research and writing, this book is the end result of all who devoted their time and efforts in the initiation and progress of this book. It will surely be a source of reference in enhancing the required knowledge of the new developments in the area. During the course of developing this book, certain measures such as accuracy, authenticity and research focused analytical studies were given preference in order to produce a comprehensive book in the area of study.

This book would not have been possible without the efforts of the authors and the publisher. I extend my sincere thanks to them. Secondly, I express my gratitude to my family and well-wishers. And most importantly, I thank my students for constantly expressing their willingness and curiosity in enhancing their knowledge in the field, which encourages me to take up further research projects for the advancement of the area.

Editor

1

Critical Molecular and Genetic Markers in Primary Brain Tumors with their Clinical Importance

Ilhan Yaylim, Sumeyya Azam,
Ammad Ahmad Farooqi, Özlem Küçükhüseyin,
Muhammad Ismail and Ali Metin Kafadar

Abstract

Classification of primary brain tumors is based mainly on histopathological characteristics. Due to the peculiarity of the central nervous system (CNS), the location of the tumor is also used in the naming of the CNS tumors. These features, histopathology, and location determine the main prognostic factors in these tumors. Updated molecular and genetic findings in the last two decades accumulated vast amount of knowledge about the biological behavior, response to the treatment, and consequently the prognosis of CNS tumors. After the clinical use of these data, a recent classification is proposed by the International Society of Neuropathology named as "integrated diagnosis."

This classification considers the histopathological classification, World Health Organization (WHO) grade along with the molecular information. The emerging molecular-genetic data about the CNS tumors will allow the translational researchers to deliberately understand the oncogenic mechanisms involved in the evolution of these tumors and judge the optional treatment strategies.

Evaluating the check points of cell cycle and apoptosis provides valuable information about the tumor biology (tumorigenesis). These mechanisms (pathways) also play an exclusive role in CNS tumors. Knowledge concerning the gene repressors and gene activators or some epigenetic changes in proliferative and antiproliferative pathways that regarded gliomas may yield new individualized treatment options.

In this chapter, we will review the basic and translational research molecular-genetic data of gliomas with special interest on proliferative and antiproliferative pathways. Further emerging treatment options and treatment responses in gliomas will be critically evaluated with regard to their histopathology, anatomical location, and molecular-genetic fingerprints.

Keywords: gliomas, proliferation, apoptosis, cell cycle, gene

1. Introduction

Primary brain tumors are a distinct group of pathologies due to their location, low incidence compared to other human tumors, histopathologic diversities, and unexpected response to treatment methods mainly caused by their peculiar genetic and molecular characteristics. Evaluating new important biomarkers which affect the etiopathogenesis of brain tumors may also help clinicians in consulting patients about prognosis, potential clinical studies, and following response to the treatment strategies [1]. Nowadays, the value of early detection of various types of cancer before metastasis has become a very significant issue. This approach may increase life expectancy and the quality of life in these patients [2]. It is known that one of the best management strategies of cancer is to predict its prognosis and response to the updated therapeutic procedures. In order to achieve this, it is significant to consider the blood, serum, plasma, or tissue biomarkers. Although the value of liquid biopsy in different human tumors is established, there is a lack of data regarding primary brain tumors [3]. Confluence of information suggested that genetic, epigenetic, functional or compositional heterogeneity of diseased and healthy tissues presented a major challenge to strategies to improve clinical outcome. [4]. Many molecules found in various fluids, tissues, and cell lines are produced either by the tumor itself, other tissues, or tumor microenvironment, in response to the presence of cancer or other associated conditions including inflammation. The scientists study on cancer search for proper candidate tumor markers and for identifying patients who face different diagnosis or clinical stages of cancer. This type of biomarkers must have some characteristics which can be used to estimate tumor volume, determine response to treatment, and assess disease recurrence through monitoring. Recent advancements have shown that amplifications/translocations, genetic mutations and changes in microarray-generated profiles (genetic signatures) are contributory in cancer development, metastasis and development of resistance against different therapeutics. These genetic signatures are referred according to the type of tumor marker or profile and may be associated with clinical outcomes or good prognosis or enhanced quality of life [3,4]. An ideal tumor marker is described as easily measurable, reliable, and cost-effective by use of an assay with high analytical sensitivity and specificity. Although we have developed a deeper understanding of the underlying mechanisms, there are only a few markers which have been used in routine applications and only a limited number of them can be used to identify patients or monitor progression of cancer types and clinical staging.

Gene overexpression is described as increase in copy number of genes or chromosomes (i.e., gene amplification) through increased transcriptional activity. It is known that imbalance between the gene repressors and gene activators or some epigenetic changes as DNA methylation or chromosomal translocations can alter transcriptional activity of the gene [3,4].

2. Defined molecular markers which changed our clinical attitude

The use of biomarkers in glioblastoma (GBM) has been evaluated in a recent survey by neuro-oncologists [5]. Current evidences indicate that MGMT, EGFR, 1p/19q, EGFR, p53, phosphatase and tensin homolog (PTEN) mutation or deletion, EGFRvIII, IDH1/2, PDGFR, and PIK3CA are the most commonly used markers. But, use of these biomarkers claimed to be prognostic in GBM cases is still debated. There exist significantly varying clinical representations and cases of GBM, and the structure of the signaling molecules is highly complex, and therefore, use of these markers is not very common as of now. In addition, glioblastoma, still a heterogeneous disease, also possesses additional difficulties such as having limited biomarkers to diagnosis and monitoring and therapeutic options, having poorly understood pathogenesis, and requiring individualized treatments. On the other hand, the discovery of new biomarkers together with currently used markers can enable us to better stratify patients regarding treatment paradigms and clinical trials (**Figure 1**) [6,7].

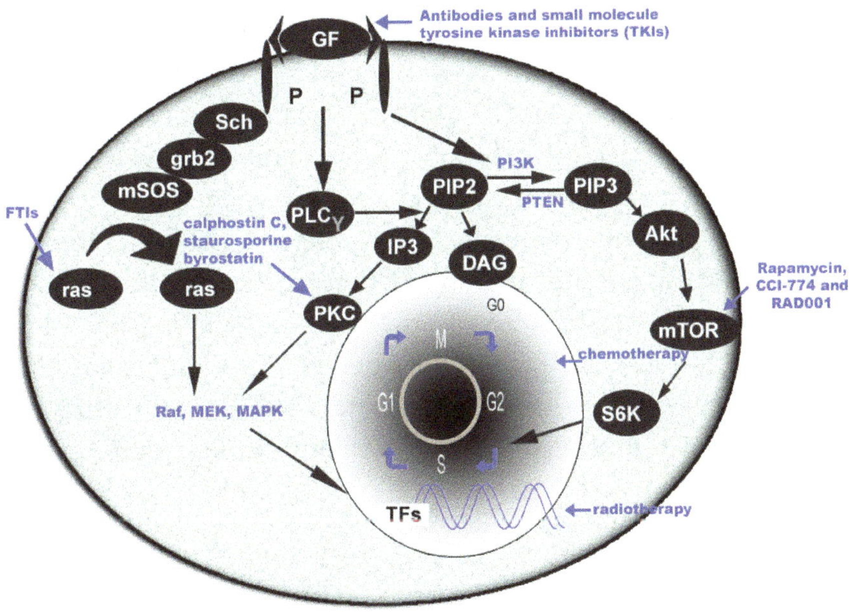

Figure 1. Some signaling pathways with therapeutic implications in gliomas [7]. Some abbreviations are shown below. EGF: epidermal growth factor; PIP2, phosphatidylinositol phosphate-2; PIP3, phosphatidylinositol phosphate-2; PKC, protein kinase C; Grb2, growth factor receptor-bound protein-2; VEGF, vascular endothelial growth factor; S6K, p70 S6 kinase; mTOR, mammalian target of rapamycin; TF, transcription factors; SOS, son of sevenless molecule.

3. Proliferative and antiproliferative pathways and their roles in gliomas

As more and more detailed studies into intracellular signaling cascades and modulators that regulate these pathways are published, intricacy of the fine-balance between celluar survival and death is revealed. A revolution in the signaling cascades has provided near complete resolution of how physiologically important signaling proteins interact with extracellular cues to trigger proliferation. More detailed understanding of the regulatory and activation processes of uncontrolled cellular proliferation is proving to be a key in identification of newer approaches to improve the efficacy of existing therapeutics. The homeostasis of mitogenic signaling is tactfully controlled by multiple mechanisms. The past several years have seen a dramatic leap in our understanding of how Receptor tyrosine kinase (RTK) mediated signaling is rewired during tumorigenesis to support the transformed phenotype. Activation of RTK results in receptor dimerization and autophosphorylation. More importantly, docking sites are created for different adaptor protein complexes such as Grb2/SOS. Mutant Ras is reportedly involved in 50% of all human tumors. There are direct pieces of evidence emphasizing on role of mutant Ras in gliomas. High Ras-GTP levels in advanced astrocytomas have been reported [8, 9].

Epidermal growth factor receptor (EGFR), coded as a cell-surface-bound receptor, is another important molecule involved in cell proliferation with potential effects on clinical prognosis of GBM. It is known that approximately <10% of secondary GBMs and 50% of primary GBMs have EGFR mutations [10]. The presence of EGFR variant III mutation (EGFRvIII) is known to upregulate mitogenic signaling pathways. There is a deletion of the regulator N-terminal domain (▪ 6–273) of EGFR in this pattern of EGFR. About 10–60% of the patients with GBM have EGFRvIII which can be detected in the peripheral blood of brain tumors. The detection of this mutation in brain cancer patients has great importance for anti-EGFRvIII therapies and patients can be monitored to track their response to these therapies [11,12]. Better and deeper knowledge of mechanistic insights that cause EGFR heterogeneity in GBM will prove to be helpful in identification of drugs with maximum efficacy. *EGFRvIII* mutation to identify patients for treatments such as erlotinib therapy for non-small cell lung cancer or RNA-directed treatments and vaccine therapies [13]. As of now, we still have a limited knowledge about downstream signaling pathways for EGFR and whether *EGFR* mutations affect these downstream signaling pathways, such as AKT, MAPK, and STAT3. On the other hand, it has been suggested that the clinical utility of this biomarker and its use for targeted treatment are complicated [1].

Platelet-derived growth factor receptor (PDGFR), a cell-surface tyrosine kinase, plays role in GBM proliferation and stem cell renewal. There are multiple isoforms of PDGFR, mutated in up to 30% of GBMs. One of them, the most significant one regarding GBM, is PDGFRA. The other isoform is also PDGFRAD (with a deletion of exons 8 and 9), seen in 40% of GBMs, and leads to constitutive activation [14,15]. According to the Cancer Genome Atlas, PDGFRA has a crucial role in the proneural subtype of GBM; however, no changes were observed in prognosis of the evaluated patients [16].

The phosphatidylinositol 3-kinase (PI3K)/AKT (PI3K/AKT) pathway is known as a crucial intracellular signaling pathway, taking role in regulating cell proliferation, migration, quiescence, proliferation, cancer, and longevity [17]. PI3K is an enzyme which phosphorylates phosphatidylinositol-4,5-bisphosphate (PIP2) to phosphatidylinositol-3,4,5-trisphosphate (PIP3) at the cell inner membrane. This activation process leads to recruit and upregulate various downstream pathways including AKT, a molecule localized in the plasma membrane [18].

Phosphatase and tensin homolog (PTEN) is known as a natural inhibitor of PI3K/AKT pathway. It has been shown to inhibit transduction of signals to downstream effectors via dephosphorylation of PIP_3 to PIP_2 [19]. It has been reported that an increased PI3K/Akt/mTOR signaling is seen in ~88% of all glioblastomas [20,21]. All of these biological pathways has been related to genetic alterations of key regulatory molecules involved in mitogenic signaling in RTKs and also in the PI3K-PTEN-Akt signaling axis.

Some regulatory and effector molecules play important role in classical cell death networks of both extrinsic (death receptor-mediated) and intrinsic (mitochondria-dependent) apoptosis signaling pathways [22]. Since the discovery of TNF (Tumor Necrosis Factor) family members, a new milestone in apoptosis-inducing cancer therapies has emerged. TRAIL (tumor necrosis factor-related apoptosis-inducing ligand) is a protein reportedly involved in selective killing of cancer cells while leaving normal cells intact. The major biological role of this 281-amino acid-type II transmembrane protein is apoptosis induction after interacting with its receptors to trigger extrinsically and intrinsically controlled pathways. Four different homologous human TRAIL receptors have been categorized into TRAIL-R1/DR4, TRAIL-R2/DR5 also known as Killer, TRAIL-R3 or DcR1, and TRAIL-R4 or DcR2. Substantial fraction of information has been added into the existing pool of knowledge related to TRAIL biology and known that different cancers are resistant to TRAIL-based therapeutics. Mechanistically it has been shown that downregulation of death receptors considerably impaired TRAIL-induced apoptosis in cancer cells. In the upcoming section, we briefly summarize advancements in our understanding related to the underlying mechanisms of resistance against TRAIL-induced apoptosis. We also discuss how TRAIL has shown as a potent anticancer agent in xenografted mice. Natural products have also added more options in the armory against brain tumor. Detailed mechanistic insights have provided a near complete resolution of protein network TRAIL-resistant glioblastoma and increasingly it is being realized that imbalance of stoichiometric ratios of proapoptotic and antiapoptotic proteins modulates response of cancer cells to TRAIL. Previously, it has been convincingly revealed that Znf domain of A20 E3 ligase ubiquitinated RIP1 through a K63-linked polyUB chain that structurally interacted with p18 domain of caspase-8 and blocked its dimerization and cleavage. Functionally inactive caspase-8 was unable to proteolytically process downstream effectors that resulted in impairment of TRAIL-induced apoptosis in glioblastoma [23]. Adeno-associated virus (AAV) vectors are being used to efficiently deliver secreted, soluble TRAIL in different preclinical studies. Additionally, these are also used in combination with TRAIL-sensitizing cardiac glycoside, lanatoside C (lan C). Tumor growth was considerably reduced in intracranial U87 tumor-bearing mice treated with AAV-sTRAIL and lanatoside C [24]. Mesenchymal stem cells (MSCs) have the ability to migrate toward intracranial glioma xenografts. Experimentally verified data indicated that MSCs expressing firefly luciferase (fluc) injected into the left hemisphere migrated rapidly toward right, tumor-bearing region of the brain. Results revealed that 11% of implanted MSCs were noted to be localized in right hemisphere within 2 hours after MSC inoculation. Coculture of GBM43 and U87 glioma cells with MSCs-TRAIL displayed notable rise in caspase-3 activity. Survival rate of tumor-bearing mice was enhanced intranasally delivered with MSCs-TRAIL [25]. Carbenoxolone (CBX), a derivative of 18-glycyrrhetinic acid, has been shown to effectively enhance killing activity of TRAIL-expressing MSCs. CBX considerably upregulated cell-surface expression of DR5 in CBX-treated ΔGli36 and U87MG cells. CBX also inhibited gap junction (GJ) communication via modulation of connexin (Cx43). CBX remarkably reduced expression levels of Cx43 in U87MG and ΔGli36 cells after 72 hours. Results revealed that TRAIL-induced apoptosis was markedly higher in cells transfected with Cx43-siRNA [26] .

Antibody-based anticancer therapies have attracted considerable attention and different structural variations are being tested for efficacies which involve smaller antibody fragments such as ScFvs, Fabs, and nanobodies. Single-chain Fv fragment (scFv) consists of a variable light-chain (VL) and variable heavy-chain (VH) domains, which contains whole antigen-binding site.

Multidrug resistance protein 3 (MRP3) is frequently overexpressed in glioblastoma multiforme cells. scFvM58-sTRAIL is an engineered protein formed by fusion of MRP3-specific scFv antibody M58 with N-terminus of soluble TRAIL. scFvM58-sTRAIL was effective against MRP3-positive GBM cells. Expectedly, scFvM58-sTRAIL did not show significant activity against MRP3-negative Jurkat cells. These results indicated that scFvM58-sTRAIL was effective against MRP3-positive cancer cells [27].

Various bivalent EGFR-targeting nanobodies (ENbs) have been designed and noted to be effective. Neural stem cells (NSC) are potent agents to deliver ENbs. Preclinical study revealed that tumor regression was significantly higher in xenografted mice treated with NSC-ENb2-TRAIL. Xenografted mice survived for 51 days upon treatment with control NSC-ENb2 and 80% of mice survived for 80 days after treatment with NSC-ENb2-TRAIL. These findings indicated that tumoritropic NSC-releasing ENb2 inhibited growth of glioblastoma and effectiveness of ENb2-based therapy was markedly improved by NSC-releasing ENb2-TRAIL [28].

Diethylamino-curcumin mimics with substituted triazolyl groups have previously been synthesized and reported to effectively sensitize resistant CRT-MG astroglioma cells to TRAIL [29].

Gingerol, a major bioactive component of ginger, has been shown to trigger expression of DR5 in a p53-dependent manner in U87 glioblastoma cells. Digitoxin (DT), a clinically approved cardiac glycoside, has been observed to overcome resistance against TRAIL in resistant U87MG glioblastoma cells. Digitoxin effectively enhanced DR5 expression on cell surface of resistant cancer cells [30].

4. Natural products mediated targeting of proliferative protein network in glioblastoma

Crude hydromethanolic extracts produced by maceration of *Spartium junceum* flowers and *Onopordum acanthium* leaves were tested for anticancer activity against glioblastoma U-373 cancer cells. *O. acanthium* was effective against glioblastoma cells and induced apoptosis [31] .

Aqueous extract of *Ruta graveolens* L. notably enhanced phosphorylated ERK1/2 and Akt levels in glioma cells. The results indicated that *Ruta graveolens* exerted inhibitory effects via activation of ERK1/2 and Akt-induced signaling pathways [32].

Triterpenoid saponins from *Albizia lebbeck* (L.) showed activity against TG1 and U-87 MG cancer cells with IC_{50} values of 2.10 and 2.24 μM for compound 2 and 3.46 and 1.36 μM for compound 1 [33].

Isocitrate Dehydrogenase 1 and 2 (IDH1/2) are two important enzymes involved in the Krebs cycle and oxidatively decarboxylate isocitrate to produce a-ketoglutarate and CO_2. IDH1 is a cytosolically located protein. IDH2 encodes a mitochondrial protein. Parsons et al. reported that IDH1/2 was mutated in approximately 60–80% of secondary gliomas and 5% of primary gliomas [34]. There are two common IDH mutation (IDH1R132H and IDH2172 mutations) types. It has been reported that these mutations are seen in GBM (>90% samples with IDH1/2 mutation). These mutations lead to increased production of the oncometabolite D-2-hydroxyglutarate. This metabolite has previously been noted to modify DNA methylation patterns in GBM and transcriptional activity of different target genes [35]. *IDH1* mutation may be correlated with several clinical factors such as younger patient age and frontal location. It has also been reported that additional survival benefit (median survival 9.75 years) was achieved from greater tumor resection (<5 cm^3 residual) in *IDH1* mutants, except for wild-type *IDH1*. It has also been suggested that the presence of *IDH1/2* mutation supports increased therapeutic efficacy with chemoradiotherapy and greater resection [1]. When IDH mutations occur, enzymatic activities of some important molecules can be altered. While alpha-ketoglutarate (α-KG) is decreased, produced 2-hydroxyglutarate (2-HG) can inhibit the activity of some enzymes. These enzymes play a significant role in regulating DNA and histone methylation (α-KG-dependent dioxygenase), including histone demethylases and the TET family of 5mC hydroxylases [36–38].

TET proteins are described as a new class of enzymes which can alter the methylation status of the DNA by converting 5-methylcytosine (5mC) to 5-hydroxymethylcytosine (5hmC). The biological function of 5hmC is not clear. It has been suggested that it is an intermediate in DNA demethylation process. 5hmC offers remarkable reduction in human gliomas as compared to normal brain. An inverse relationship has been reported between 5hmC levels and cell proliferation [39,40].

p53 is a very important protein involved in many physiological and pathological process in the regulation of cell viability in terms of cell cycle, apoptosis, cell differentiation, and other mechanisms of cell regulation during exposure to DNA-damaging agents (e.g., ultraviolet radiation, toxins, chemotherapeutic agents) [1]. It has been reported that P53 gene is mutated in 28% of primary GBMs [41]. There are three patterns regarding p53 dysfunction. One is called loss of function. This pattern may describe a lot of endogenous growth inhibitor effects of wild-type p53. The other is gain of function. This means that mutant p53 upregulates a distinct subset of genes from wild-type p53. The last one is dominant-negative effects of p53. It is associated with a tetramer pattern of mutant p53/wild-type p53 and leads to downregulate activity [42]. It is known that some other mechanisms of p53 inactivation include mutations of its modulators including MDM2 inhibitor or deletion of p14ARF [43,44]. Whether there is a correlation between p53 and GBM prognosis is still unclear due to the complexity of the p53 signaling pathway. P53 pathway includes many important regulators and the heterogeneity of p53 mutation types can also affect the p53 molecule. Because of those mentioned, therapies targeting P53 have been limited in this field [42].

The deletion of 1p and 19q, occurring early in tumorigenesis, is known as an important genetic signature. The deletion is seen in 50–70% of patients with low-grade oligodendrogliomas. This can be predictive for the tumor's chemosensitivity to some agents [46,47]. It has been reported that *P190RhoGAP*, localized on 19q13.3, can be one of the candidate genes as a tumor suppressor [48]. A large-scale genomic analysis by array CGH has reported two different patterns about 1p deletion for prognostic factors. One of them is the whole 1p (associated with the deletion of the whole 19q). This may be associated with a good prognosis for oligodendrogliomas. Another is 1p deletion (not associated with 19q loss). This deletion has a negative prognostic value and improves progression-free survival (PFS) and overall survival (OS). It is mostly associated with astrocytomas [49]. It is also related to the response to chemotherapy and radiation in oligodendroglioma. Data obtained from EORTC 26951 and RTOG 9402 trials showed an improvement in OS with the addition of radiation to procarbazine/lomustine/vincristine chemotherapy in anaplastic oligodendroglioma with 1p/19q mutation [50]. There are some studies correlated with these similar findings, In GBM, similar findings have been demonstrated in some studies [51,52], but not in others [53,54]. It has also been reported that codeletion of 1p and 19q is related with *IDH1* mutation and *MGMT* hypermethylation [47,55].

O-6-Methylguanine-DNA-methyltransferase (MGMT) is involved in removal of alkylation at the O6 position of guanine. Hypermethylation of *MGMT* transcriptionally down-regulated its expression. This situation results in impaired repair capability response to chemotherapeutic agents and radiation. Some clinical trials have confirmed the prognostic and predictive roles of *MGMTm* [56]. It has been suggested that patients with *MGMTm* are responsive to chemotherapy. However, *MGMT* status was not distinguished between patients with glioblastoma (GBM) and those with anaplastic astrocytoma (AA) and this restricts interpretation of the study. The European Organisation for Research and Treatment of Cancer (EORTC) 26981/22981 and National Cancer Institute of Canada (NCIC) trials also indicates increased responsiveness to temozolomide for patients with MGMTm [57]. It has been suggested that a standard marker both following prognosis and identifying patients for clinical trials, in which alkylation therapies and/or radiation therapy are applied, may be used for MGMTm [1].

5. Epigenetics in human gliomas with some details

Acetylation of lysine residues is a post-tranlational modification controlled by the opposing action of histone deacetylases (HDACs) and histone acetyl transferases (HATs) [58–60]. Histone methylation may generally occur on the side chains of lysines and arginines, which can alter the activity of effector proteins of the transcriptional machinery [58–60]. It has been reported that some mutations in some regulatory genes such as HDACs (HDAC2 and HDAC9), histone demethylases (JMJD1A and JMJD1B), and histone methyltransferases (SET7, SETD7, MLL, MLL3, and MLL4) have been detected to a large extent in genomic analysis of GBM samples [34]. However, it is still unclear whether histone modifications play significant roles in gliomas and their potential can serve as biomarkers and/or therapeutic targets. Noncoding RNAs are known to play an important role in the epigenetic regulation of gene expression [61,62].

One group of RNAs are described as microRNAs (miRNAs). miRNAs are important regulators for gene expression. miRNAs post-transcriptionally regulate expression of target genes. miRNAs are double-stranded RNA molecules of approximately 22 nucleotides (nt) in length. miRNA binds to specific recognition sequences within the 3′-untranslated region (3′-UTR) of target mRNAs [61–63]. miRNAs are characterized functionally into tumor suppressors and oncogenic miRNAs. Tumor suppressor miRNAs are frequently down-regulated in gliomas as compared to normal brain [64–67]. In contrast, some miRNAs are defined as oncogenes with enhanced expression in glioma such as miR-21, targeting regulators, miR-10b and miR-221, targeting cell cycle inhibitors, miR-30e, and targeting IjBa [68–71]. It has been suggested that there is a link between miRNAs and well-known stem cell-regulating proteins [72]. It has also been reported that miR-17-92 plays a critical role in regulation of glioma stem cell (GSC) differentiation, apoptosis, and proliferation [73]. miR-451 expression reduced notably in cancer cells kept in low glucose conditions. Results revealed that cancer cells kept in low glucose conditions had reduced cell proliferation but an enhanced rate of cell migration and survival in glioblastomas. Glucose sufficiency induced upregulation of miR-451 notably inhibited LKB1/AMPK pathway activation [74]. miR-128, downregulated in glioblastoma tissue, has a tumor-suppressive function. Both in vitro and in vivo, miR-128 expression significantly reduces glioma cell proliferation via downregulation of *Bmi-1 oncogene,* a component of the polycomb repressor complex (PRC). In addition, miR-128 inhibits GSC self-renewal [75]. The PRC has been shown to induce normal and cancer stem cell self-renewal and plays role in GSC regulation [76]. When miR-124 has overexpression, it can inhibit the CD133+ cell subpopulation of the neurosphere and downregulate stem cell markers, such as *BMI1, Nanog,* and *Nestin* [77]. Both miR-124 and miR-137 are up-regulated during adult neural stem cell differentiation and down-regulated in high-grade gliomas [78]. Although there are comprehensive studies about miRNa in gliomas, it should not be forgotten that one miRNA can affect the expression of various target genes. It must be reconsidered in terms of several important aspects before miRNAs may be used therapeutically [79].

LncRNAs which have more than 200 nucleotides and are up to 100 kb in length are described as an important RNA molecule that plays role in some biological cellular actions such as stemness, development, and cell survival [80–82]. Maternally expressed gene 3 (*MEG3*) is a maternally expressed imprinted gene that can also act as an lncRNA. Its expression in glioma tissues is lower than that in normal adjacent tissues [83]. The tumor-suppressive role of *MEG3* is confirmed by the fact that it can associate with p53. It is known that this association is needed for p53 activation [84].

6. Possible relationships between location and genetic signature in primary brain tumors

A unique finding is that the location of certain primary brain tumors determines their genetic characteristics. Cranial base meningiomas are less malignant compared to the non-cranial base meningiomas [85]. The frequencies of grade II and III cranial base and non-cranial base meningiomas are 3.5 and 12.1%, respectively. These findings origin from a clinical-pathological observation. The biological, molecular, and genetic basis of this fact requires further explanation. A simple answer would be the diverse embryological origins of the dura mater in various locations of human skull [86]. A recently published paper showed (utmost) intriguing data about meningioma biology, which is going to help our understanding of this tumor, of which 85–90% is classified as benign (grade I), but has in certain locations an aggressive course. Meningiomas regarding their genetic origin are divided as NF2 and non-NF2 meningiomas. The non-NF2 meningiomas behave clinically different and are generally always benign, with chromosomal stability, and originate from the medial skull base. In contrast to these findings, meningiomas with mutant NF2 and/or chromosome 22 loss are more likely to be atypical and demonstrate genomic instability and are localized to the cerebral and cerebellar hemispheres. This group concludes their study: "Collectively, these findings identify distinct meningioma subtypes, suggesting avenues for targeted therapeutics" [87]. There is a mutational profile of a meningioma, which can be predicted based on its anatomical location in human calvarium. This finding may provide a unique treatment strategy for midline tumors, which may have a response to medical treatment like hedgehog inhibitors. There are treatment-resistant meningiomas, which are surgically unresectable, recurrent, or invasive. In these patients one can reserve surgery or irradiation, bearing in mind that there is an independent risk factor for progression of these generally benign considered primary brain tumors. This location-based molecular and genetic data provides an updated information about prognosis and treatment response of meningiomas. This update research, which is collected over 300 meningiomas, is a valuable finding, regarding designing personalized management strategies for meningiomas.

Another fact about meningioma is that there is a subgroup of meningiomas, which are histopathologically classified as grade I meningioma, but recurs during follow-up in a short distance unexpectedly as grade II and later as grade III meningiomas. Although the malignant progression of gliomas is considerably well defined and researched entity, there is lack of scientific data about meningiomas, regarding which one is going to transform malignantly. Al-Mefty et al. explained this clinical observation with their FISH analysis of primary and recurring meningiomas with malignant progression in their series. They studied 175 recurrent meningiomas and found that 11 tumors showed histopathologically verified progression to a higher grade. In this study, the cytogenetic analysis with FISH showed deletions of 22, 1p, and 14q. The interesting finding was that in all but one case, these aberrations have been shown to be also present in the previous specimen despite their lower histopathological grades [88].

The conclusion of this translational paper from 2004 was defined: "Tumors that present with complex genetic alterations, even those with a benign histopathological grade are potentially aggressive and require closer follow-up." After 12 years this sentence is still valid for meningiomas and other primary brain tumors, which are genetically prone to upgrade. The designated malignant progression of primary brain tumors is an important issue for designing molecular-genetic-based therapeutic approaches in the near future. The finding that oligodendrogliomas show allelic deletions on 19q and 1p has been defined in 1994 by Reifenberger et al. [89]. Clinical relevance and its implication in changing management strategies followed this genetic finding. The chemotherapeutic response and survival in patients with anaplastic oligodendrogliomas were explained with the over-mentioned genetic background [90]. Its relationship with better prognosis and response to chemotherapy is today an established fact and will be considered in the update "integrated-layered" classification of central nervous system tumors after Haarlem consensus [91]. The location of oligodendrogliomas and its relationship with 1p19q deletion further changed our direction in a phylogenetic explanation of primary brain tumor development and coexisting molecular-genetic mechanisms. Frontal location of oligodendroglioma was suggested to be a favorable prognostic factor. The accumulated data clearly demonstrated that frontal location was strongly correlated with 1p19q deletion [92]. Prognostic variables in oligodendroglial tumors: a single-institution study of 95 cases. This translational information eased (helped) to predict the prognosis of these peculiar tumors. The embryological developmental basis of oligodendroglioma and its molecular-genetic relationship are other issues, which require further investigation.

Lucius Annaeus Seneca, known as Seneca the Younger (c. 4 BC–AD 65), stated: "No one can wear a mask for very long." We can further apply this wise quote to our update neuro-oncological approach, which requires redefinition in the coming decades: "No tumor can wear a mask for very long." The molecular-genetic data and determining its relationship with primary brain tumors will further relieve "the mask" of the primary brain tumors. The upcoming new WHO classification of central nervous system tumors will consider this issue.

Author details

Ilhan Yaylim[1], Sumeyya Azam[2], Ammad Ahmad Farooqi[3], Özlem Küçükhüseyin[1], Muhammad Ismail[3] and Ali Metin Kafadar[4*]

*Address all correspondence to: ctfkafadar@gmail.com

1 Institute of Experimental Medicine, Department of Molecular Medicine, Istanbul University, Istanbul, Turkey

2 First Affiliated Hospital of Xinjiang Medical University, Xinjiang, Urumqi, PR China

3 Institute of Biomedical and Genetic Engineering (IBGE), Islamabad, Pakistan

4 Department of Neurosurgery, Cerrahpaşa Medical Faculty, Istanbul University, Istanbul, Turkey

References

[1] Karsy M, Neil JA, Guan J, Mahan MA, Colman H, Jensen RL: A practical review of prognostic correlations of molecular biomarkers in glioblastoma. Neurosurg Focus. 2015;38(3):E4. doi: 10.3171/2015.1.FOCUS14755.

[2] Etzioni R, Urban N, Ramsey S, McIntosh M, Schwartz S, Reid B, Radich J, Anderson G, Hartwell L: The case for early detection. Nat Rev Cancer. 2003;3(4):243–252.

[3] Kulasingam V, Diamandis EP: Strategies for discovering novel cancer biomarkers through utilization of emerging technologies. Nat Clin Pract Oncol. 2008;5:588–599.

[4] Hayes DF, Bast RC, Desch CE, Fritsche H Jr, Kemeny NE, Jessup JM, Locker GY, Macdonald JS, Mennel RG, Norton L, Ravdin P, Taube S, Winn RJ: Tumor marker utility grading system: a framework to evaluate clinical utility of tumor markers. J Natl Cancer Inst. 1996;88(20):1456–1466.

[5] Holdhoff M, Ye X, Blakeley JO, Blair L, Burger PC, Grossman SA, et al: Use of personalized molecular biomarkers in the clinical care of adults with glioblastomas. J Neurooncol. 2012;110:279–285.

[6] Westhoff MA, Karpel-Massler G, Brühl O, Enzenmüller S, La Ferla-Brühl K, Siegelin MD, Nonnenmacher L Debatin KM: A critical evaluation of PI3K inhibition in glioblastoma and neuroblastoma therapy. Mol Cell Ther. 2014;2:32.

[7] Rao RD, James CD: Altered molecular pathways in gliomas: an overview of clinically relevant issues. Semin Oncol. 2004;31(5):595–604

[8] Guha A, Feldkamp MM, Lau N, Boss G, Pawson A: Proliferation of human malignant astrocytomas is dependent on Ras activation. Oncogene. 1997;15:2755–2765.

[9] Pandey V, Bhaskara VK, Babu PP: Implications of mitogen-activated protein kinase signaling in glioma. J Neurosci Res. 2016;94:114–127. doi: 10.1002/jnr.23687.

[10] Wong AJ, Ruppert JM, Bigner SH, Grzeschik CH, Humphrey PA, Bigner DS, et al: Structural alterations of the epidermal growth factor receptor gene in human gliomas. Proc Natl Acad Sci U S A. 1992;89:2965–2969.

[11] Frederick L, Wang XY, Eley G, James CD: Diversity and frequency of epidermal growth factor receptor mutations in human glioblastomas. Cancer Res. 2000;60:1383–1387.

[12] Salkeni MA, Zarzour A, Ansay TY, McPherson CM, Warnick RE, Rixe O, et al: Detection of EGFRvIII mutant DNA in the peripheral blood of brain tumor patients. J Neurooncol. 2013;115:27–35

[13] Taylor TE, Furnari FB, Cavenee WK: Targeting EGFR for treatment of glioblastoma: molecular basis to overcome resistance. Curr Cancer Drug Targets. 2012;12:197–209.

[14] Brennan C, Momota H, Hambardzumyan D, Ozawa T, Tandon A, Pedraza A, et al: Glioblastoma subclasses can be defined by activity among signal transduction pathways and associated genomic alterations. PLoS ONE. 2009;4:e7752.

[15] Ozawa T, Brennan CW, Wang L, Squatrito M, Sasayama T, Nakada M, et al: PDGFRA gene rearrangements are frequent genetic events in PDGFRA-amplified glioblastomas. Genes Dev. 2010;24:2205–2218.

[16] Verhaak RGW, Hoadley KA, Purdom E, Wang V, Qi Y, Wilkerson MD, et al: Integrated genomic analysis identifies clinically relevant subtypes of glioblastoma characterized by abnormalities in PDGFRA, IDH1, EGFR, and NF1. Cancer Cell. 2010;17:98–110.

[17] Sami A, Karsy M: Targeting the PI3K/AKT/mTOR signaling pathway in glioblastoma: novel therapeutic agents and advances in understanding. Tumour Biol. 2013;34:1991–2002.

[18] King D, Yeomanson D, Bryant HE: PI3King the lock: targeting the PI3K/Akt/mTOR pathway as a novel therapeutic strategy in neuroblastoma. J Pediatr Hematol Oncol. 2015;37:245–251.

[19] Rafalski VA, Brunet A: Energy metabolism in adult neural stem cell fate. Prog Neurobiol. 2011;93(2):182–203. doi: 10.1016/j.pneurobio.2010.10.007. PMID 21056618.

[20] Network CGAR: Comprehensive genomic characterization defines human glioblastoma genes and core pathways. Nature. 2008;455:1061–1068.

[21] Fan QW, Weiss WA: Targeting the RTK–PI3K–mTOR axis in malignant glioma: overcoming resistance. Curr Top Microbiol Immunol. 2010;347:279–296.

[22] Lavrik IN, Golks A, and Krammer PH: Caspases: pharmacological manipulation of cell death. J Clin Invest. 2005;115:2665–2672.

[23] Bellail AC, Olson JJ, Yang X, Chen ZJ, Hao C: A20 ubiquitin ligase-mediated polyubiquitination of RIP1 inhibits caspase-8 cleavage and TRAIL-induced apoptosis in glioblastoma. Cancer Discov. 2012;2(2):140–155.

[24] Crommentuijn MH, Maguire CA, Niers JM, Vandertop WP, Badr CE, Würdinger T, Tannous BA: Intracranial AAV–sTRAIL combined with lanatoside C prolongs survival in an orthotopic xenograft mouse model of invasive glioblastoma. Mol Oncol. 2015;11. pii: S1574-7891(15)00226-4.

[25] Balyasnikova IV, Prasol MS, Ferguson SD, Han Y, Ahmed AU, Gutova M, Tobias AL, Mustafi D, Rincón E, Zhang L, Aboody KS, Lesniak MS: Intranasal delivery of mesenchymal stem cells significantly extends survival of irradiated mice with experimental brain tumors. Mol Ther. 2014;22(1):140–148.

[26] Yulyana Y, Endaya BB, Ng WH, Guo CM, Hui KM, Lam PY, Ho IA: Carbenoxolone enhances TRAIL-induced apoptosis through the upregulation of death receptor 5 and

inhibition of gap junction intercellular communication in human glioma. Stem Cells Dev. 2013;22(13):1870–1882.

[27] Wang LH, Ni CW, Lin YZ, Yin L, Jiang CB, Lv CT, Le Y, Lang Y, Zhao CY, Yang K, Jiao BH, Yin J: Targeted induction of apoptosis in glioblastoma multiforme cells by an MRP3-specific TRAIL fusion protein in vitro. Tumour Biol. 2014;35(2):1157–1168.

[28] van de Water JA, Bagci-Onder T, Agarwal AS, Wakimoto H, Roovers RC, Zhu Y, Kasmieh R, Bhere D, Van Bergen en Henegouwen PM, Shah K: Therapeutic stem cells expressing variants of EGFR-specific nanobodies have antitumor effects. Proc Natl Acad Sci U S A. 2012;109(41):16642–16647

[29] Ahn Y, Oh S, Lee SJ, Park BG, Park YS, Shin WS, Jang HJ, Park JH, Kwon D, Lee S: Synthesis of diethylamino-curcumin mimics with substituted triazolyl groups and their sensitization effect of TRAIL against brain cancer cells. Bioorg Med Chem Lett. 2014;24(15):3346–3350.

[30] Lee DH, Lee CS, Kim DW, Ae JE, Lee TH: Digitoxin sensitizes glioma cells to TRAIL-mediated apoptosis by upregulation of death receptor 5 and downregulation of survivin. Anticancer Drugs. 2014;25(1):44–52.

[31] Abusamra YA, Scuruchi M, Habibatni S, Maammeri Z, Benayache S, D'Ascola A, Avenoso A, Campo GM, Spina E: Evaluation of putative cytotoxic activity of crude extracts from *Onopordum acanthium* leaves and Spartium junceum flowers against the U-373 glioblastoma cell line. Pak J Pharm Sci. 2015;28(4):1225–1232.

[32] Gentile MT, Ciniglia C, Reccia MG, Volpicelli F, Gatti M, Thellung S, Florio T, Melone MA, Colucci-D'Amato L: *Ruta graveolens* L. induces death of glioblastoma cells and neural progenitors, but not of neurons, via ERK 1/2 and AKT activation. PLoS One. 2015;10(3):e0118864.

[33] Noté OP, Jihu D, Antheaume C, Zeniou M, Pegnyemb DE, Guillaume D, Chneiwess H, Kilhoffer MC, Lobstein A: Triterpenoid saponins from *Albizia lebbeck* (L.) Benth and their inhibitory effect on the survival of high grade human brain tumor cells. Carbohydr Res. 2015;404:26–33.

[34] Parsons DW, Jones S, Zhang X, Lin JC, Leary RJ, Angenendt P, Mankoo P, Carter H, Siu IM, Gallia GL, Olivi A, McLendon R, Rasheed BA, Keir S, Nikolskaya T, Nikolsky Y, Busam DA, Tekleab H, Diaz LA Jr, Hartigan J, Smith DR, Strausberg RL, Marie SK, Shinjo SM, Yan H, Riggins GJ, Bigner DD, Karchin R,Papadopoulos N, Parmigiani G, Vogelstein B, Velculescu VE, Kinzler KW: An integrated genomic analysis of human glioblastoma multiforme. Science. 2008;321:1807–1812. doi: 10.1126/science.1164382.

[35] Noushmehr H, Weisenberger DJ, Diefes K, Phillips HS, Pujara K, Berman BP, et al: Identification of a CpG island methylator phenotype that defines a distinct subgroup of glioma. Cancer Cell. 2010;17:510–522.

[36] Lu C, Ward PS, Kapoor GS, Rohle D, Turcan S, Abdel-Wahab O, Edwards CR, Khanin R, Figueroa ME, Melnick A, Wellen KE, O'Rourke DM, Berger SL, Chan TA, Levine RL,

Mellinghoff IK, Thompson CB: IDH mutation impairs histone demethylation and results in a block to cell differentiation. Nature. 2012;483:474–478.

[37] Dang L, White DW, Gross S, Bennett BD, Bittinger MA, Driggers EM, Fantin VR, Jang HG, Jin S, Keenan MC, Marks KM, Prins RM, Ward PS, Yen KE, Liau LM, Rabinowitz JD, Cantley LC, Thompson CB, Vander Heiden MG, Su SM: Cancer-associated IDH1 mutations produce 2-hydroxyglutarate. Nature. 2010;465:966.

[38] Xu W, Yang H, Liu Y, Yang Y, Wang P, Kim SH, Ito S, Yang C, Wang P, Xiao MT, Liu LX, Jiang WQ, Liu J, Zhang JY, Wang B, Frye S, Zhang Y, Xu YH, Lei QY, Guan KL, Zhao SM, Xiong Y: Oncometabolite 2-hydroxyglutarate is a competitive inhibitor of alpha-ketoglutarate-dependent dioxygenases. Cancer Cell. 2011;19:17–30.

[39] Jin SG, Jiang Y, Qiu R, Rauch RA, Wang Y, Schackert G, Krex D, Lu Q, Pfeifer GP: 5-Hydroxymethylcytosine is strongly depleted in human cancers but its levels do not correlate with IDH1 mutations. Cancer Res. 2011;71:7360–7365.

[40] Kraus TF, Globisch D, Wagner M, Eigenbrod S, Widmann D, Munzel M, Muller M, Pfaffeneder T, Hackner B, Feiden W, Schuller U, Carell T, Kretzschmar HA: Low values of 5-hydroxymethylcytosine (5hmC), the "sixth base," are associated with anaplasia in human brain tumors. Int J Cancer. 2012, http://dx.doi.org/10.1002/ijc.27429.

[41] Ohgaki H, Kleihues P: Genetic profile of astrocytic and oligodendroglial gliomas. Brain Tumor Pathol. 2011;28:177–183.

[42] England B, Huang T, Karsy M: Current understanding of the role and targeting of tumor suppressor p53 in glioblastoma multiforme. Tumour Biol. 2013;34:2063–2074.

[43] Biernat W, Kleihues P, Yonekawa Y, Ohgaki H: Amplification and overexpression of MDM2 in primary (de novo) glioblastomas. J Neuropathol Exp Neurol. 1997;56:180–185.

[44] Nakamura M, Watanabe T, Klangby U, Asker C, Wiman K, Yonekawa Y, et al: p14ARF deletion and methylation in genetic pathways to glioblastomas. Brain Pathol. 2001;11:159–168.

[45] Blough MD, Beauchamp DC, Westgate MR, Kelly JJ, Cairncross JG: Effect of aberrant p53 function on temozolomide sensitivity of glioma cell lines and brain tumor initiating cells from glioblastoma. J Neurooncol. 2011;102:1–7.

[46] Ino Y, Betensky RA, Zlatescu MC, Sasaki H, Macdonald DR, Stemmer-Rachamimov AO, Ramsay DA, Cairncross JG, Louis DN: Molecular subtypes of anaplastic oligodendroglioma: implications for patient management at diagnosis. Clin Cancer Res. 2001;7:839–845.

[47] Jeuken JW, von Deimling A, Wesseling P: Molecular pathogenesis of oligodendroglial tumors. J Neurooncol. 2004;70:161–181.

[48] Wolf RM, Draghi N, Liang X, Dai C, Uhrbom L, Eklof C, Westermark B, Holland EC, Resh MD: p190RhoGAP can act to inhibit PDGF induced gliomas in mice: a putative

tumor suppressor encoded on human chromosome 19q13.3. Genes Dev. 2003;17:476–487.

[49] Idbaih A, Marie Y, Pierron G, Brennetot C, Hoang-Xuan K, Kujas M, Mokhtari K, Sanson M, Lejeune J, Aurias A, Delattre O, Delattre JY: Two types of chromosome 1p losses with opposite significance in gliomas. Ann Neurol. 2005;58:483– 487.

[50] Cairncross G, Wang M, Shaw E, Jenkins R, Brachman D, Buckner J, et al: Phase III trial of chemoradiotherapy for anaplastic oligodendroglioma: long-term results of RTOG 9402. J Clin Oncol. 2013;31:337–343.

[51] Boots-Sprenger SHE, Sijben A, Rijntjes J, Tops BBJ, Idema AJ, Rivera AL, et al: Significance of complete 1p/19q codeletion, IDH1 mutation and MGMT promoter methylation in gliomas: use with caution. Mod Pathol. 2013;26:922–929.

[52] Schmidt MC, Antweiler S, Urban N, Mueller W, Kuklik A, Meyer-Puttlitz B, et al: Impact of genotype and morphology on the prognosis of glioblastoma. J Neuropathol Exp Neurol. 2002;61:321–328.

[53] Hartmann C, Hentschel B, Simon M, Westphal M, Schackert G, Tonn JC, et al: Long-term survival in primary glioblastoma with versus without isocitrate dehydrogenase mutations. Clin Cancer Res. 2013;19:5146–5157.

[54] Laxton RC, Popov S, Doey L, Jury A, Bhangoo R, Gullan R, et al: Primary glioblastoma with oligodendroglial differentiation has better clinical outcome but no difference in common biological markers compared with other types of glioblastoma. Neuro Oncol. 2013;15:1635–1643.

[55] SongTao Q, Lei Y, Si G, YanQing D, HuiXia H, XueLin Z, et al: IDH mutations predict longer survival and response to temozolomide in secondary glioblastoma. Cancer Sci. 2012;103:269–273.

[56] Wick W, Hartmann C, Engel C, Stoffels M, Felsberg J, Stockhammer F, Sabel MC, Koeppen S, Ketter R, Meyermann R, Rapp M, Meisner C, Kortmann RD,Pietsch T, Wiestler OD, Ernemann U, Bamberg M, Reifenberger G, von Deimling A, Weller M: NOA-04 randomized phase III trial of sequential radiochemotherapy of anaplastic glioma with procarbazine, lomustine, and vincristine or temozolomide. J Clin Oncol. 2009;27(35):5874–5880. doi: 10.1200/JCO.2009.23.6497.

[57] Gorlia T, van den Bent MJ, Hegi ME, Mirimanoff RO, Weller M, Cairncross JG, Eisenhauer E, Belanger K, Brandes AA, Allgeier A, Lacombe D, Stupp R.: Nomograms for predicting survival of patients with newly diagnosed glioblastoma: prognostic factor analysis of EORTC and NCIC trial 26981-22981/CE.3. Lancet Oncol. 2008;9:29–38.

[58] Karlic R, Chung HR, Lasserre J, Vlahovicek K, Vingron M: Histone modification levels are predictive for gene expression. Proc Natl Acad Sci U S A. 2010;107:2926–2931.

[59] Bannister AJ, Kouzarides T: Regulation of chromatin by histone modifications. Cell Res. 2011;21:381–395.

[60] Santos-Rosa H, Schneider R, Bannister AJ, Sherriff J, Bernstein BE, Emre NC, Schreiber SL, Mellor J, Kouzarides T: Active genes are tri-methylated at K4 of histone H3. Nature. 2002;419:407–411.

[61] Costa FF: Non-coding RNAs, epigenetics and complexity. Gene. 2008;410:9–17.

[62] Esteller M: Non-coding RNAs in human disease. Nat Rev Genet. 2011;12:861–874.

[63] Mendell JT: MicroRNAs: critical regulators of development, cellular physiology and malignancy. Cell Cycle. 2005;4:1179–1184.

[64] Li Y, Guessous F, Zhang Y, diPierro C, Kefas B, Johnson E, Marcinkiewicz L, Jiang J, Yang Y, Schmittgen TD, Lopes B, Schiff D, Purow B, Abounader R: MicroRNA-34a inhibits glioblastoma growth by targeting multiple oncogenes. Cancer Res. 2009;69:7569–7576.

[65] Mei J, Bachoo R, Zhang CL: MicroRNA-146a inhibits glioma development by targeting Notch1. Mol Cell Biol. 2011;31:3584–3592.

[66] Kefas B, Godlewski J, Comeau L, Li Y, Abounader R, Hawkinson M, Lee J, Fine H, Chiocca EA, Lawler S, Purow B: MicroRNA-7 inhibits the epidermal growth factor receptor and the Akt pathway and is down-regulated in glioblastoma. Cancer Res. 2008;68:3566–3572.

[67] Zhang QQ, Xu H, Huang MB, Ma LM, Huang QJ, Yao Q, Zhou H, Qu LH: MicroRNA-195 plays a tumor-suppressor role in human glioblastoma cells by targeting signaling pathways involved in cellular proliferation and invasion. Neuro Oncol. 2012;14:278–287.

[68] Gabriely G, Yi M, Narayan RS, Niers JM, Wurdinger T, Imitola J, Ligon KL, Kesari S, Esau C, Stephens RM, Tannous BA, Krichevsky AM: Human glioma growth is controlled by microRNA-10b. Cancer Res. 2011;71;3563–3572.

[69] Gabriely G, Wurdinger T, Kesari S, Esau CC, Burchard J, Linsley PS, Krichevsky AM: MicroRNA 21 promotes glioma invasion by targeting matrix metalloproteinase regulators. Mol Cell Biol. 2008;28:5369–5380.

[70] Jiang L, Lin C, Song L, Wu J, Chen B, Ying Z, Fang L, Yan X, He M, Li J, Li M: MicroRNA-30e_ promotes human glioma cell invasiveness in an orthotopic xenotransplantation model by disrupting the NF-kappaB/IkappaBalpha negative feedback loop. J Clin Invest. 2012;122:33–47.

[71] Zhang CZ, Zhang JX, Zhang AL, Shi ZD, Han L, Jia ZF, Yang WD, Wang GX, Jiang T, You YP, Pu PY, Cheng JQ, Kang CS: MiR-221 and miR-222 target PUMA to induce cell survival in glioblastoma. Mol Cancer. 2010;9;229.

[72] Piccirillo SG, Reynolds BA, Zanetti N, Lamorte G, Binda E, Broggi G, et al: Bone morphogenetic proteins inhibit the tumorigenic potential of human brain tumour-initiating cells. Nature. 2006;444:761–765. doi: 10.1038/nature 05349.

[73] Ernst A, Campos B , Meier J, Devens F, Liesenberg F, Wolter M, et al: De-repression of CTGF via the miR-17-92 cluster upon differentiation of human glioblastoma spheroid cultures. Oncogene. 2010;29:3411–3422. doi: 10.1038/onc.2010.83.

[74] Godlewski J, Nowicki MO, Bronisz A,Nuovo G, Palatini J, DeLay M, et al: MicroRNA-451regulates LKB1/AMPKsignalingandallows adaptation to metabolic stress in glioma cells. Mol Cell. 2010;37:620–632. doi: 10.1016/j.molcel.2010.02.018.

[75] Godlewski J, Nowicki MO, Bronisz A, Williams S, Otsuki A, Nuovo G, et al: Targeting of the Bmi-1 oncogene/stemcell renewal factor by microRNA-128 inhibits glioma proliferation and self-renewal. Cancer Res. 2008;68:9125–9130. doi: 10.1158/0008-5472.CAN-08-2629.

[76] Natsume A, Ito M, Katsushima K,Ohka F, Hatanaka A,Shinjo K, et al: Chromatin regulator PRC2Is a key regulator of epigenetic plasticity in glioblastoma. Cancer Res. 2013;73:4559–4570.

[77] Xia H, Cheung WK, Ng SS, Jiang X, Jiang S, Sze J, et al: Loss of brain-enriched miR-124 microRNA enhances stem-like traits and invasiveness of glioma cells. J Biol Chem. 2012. 287:9962–9971. doi: 10.1074/jbc.M111.332627

[78] Silber J, Lim DA,Petritsch C, Persson AI, Maunakea AK, Yu M, et al: miR-124 and miR-137 inhibit proliferation of glioblastoma multiforme cells and induce differentiation of brain tumor stem cells. BMC Med. 2008;6:14. doi: 10.1186/1741-7015-6-14.

[79] Kreth S, Thon N, Kreth FW: Epigenetics in human gliomas. Cancer Lett. 2014;342:185–192

[80] Mercer TR, Dinger ME, Mattick JS: Long non-coding RNAs: insights into functions. Nat Rev Genet. 2009;10:155–159. doi: 10.1038/nrg2521

[81] Koziol MJ, Rinn JL: RNA traffic control of chromatin complexes. Curr Opin Genet Dev. 2010;20:142–148. doi: 10.1016/j.gde.2010.03.003.

[82] Zhang H, Chen Z, Wang X, Huang Z, He Z, Chen Y. Long non-coding RNA:a new player in cancer. J Hematol Oncol. 2013;6:37. doi: 10.1186/1756-8722-6-37.

[83] Wang P, Ren Z, Sun P: Overexpression of the long non-coding RNA MEG3 impairs in vitro glioma cell proliferation. J Cell Biochem. 2012;113:1868–1874. doi: 10.1002/jcb.24055

[84] Lu KH, Li W, Liu XH, Sun M, Zhang ML, Wu WQ, et al: Long non-coding RNA MEG3 inhibits NSCLC cells proliferation and induces apoptosis by affecting p53 expression. BMC Cancer. 2013;13:461. doi: 10.1186/1471-2407-13-461.

[85] Sade B, Chahlavi A, Krishnaney A, Nagel S, Choi E, Lee JH: World Health Organization grades II and III meningiomas are rare in the cranial base and spine. Neurosurgery. 2007;61:1194–1198.

[86] O'Rahilly R, Muller F: The meninges in human development. J Neuropathol Exp Neurol. 1986;45:588–608.

[87] Clark VE, Erson-Omay EZ, Serin A, Jun Yin J, Cotney J, Ozduman K, et al: Genomic analysis of non-NF2 meningiomas reveals mutations in TRAF7, KLF4, AKT1, and SMO. Science. 2013;339(6123)1077–1080.

[88] Al-Mefty O, Kadri P, Pravdenkova S, Sawyer JR, Stangeby C, Husain M: Malignant progression in meningioma: documentation of a series and analysis of cytogenetic findings. J Neurosurg. 2004;101:210–218.

[89] Reifenberger J, Reifenberger G, Liu L, James CD, Wechsler W, Collins VP: Molecular genetic analysis of oligodendroglial tumors shows preferential allelic deletions on 19q and 1p. Am J Pathol. 1994;145(5):1175–1190.

[90] Cairncross JG, Ueki K, Zlatescu MC, Lisle DK, Finkelstein DM, Hammond RR, Silver JS, Stark PC, Macdonald DR, Ino Y, Ramsay DA, Louis DN: Specific genetic predictors of chemotherapeutic response and survival in patients with anaplastic oligodendrogliomas. J Natl Cancer Inst. 1998;90:1473–1479.

[91] Louis DN, Perry A, Burger P, Ellison DW, Reifenberger G, von Deimling A, Aldape K, Brat D, Collins VP, Eberhart C et al.International society of neuropathology-haarlem consensus guidelines for nervous system tumor classification and grading. Brain Pathol. 2014;24:429–435.

[92] Scheie D, Meling TR, Cvancarova M, Skullerud K, Mørk S, Lote K, Eide TJ, Helseth E, Beiske K. Prognostic variables in oligodendroglial tumors: a single-institution study of 95 cases. Neuro Oncol. 2011;13:1225–1233.

2

Diffuse Intrinsic Pontine Glioma

Santosh Valvi and Nicholas G. Gottardo

Abstract

Diffuse intrinsic pontine glioma (DIPG) is a leading cause of brain cancer-related death in children. These aggressive high-grade gliomas cannot be effectively treated and are associated with dismal prognosis. Whilst radiation therapy (RT) prolongs survival, it is a palliative therapy, as half of children with DIPG die within 1 year of diagnosis and almost all are dead by 2 years. These statistics have not changed for decades, despite a multitude of clinical trials. No chemotherapeutic regimen has been shown to improve survival, emphasizing the need to find novel and effective treatments. One of the principal reasons for this poor outcome was our limited knowledge of the biology of DIPG's. Due to their location in brainstem, surgical resection is not feasible and up until recently, even performing a limited biopsy was considered too dangerous. In the last decade, DIPG tumor tissue has become available through autopsies and biopsies. This combined with the genome revolution has resulted in a transformation in our understanding of the underlying biology of this disease. Moreover, viable DIPG cells can now be grown in the laboratory which have allowed development of *in-vitro* (neurospheres) and *in-vivo* models (allograft and xenograft). This chapter summarizes recent advances in DIPG and potential novel therapies.

Keywords: diffuse intrinsic pontine glioma (DIPG), advances in biology, novel therapies

1. Introduction

Diffuse intrinsic pontine glioma (DIPG) is a high-grade glioma originating in the pons and occurs predominantly in children. It is one of the most dreaded pediatric cancers as they are essentially incurable. At the same time, it has become one of the most intense areas of research in the past few years. Due to the lack of tumor samples, there was limited information available about the genetic and molecular abnormalities in DIPG. These tumors were considered to mimic other pediatric and adult high-grade gliomas and therapies were based on these inaccurate assumptions. Radiation therapy (RT) is the only treatment modality available, that has been demonstrated to prolong survival and improve quality of life (ref) but is not curative. Almost all children die with a median survival of 1 year. Indeed, 50% of children with DIPG die within 1 year of diagnosis and almost all are dead by 2 years (ref). Despite a myriad of clinical trials, no effective treatment has been identified so far. But recently, there has been an exponential increase in the pre-clinical research involving DIPG and many, previously unknown, abnormalities contributing to DIPG pathogenesis have been identified. These may provide treatable targets and help improve the outcome of patients with DIPG.

2. Epidemiology

Tumors of the central nervous system (CNS) constitute the largest group of solid tumors and the second most common pediatric cancer [1, 2]. Around 20% of CNS tumors are brainstem gliomas [3] of which 80% arise within the pons as DIPG [4] with approximately 200–300 children in the United States [5] being diagnosed each year. Survival rates for children with cancer have improved dramatically since the 1960s; from an estimated 5-year survival of 28% to approximately 80–85% at present [6]. The outcome for patients diagnosed with brain tumors has also improved with more than 70% expected to survive at least 5 years from the diagnosis [7]. Pediatric CNS tumors are a very heterogeneous group of diseases with over 100 distinct histological types and survival differs markedly amongst the different histological types. Unlike other childhood cancers, survival for DIPG has not changed [5]. The median survival for children with DIPG is less than 1 year from the diagnosis [8] with more than 90% dying within 2 years of diagnosis [4, 9]. Although DIPG constitute only 10–15% of all pediatric brain tumors, they are the leading cause of death in this group [10]. More than three decades of research and different treatment modalities have not yielded any survival improvement.

3. Clinical features

The symptoms and signs of patients with DIPG occur secondary to the involvement of different parts of the brainstem, which include the midbrain, pons and medulla. The brainstem serves as a conduit through which axonal tracts pass to the spinal cord, cerebrum or exit as cranial nerves. Due to the diffuse nature of DIPG, the tumor infiltrates the white matter affecting the adjacent cranial nerves and white matter tracts [11]. As the pons contains important nuclei critical for life-sustaining function, any damage caused by the tumor or its treatment has devastating effects. DIPG predominantly occurs in in the middle childhood. Median age at diagnosis is 6–7 years, with males and females affected equally [11–13]. Interestingly, adults with DIPG tend to have a longer survival which may indicate a less aggressive and biologically different tumor from that in children [14]. Typically, the presentation is with neurological symptoms of less than 3 months duration [15] with the "classic" triad of cranial nerve deficits (diplopia and facial asymmetry), long tract signs (hyperreflexia, clonus, upward Babinski, increased tone and decreased strength) and cerebellar signs (ataxia, dysmetria and dysarthria), which is seen in about 50% patients [16, 17]. In most cases, abducens nerve palsy is the earliest sign and is a sensitive predictor for DIPG [17]. Obstructive hydrocephalus with signs of raised intracranial pressure are seen in <10% of patients [18]. Other symptoms for example behavioral changes, night terrors, and school difficulties may also occur.

4. Imaging characteristics

4.1. Magnetic resonance imaging (MRI)

DIPG is diagnosed clinically on the basis of history, clinical signs and MRI findings [18]. The classic MRI appearance is of an expansile lesion centred in the pons that frequently extends laterally into the cerebellar peduncles and hemispheres and often extends vertically into the midbrain and medulla (**Figure 1A**). It is poorly marginated, occupying more than 50% of the axial diameter of the pons [11]. Necrosis can be seen but cysts are rare [14]. The tumors are hypointense with indistinct margins on T1-weighted images (**Figure 1B**) and hyperintense on T2-weighted/fluid-attenuated inversion recovery (FLAIR) images (**Figure 1C** and **D**) [4]. Post-gadolinium enhancement as commonly seen in pilocytic astrocytomas is often minimal or absent in DIPG (**Figure 1E**) [19, 20]. With an average molecular weight of 545 kDa, gadolinium largely exceeds the penetration cut-off of the blood brain barrier (BBB) (400–600 Da) with limited contrast enhancement in DIPG suggesting a largely intact BBB [14, 21]. Other MRI features typical of DIPG include ventral involvement of the pons and encasement of the basilar artery (**Figure 1F**) [5].

4.2. New imaging techniques

4.2.1. MR spectroscopy (MRS)

MRS provides a measure of brain chemistry. The most prominent peaks in the brain spectrum on Proton MRS are N-acetyl aspartate (NAA), creatine, and choline. NAA is a neuronal marker which is usually decreased in tumors. Choline is associated with the metabolism of membrane turnover and is generally increased in tumors. In DIPG, MRS shows a modest increase in choline levels and a decrease in NAA levels [14]. Additionally, peaks from lactate and mobile lipids are often elevated [11]. The abnormalities in these normally occurring brain metabolites may provide insight into the biology of DIPG and become invaluable tools in DIPG radiodiagnosis.

4.2.2. Perfusion and diffusion techniques

Some of the newer perfusion and diffusion MRI techniques are being tested in prospective trials and although not a standard for DIPG diagnosis currently, may prove beneficial in the future.

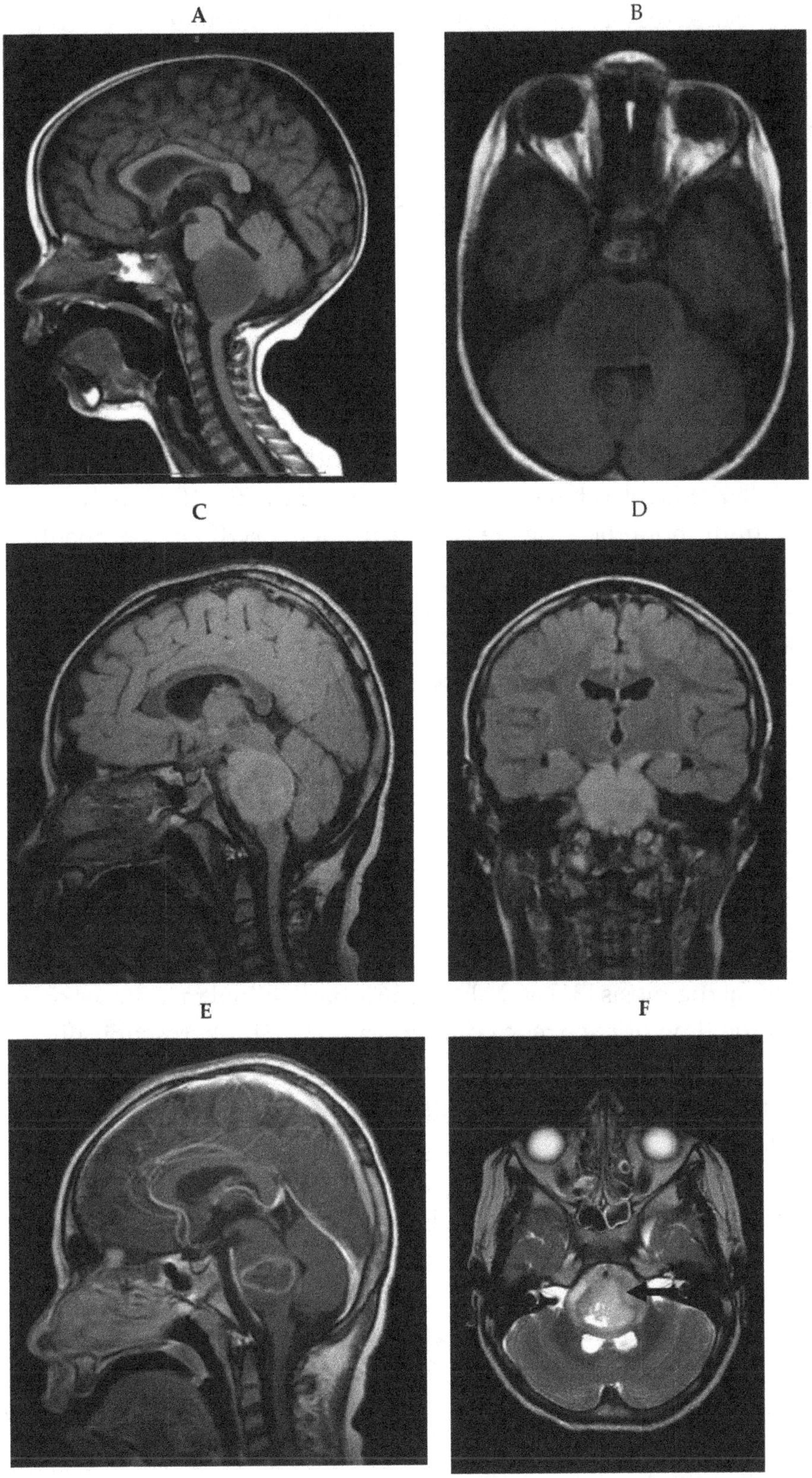

Figure 1. T1-weighted pre-contrast sagittal (A) and axial (B) MRI pictures showing poorly marginated, expansile and hypointense pontine mass. It is hyperintense onT2-weighted/FLAIR sagittal (C) and coronal (D) images. (E) There is minimal post-gadolinium enhancement. (F) Basilar artery encasement by DIPG (black arrow).

MR perfusion measures regional blood volume and flow reflecting the vascular nature of neoplasms [22]. Serial changes in tumor vascularity may be useful to monitor the effectiveness of therapy. Diffusion tensor imaging may provide visualization and quantitative characterization of the major white matter pathways in DIPG [23, 24]. This superior delineation between tumor and normal brain compared to the conventional MRI techniques may prove useful, especially to perform biopsies and obtain DIPG samples. Specific MRI sequences, including single-voxel spectroscopy (SVS), multi-voxel MRS and dynamic susceptibility contrast (DSC) MRI may help in predicting short or long survival interval from diagnosis in patients with DIPG [25].

4.2.3. Molecular drug imaging

Imaging of radiolabeled drugs like monoclonal antibodies and tyrosine kinase inhibitors can be achieved by using PET technology [26]. A recently introduced PET imaging technique of zirconium-89 (89Zr)-labeled bevacizumab in children with DIPG demonstrated considerable inter-and intra-tumoral heterogeneity in drug delivery [27]. Therapeutic potential and toxicity both can be quantified by such non-invasive, in patient techniques of tumor imaging and drug distribution [28]. Thus, these newer imaging modalities provide quantitative physiologic and functional information to complement the anatomic visualization provided by conventional imaging. However, these techniques need further validation and have yet to impact treatment decisions [11].

5. Pathology

Grossly, DIPG tumors tend to spread contiguously, extending to involve the midbrain, medulla, and cerebellar peduncles [29, 30]. Up to 20% of patients are reported to have leptomeningeal disease at diagnosis [31] and almost 56% have spinal metastases or leptomeningeal dissemination at the time of recurrence or autopsy [32, 33]. Microscopically, the majority of tumors resemble malignant gliomas in other regions. Tumor cells appear relatively small, with prominent cytoplasmic intermediate filaments and cell processes [34]. Tumor cells pervade normal cells (**Figure 2A** and **B**), diffusely expanding the pons and distorting, displacing and destroying nerve fiber tracts that normally course through it [34]. Anaplasia, increased mitotic activity (**Figure 2C**), tumor necrosis (**Figure 2D**) and vascular proliferation (**Figure 2E**) are often present [5]. A histopathological hallmark is perineuronal satellitosis in which collection of tumor cells are found around pontine neurons [35]. DIPG is histologically classified as fibrillary astrocytoma, World Health Organization (WHO) Grades II–IV [36] but the prognosis is not associated with histological grade [37, 38]. There can be marked intratumoral heterogeneity with a high proportion of samples showing focal areas of WHO grade I phenotype [39].

5.1. Diffuse midline glioma, H3K27M-mutant

In the latest WHO classification, DIPG have been grouped with other midline gliomas (thalamus, spinal cord) forming a new diagnostic entity. These tumors are characterized by a

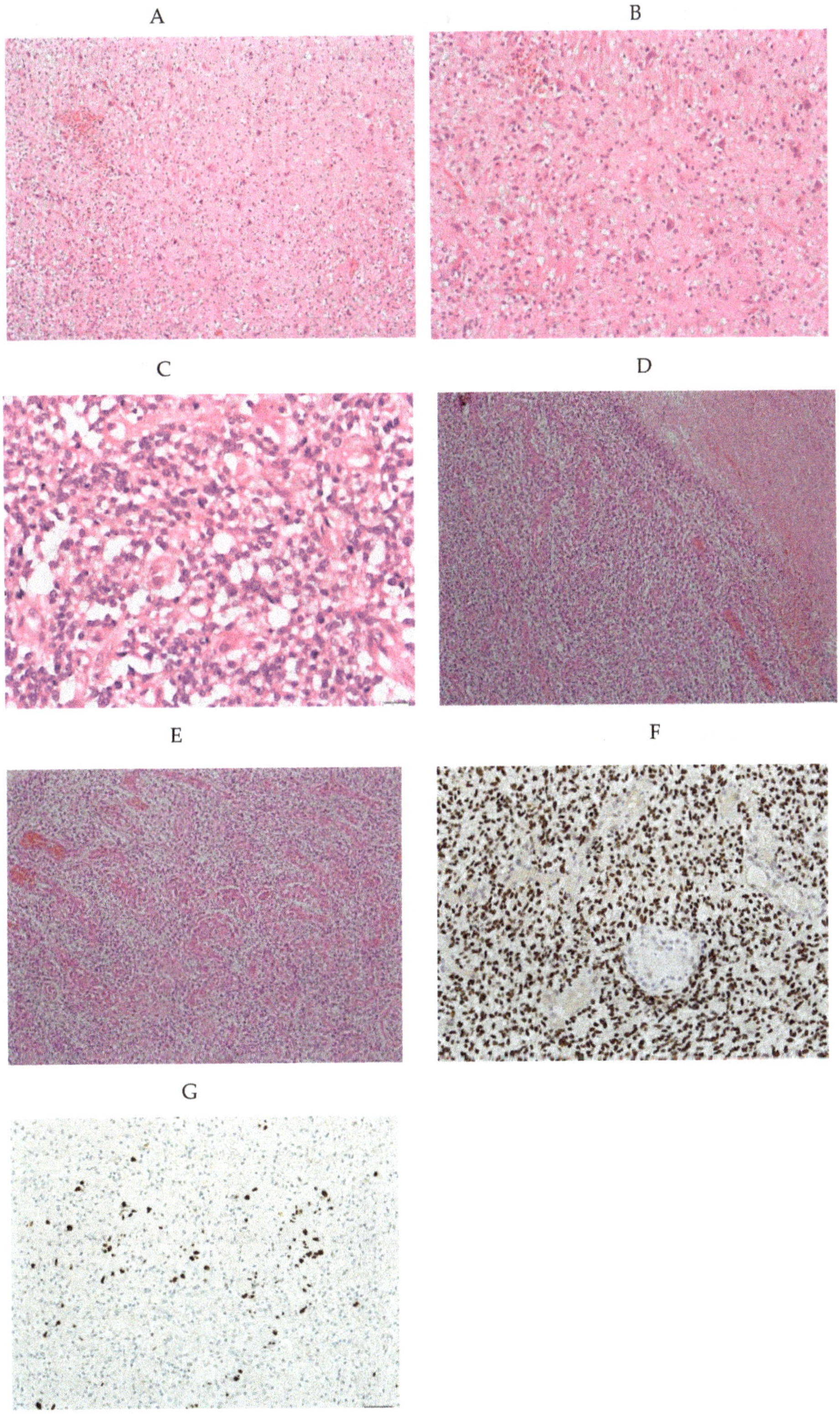

Figure 2. Histologic features of DIPG. Tumor infiltrating medullary neurons, H & E 100× (A) and 200× (B). (C) Tumor showing mitotic figures, H & E 400×. (D) Tumor/necrosis interface showing pseudo-palisading tumor necrosis. (E) Exuberant tumor-associated microvascular proliferation. (F) Tumor cells showing positive nuclear H3K27 M staining with sparing of the endothelial nuclei of admixed blood vessels H3K27 M 200×. (G) Loss of staining of tumor cell nuclei with the trimethylated antibody with retained staining in the endothelial cells, H3K27me3 200×. Images courtesy of Dr. Jason Dyke (Royal Perth Hospital, Australia).

specific histone mutation (H3K27 M) and are called diffuse midline glioma, H3K27M-mutant [40]. A mutation-specific antibody can be used to detect this mutation on immunohistochemistry (**Figure 2F**).

6. The role of biopsy in diagnosis

Prior to the routine MRI use, it was estimated that up to 15% of patients diagnosed with DIPG had a non-glial tumor or non-tumor process [41, 42]. The role of surgical intervention was controversial and, in some centres, biopsy procedures were frequently undertaken for histological confirmation. Although it is not 100% specific, with the wide availability in the early 1990s MRI became the modality of choice for DIPG diagnosis. Biopsy confirmation was thought to be an unnecessary risk as it did not alter the management [43]. The lack of clear biopsy benefit combined with improved diagnostic imaging capabilities led to MRI scans becoming the diagnostic standard of care for DIPG in the United Sates [18, 44]. More recently, there has been a renewed interest in performing stereotactic biopsies in patients with DIPG [45]. In France, biopsies were routinely performed with minimal morbidity and high diagnostic yield [46], nonetheless, it was not a common practice. The increase in the available DIPG tumor samples has yielded valuable data toward improving our understanding of the biology of DIPG [45, 47, 48]. Some of the identified biologic markers have been shown to correlate with progression-free survival (PFS) and may be useful to stratify patients in future clinical trials [49]. Considering the potential for new diagnostic and therapeutic methods combined with low morbidity associated with surgical procedures [50], the option of biopsy is being reconsidered and may eventually be included as part of the routine diagnostic evaluation for DIPG [51]. The second Consensus Conference on Pediatric Neurosurgery recommended biopsy in DIPG to ascertain biological characteristics to enhance understanding and targeting of treatment, especially in the setting of clinical trials [52]. Biopsy from a single area may not be representative of the entire tumor [53] but it may still provide important molecular information.

7. Treatment

More than 250 clinical trials in the last three decades have failed to improve the poor outcome of DIPG [20]. Due to the location it is not amenable to the surgery and chemotherapy agents are yet to show any response. Radiation therapy remains the standard of care at present. The barriers to achieve a cure for DIPG may include the inability of the surgical resection, drug delivery difficulties secondary to the blood-brain barrier (BBB) and intra- and inter-tumoral heterogeneity in the identified molecular aberrations [54].

7.1. Surgery

Surgical resection of DIPG is not feasible due to the presence of vital structures where the tumor is located. Rarely, surgical intervention like ventriculoperitoneal shunt or endoscopic third ventriculostomy may be necessary to relieve raised intracranial pressure secondary to hydrocephalus. Many patients benefit from steroids which help by reducing peritumoral edema.

7.2. Radiation therapy (RT)

Conventional RT in a dose of 54–60Gy over a 6 week period is commonly utilized in the treatment of DIPG [9]. Temporary improvement or stabilization of symptoms is seen in 70% of patients, but almost all patients have progressive disease. The mean progression-free survival (PFS) is 5.8 months with radiotherapy and 5 months without it [4]. As RT is effective temporarily, non-conventional doses and delivery schedules were investigated. In hyperfractionated RT, the total dose is divided into smaller doses and given more than once a day. Hyperfractionated RT in the form of 1Gy twice a day, to the total dose of 72Gy failed to improve the outcome [37]. Hypofractionated RT is given over a smaller period of time than standard RT by dividing the total RT dose into larger doses and treatments given once a day or less often. Studies investigating the role of hypofractionated RT with 39Gy [55] or 45Gy [56] delivered over 3 weeks have revealed similar survival outcomes, but may be more acceptable to fami9lies due to the shorter delivery times.

7.3. Chemotherapy

Various chemotherapy and targeted agents have been used to potentiate the beneficial effects of RT. These agents were combined before, with, and after RT without much success [9, 10].

7.3.1. Intensive chemotherapy

Chemotherapy combinations used with RT in the setting of phase I–III clinical trials. These include lomustine, vincristine and prednisone [41], cisplatin, etoposide, vincristine, ifosfamide and oral valproic acid [57], myeloablative thiotepa, isotretinoin and vinorelbine [58] and multiple other agents at relapse [59]. One trial evaluated the role of preradiation chemotherapy [60]. The outcome was uniformly poor.

7.3.2. Radiosensitizing agents

i. Temozolomide (TMZ): TMZ is an alkylating prodrug which is converted into its active metabolite monomethyl 5-triazeno imidazole carboxamide. TMZ causes DNA damage by alkylating O^6-guanine, N^7-gaunine and N^3-adenine resides [61]. Due to its proven efficacy in high grade gliomas, low toxicity and radiosensitization potential, temozolomide was trialed to potentiate RT efficacy without much success [8, 62, 63]. Addition of lomustine to adjuvant temozolomide [64] was not beneficial. O6-methylguanine DNA methyltransferase (MGMT) contributes to TMZ resistance by repairing alkylated O^6-guanine nucleotides. But this does not appear to be the cause of TMZ resistance as MGMT is not expressed in DIPG [47]. However, 3-methylpurine-DNA glycosylase (MPG), enzyme responsible for repair of N^7-gaunine and N^3-adenine nucleotides, and its ATM-dependent regulation may play a role in TMZ resistance in DIPG [65]. A recently closed phase II study stratified patients to receive TMZ and erlotinib based on MGMT methylation and EGFR expression status [66].

ii. Topotecan: topotecan acts as a radiosensitizing agent by stabilizing the DNA topoisomerase I complex, interfering with DNA replication and DNA repair. Concurrent administration of topotecan with RT was found to be ineffective [67, 68].

iii. Other radiosensitizing agents like motexafin-gadolinium [69] and carbogen [70] also showed similar poor results.

8. Biology

More than 250 therapeutic clinical trials including several targeted agents have not improved the dismal prognosis of DIPG [10]. The reason for this, at least in part, has been attributed to our lack of understanding of the biology of this disease. More has been published on the biology and pathophysiology of DIPG in the past 10 years than in all prior years combined [5]. A more recent and significant achievement in DIPG research is sample collection at autopsy. This has provided invaluable insights into understanding of the biology [71, 72]. Both autopsy and biopsy samples have allowed development of *in-vitro* (neurospheres) and *in-vivo* models (allograft and xenograft) [73–75].

8.1. Cell of origin

Pontine precursor-like cells (PPC), found in the ventral pons region, which are positive for the markers for the primitive neural precursor cells, nestin and vimentin, are postulated as the candidate cell of origin for DIPG [35]. Approximately half of PPC also expressed Olig2, a transcription factor which is associated with oligodendroglial precursors. This cell type was morphologically distinct from the nestin positive cells seen in the dorsal brainstem. PPC are present in all ventral brainstem structures during infancy and wane by 2 years of age. The ventral pontine and medullary nestin$^+$ cells show a second peak at 6 years, corresponding to the age of presentation of DIPG. Thus, temporal and spatial distribution of these cells correlates closely with the incidence of DIPG suggesting that tumors arise secondary to dysregulation of a postnatal neurodevelopmental process [35]. Expression of SOX2, a transcription factor with activity during embryogenesis, and Olig2 in another model supports the disordered neurodevelopmental origin of DIPG [76].

8.2. The genomic landscape

DIPG biopsy and autopsy samples have undergone extensive genomic profiling and major breakthroughs have been achieved in identifying key oncogenic pathways [77]. The drivers for DIPG tumorigenesis include epigenetic changes, gene mutations, deletions or overexpression and chromosomal number changes.

8.3. Epigenetic changes

8.3.1. Histone mutations

The DNA is packaged by histone proteins into a chain of nucleosomes which are the basic building blocks of the chromatin fiber [78]. In a single nucleosome, 147 base pairs (bp) of DNA wrap around histone octamers containing two copies each of histones H2A, H2B, H3 and H4 [79]. The N-terminal ends of histones containing lysine (K) and arginine (R) residues are post-translationally modified by acetylation or methylation and regulate DNA repair, replication and transcription. The histone H3 family consists of a number of related proteins. Histone H3 isoforms H3.1 and H3.2 (also called as canonical H3) help in packaging newly replicated DNA. While H3.3 can function much the same as canonical H3 as a core part of the nucleosome, it is also deposited into transcriptionally active regions to replace histones lost during processes disrupting nucleosomes [80].

8.3.1.1. H3 mutations and DIPG

8.3.1.1.1. H3K27M mutations

H3F3A and *H3F3B* produce identical H3.3 proteins whereas *HIST1H3B* is one of the many genes encoding H3.1 [81, 82]. Distinct and recurrent mutations in H3 have been implicated in 70–80% of pediatric gliomas [83]. Lysine to methionine missense mutation at position 27 (K27M) was present in 78% of DIPG patients, with most of these mutations in *H3F3A* and up to 25% in *HIST1H3B* [84, 85]. H3K27M mutations are restricted to the midline structures [86] and H3.1 and H3.3 mutations involve two different oncogenic pathways resulting in distinct clinicopathological variants. H3.1 mutated tumors are exclusively linked to DIPG and exhibit a mesenchymal/astrocytic phenotype, a pro-angiogenic/hypoxic signature and are co-segregated with *ACVR1* mutations. Clinically, these tumors are less aggressive when compared to H3.3 mutant tumors, metastasize less frequently and respond better to radiation therapy (RT) with a median overall survival (OS) of 15 months. H3.3 mutated tumors are located in the midline structures including the brainstem, thalamus and spinal cord. They have a proneural/oligodendroglial phenotype, a pro-metastatic gene expression signature with *PDGFRA* activation. They behave more aggressively, responding poorly to RT with a median OS of 9 months and metastasize more frequently [87]. The gain-of-function H3K27M alterations are exclusive to pediatric high-grade gliomas and any H3 mutation is associated with a dismal outcome but identification of a specific mutation may help in developing specific therapeutic targets.

8.3.1.1.2. G34R/V mutations

H3F3A mutations encoding a glycine 34 to arginine or valine G34R/V comprise a smaller proportion of H3.3 mutations [88]. G34R/V mutations are seen in cerebral hemispheres of slightly older patients (9–42 years) as compared to K27M mutations (5–29 years) [86, 88, 89].

K27M and G34R/V mutations are mutually exclusive and heterozygously expressed, with one wild-type *H3F3A* allele [89].

8.3.1.1.3. Other novel mutations

H3F3A mutation resulting in lysine-to isoleucine substitution at K27 has been rarely seen in DIPG [87]. A mutation in the gene encoding the H3.2 variant, HIST2H3C, resulting in a novel K27 M mutation has been described [87].

8.3.1.2. Downstream effects of H3 mutations and gliomagenesis

8.3.1.2.1. K27 M mutations

K27M (and to a lesser extent K27I) is the only amino acid substitution which can ablate tri-methylation (H3K27me3) [90]. The mutant H3K27M binds to the enhancer of zeste homolog 2 (EZH2) component of PRC2 interfering with methyltransferase activity of EZH2 which results in generalized hypomethylation. The downstream effect is derepression of targets of PRC2, upregulation of gene expression and gliomagenesis [91]. In addition, K27M mutation contributes to altered cell cycle control, inhibition of autophagy pathways and potentially increased resistance to radiotherapy [92]. Even though the mutant histone forms only 3.6–17.6% of the total cellular H3 pool, there is a near-absolute loss of H3K27me3. This represents a *trans*-dominant-negative effect across all three isoforms of the wild-type H3 protein [90, 91, 93, 94]. However, the exact role of H3K27M in DIPG tumorigenesis remains unknown as it does not induce the tumors on its own *in vivo* [95]. One of the postulates of gliomagenesis is H3.3 K27M and G34R/V acting as driver mutations followed by a second hit by another mutation like *TP53, PPM1D, ACVR1 or PI3KR1* [83, 95, 96].

In summary, H3K27 mutations have a great significance irrespective of whichever histone H3 variant (H3.1-HIST13B, H2-HIST2H3C and H3.3-H3F3A) is targeted and will result in loss of H3K27me3 and development of DIPG.

8.3.1.2.2. G34R/V mutations

The role of H3.3G34R/V in gliomagenesis is less clear. It may act by disrupting K36me3 levels and activating potential oncogenes [90, 93]; inducing *MYCN* upregulation [97, 98] and disrupting interaction between H3.3 and ATRX/DAXX leading to aberrant deposition of H3.3 near telomeric regions and leading to alternate lengthening of telomerase [88, 89, 99].

8.3.1.3. Co-mutations associated with H3 mutations in DIPG

Other mutations associated with H3K27M mutation include α thalassemia/mental retardation syndrome X-linked *(ATRX)* or death-domain associated protein *(DAXX)* (30%), *TP53* (60%) and *NF-1, PDGFRA, BRAF, KRAS,* and *FGFR1* at lower frequencies [88, 99, 100]. G35R/V mutations coexpress with mutations in *TP53, ATRX/DAXX* and *PDGFRA* [83].

8.3.1.4. Mutations of chromatin modifiers

Chromatin writers or erasers are the enzymes which catalyze the post-translational modifications of histone tails like methylation, acetylation and ubiquitylation of lysine residues, phosphorylation of serine or threonine residues and methylation of arginine residues. The effector proteins called readers are recruited to the chromatin by the resultant histone code which helps in localization of functional complexes that affect transcriptional regulation [101]. Numerous recurrent mutations are observed in chromatin writers, erasers, readers and remodelers in DIPG and other tumors [102].

The discovery of histone mutations which are present in up to 80% of DIPG is one of the most remarkable breakthroughs in terms of understanding DIPG biology and identification of actionable targets [90, 92, 99].

8.3.2. Polycomb repressive complex (PRC) abnormalities

Polycomb group proteins remodel chromatin enabling epigenetic silencing of genes. There are two main Polycomb group complexes found in mammals-PRC1 and PRC2. PRC1 catalyzes the monoubiquitylation of histone H2A and PRC2 catalyzes the methylation of H3K27 [103]. Some PRC1 complexes also act independent of enzymatic activity to regulate gene expression by compacting chromatin [104]. PRC1 functions downstream of PRC2 by binding specifically to H3K27me3 [103]. By inducing such sequential histone modifications, PRC1 and PRC2 achieve stable silencing of gene expression [105]. Dysregulation of PRC and its downstream targets has been implicated in many cancers [83]. B cell-specific Moloney murine leukemia virus integration site 1 (BMI-1) is a component of PRC1 complex. It was found to be highly expressed in DIPG tumor cells and its downregulation inhibited various cellular processes like cell proliferation, cell cycle signaling, telomerase expression and activity, and cell migration [105].

8.4. Gene abnormalities

Molecular profiling of DIPG samples has provided new insights [61]. In the past, candidate gene approaches were utilized to identify gene abnormalities associated with adult high-grade gliomas (HGG) [106]. Although, these studies were limited in defining the biology of DIPG due to their small numbers, they still highlighted some differences between adult HGG and DIPG. Recently, studies performed with next-generation sequencing approaches have confirmed that DIPG are molecularly distinct from adult HGG and non-DIPG pediatric HGG [18]. The current technologies utilize whole-genome sequencing (WGS), whole-exome sequencing (WES), and RNA-sequencing in addition to copy number, gene expression, and methylation profiles and histopathology.

8.4.1. Mutational burden of DIPG compared to other tumors

The genomic signatures of the most pediatric HGG are complex and involve significant copy number alterations (CNAs), single nucleotide variants (SNVs) and structural variants [107–109]. HGG have a higher mutation burden than many other pediatric cancers but it is still lower than common adult cancers [77]. HGG commonly show structural variants like simple rearrangements and abnormalities caused by chromothripsis [84]. But there is a wide range of genomic complexity in pediatric HGG. At one end of the spectrum is infant non-brainstem HGG (NBS-HGG) arising in children less than 3 years old. These tumors have significantly lower mutation burden [84]. At the other end of the spectrum are HGG from patients with inherited mutations in mismatch repair genes. Germline mutations in tumor suppressor genes like *TP53* and neurofibromin 1 (*NF1*) predispose to the development of HGG [110]. The hypermutated tumors arising in the context of these germline mutations show a very high number of somatic SNVs; these may be more than 100-fold higher than in 95% of pediatric HGG [84]. DIPG show similar mutation burden as other pediatric HGG and their genomic complexity is indicative of multiple genetic mechanisms generating numerous mutations which provide the tumor with diverse potential pathways to therapeutic resistance [77].

8.4.2. Abnormalities of cellular proliferation pathways

8.4.2.1. Bone morphogenetic protein (BMP) signaling and ACVR1 mutations

ACVR1, also known as *ALK2* encodes the serine kinase, Activin receptor type 1 A (ACVR1) [111]. It is a type 1 BMP receptor which belongs to the mammalian TGF-β signaling family [112]. ACVR1 binds to a diverse set of ligands, including TGF-β, activins and multiple BMP [113]. ACVR1 is essential for signaling and after ligand it is phosphorylated by ACVR2 with formation a stable ACVR1/2 complex [114]. This results in the phosphorylation and activation of growth promoting genes through SMAD transcription factors [77]. ACVR1 mutations are constitutionally activating, leading to increased expression of activin signaling targets *ID1* and *ID2* [115].

8.4.2.1.1. ACVR1 mutations and DIPG

Germline *ACVR1* mutations cause the congenital malformation syndrome fibrodysplasia ossificans progressive (FOP) [116]. Seven somatic mutations of this gene have been identified in 13–32% of DIPG samples leading to either ligand-independent kinase activation or gain-of-function effects [84, 111, 112, 115]. However, there is no increased cancer risk in FOP despite having similar germline mutations as those seen in DIPG which suggests that *ACVR1* mutations on their own are not tumor initiating and lead to DIPG only in the presence of other mutations [77, 116].

8.4.2.1.2. ACVR1 co-mutations

ACVR1 mutant tumors commonly co-segregate with *HIST1H3B* mutations [115]. *ACVR1-HIST1H3B* co-segregating tumors do not show *TP53* loss or *PDGFRA* amplifications but around 60% have mutations in the PI3K signaling pathway [114].

8.4.2.1.3. Clinical implications

ACVR1 mutations signify a distinct subset of DIPG patients. They occurred more frequently in females (F:M ratio of 1.75:1) and are associated with younger age and longer survival (median OS of 14.9 months) [84, 111]. There was a significant pharmacologic inhibition of ACVR1 by a selective ALK2 inhibitor, LDN-193189, leading to dose-dependent cytotoxicity across all the tested DIPG cell lines [111]. Due to its role in DIPG pathogenesis and targetable potential, ACVR1 inhibition represents a novel therapeutic option.

8.4.2.2. Receptor tyrosine kinase (RTK) pathway

RTKs are transmembrane protein receptors containing intrinsic enzymatic activity. Their ligands include growth factors, hormones and cytokines [117] and they play an critical role in mediating key signaling pathways involving cell proliferation, differentiation, survival and migration [118]. The human RTK family has 20 subfamilies and 58 known members including platelet-derived growth factor receptors (PDGFR), epidermal growth factor receptors (EGFR) and fibroblast growth factor receptors (FGFR) [118–120]. Upon ligand binding, the RTKs are activated leading to signal transduction to the nucleus and subsequent protein transcription. This is achieved by downstream activation of various RTK substrates like mitogen-activated protein kinase (MAPK) and phosphatidylinositol-3-kinase (PI3K) [121].

8.4.2.2.1. RTK pathway aberrations and DIPG

Amplifications and mutations in components of RTK-RAS-PI3K pathway are seen in up to 60% of DIPG [18]. The most common affected component is *PDGFRA*. Other abnormalities involve *AKT1, AKT3, c-MET*, epidermal growth factor receptor (*EGFR*), erythroblastic leukemia viral oncogene homolog-4 (*ERBB4*), hepatocyte growth factor, Kirsten rat sarcoma viral oncogene homolog (*KRAS*), *PIK3CA, PIKC2G, PIK3R1, PTEN*, insulin-like growth factor 2, and insulin-like growth factor receptor [18, 45, 53, 111].

8.4.2.2.1.1. PDGFRA amplifications

Whole-genome profiling of DIPG tumors have identified recurrent amplifications of *PDGFA* and *PDGFRA* with overexpression of PDGFR-α in 28–50% tumors [47, 48, 122, 123].

8.4.2.2.1.2. PDGFRA mutations

Somatic activating mutations including missense mutations and in-frame deletions and insertions were identified in 4.7% DIPG tumors and were found to be oncogenic *in vivo* [124]. Concurrent amplification was seen in 40% of tumors with mutations and 60% had heterozygous mutations [124]. Similar mutations were identified in other studies in 8.8–25% samples [54, 123]. Downstream activation of the PDGFR pathway has been shown by phospho-mammalian target of rapamycin (m-TOR) immunopositivity [47] as well as activation of MAPK and PI3K pathways [124]. PDGFR-α is expressed by the oligodendrocyte precursor cell derived from the candidate cell of origin PCC [35] and hence the precursor cell may be responsive to PDGF. Also, human DIPG cell culture yield was better after the addition of PDGF [35] and upregulation of PDGF pathway was associated with dorsal pontine glioblastoma in mouse models [125, 126].

8.4.2.2.1.3. EGFR aberrations

EGFR immunopositivity and gene amplification were seen in about 27% [47] and 7–9% [48] of cases respectively.

8.4.2.2.2. RTK pathway co-mutations in DIPG

PDGFRA gains and amplifications co-segregate with H3.3 mutations [88, 99] and *TP53* mutations [124].

8.4.2.2.3. Clinical significance

RTK signaling dysregulation, particularly PDGFR pathway either overexpression or mutation, may have an important role in the pathophysiology of DIPG and provide therapeutic targets [47]. Identification of PDGFRA mutations may be beneficial in developing targeted therapies. But some particular mutations like PDGFR D842V in the gastrointestinal stromal tumors confers resistance to imatinib [127]. Others may have only cytostatic effects so they may not be effective on their own [124].

8.4.2.3. MYC and MYCN aberrations

MYCN proto-oncogene is a member of the MYC family encoding the protein MYCN. MYCN plays a critical role during embryogenesis and is involved in cellular proliferation and differentiation [128]. *MYCN* amplification is seen in DIPG [84, 92, 99] and is associated with hypermethylation, high-grade histology and chromothripsis on chromosome 2p [115]. *MYCN* amplifications are transcriptional regulators that affect the epigenetic landscape by enhancing gene expression across the whole genome [84]. MYCN pathway maybe induced by H3.3 K27 M [99] or H3.3G34V [83, 102] but may act independent of H3 mutations [92].

8.4.2.4. Hedgehog (Hh) signaling

Hh signaling pathway plays a major role in regulation of developmental processes like cell proliferation, cell differentiation, tissue polarity and stem cell maintenance. Aberrant activation of Hh pathway has been implicated in the pathogenesis of cancers like medulloblastoma. No structural mutation involving this pathway resulting in the development of DIPG has been identified so far. However, in pre-clinical murine models [35] upregulation of Hh pathway activity resulted in ventral pontine hyperplasia. Hh pathway is essential for the normal development of PPC in humans. Also, Hh pathway activation stimulates and blockade reduces the self-renewal capacity of DIPG neurosphere cells. These findings indicate that Hh signaling, which drives the development of neural precursors in the ventral pons, may play a role in tumor formation in a subset of DIPG. Patients with Gorlin syndrome, a genetic entity occurring secondary to unregulated Hh activity, usually do not develop DIPG [35]. So, in addition to unregulated Hh pathway activity, a second "hit" may be necessary for DIPG transformation. Hh signaling role in the pathogenesis of DIPG was further investigated in a study [92] which identified upregulation of Hh signaling. DIPG samples showed upregulation of Patched (PTCH) and nuclear translocation of Glioma Associated Oncogene 1 (GLI1); both PTCH and GLI1 are key Hh pathway molecules. In summary, Hh pathway may play a significant role in DIPG tumorigenesis by stimulating PPC and transforming them into potential DIPG cancer stem cells (CSC).

8.4.3. Abnormalities of cell cycle regulation pathways

8.4.3.1. TP53 pathway

The TP53 pathway is a complex network of genes which respond to diverse internal and external stress signals and have an impact on the normal cellular homeostasis [129]. The p53 protein is activated by stress signals transmitted as post-translational modifications leading to apoptosis [130]. In addition, the TP53 pathway produces proteins which aid directly in DNA repair processes and alter cellular environment enabling inter-cellular communication [131]. In the critical role of safeguarding the genomic integrity, it functions as a tumor suppression pathway [132]. *TP53* is the most commonly mutated gene found in a broad variety of human cancers [129, 133].

8.4.3.1.1. TP53 mutations and DIPG

TP53 mutations are commonly found in DIPG with the reported incidence between 9 and 77% [45, 99]. They are more common in higher grade histology tumors (grades III and IV) [53]. About 50% of *TP53* wild-type grade II DIPG show presence of *PPM1D* mutations [134]. *PPM1D* is an oncogene associated with cancers like neuroblastoma [135] and lung cancer [136] which codes for wild-type p53-induced phosphatase 1D (WIP1). WIP1 is a negative regulator of *TP53* as it inactivates p53 and promotes termination of stress-induced responses. So *PPM1D* mutations have the same functional significance as *TP53* mutations [137]. *PPM1D* and *TP53* mutations are mutually exclusive and may ultimately lead to dysregulated homeostasis and tumorigenesis [134].

8.4.3.1.2. TP53 co-mutations in DIPG

TP53 mutations more commonly co-segregate with H3.3 K27 M than H3.1 K27 M [112] and frequently occur in the setting of *PDGFRA* aberrations [124].

8.4.3.2. The RB pathway

Cyclins and cyclin-dependent kinases (CDKs) control the G_1/S transition of the cell cycle [138]. The abnormalities involving these regulators observed in DIPG include cyclin-dependent kinase inhibitor 2A or 2B (*CDKN2A* or *CDKN2B*) deletions [48, 122] and *CDK4*, *CDK6* or cyclin D1 (*CCND1*), *CCND2*, and *CCND3* amplifications [48, 122, 139].

8.4.3.3. Aurora kinase pathway

Aurora kinase family include three highly homologous serine/threonine kinases required during mitosis and which are linked to many cancers [140]. AURKB forms the catalytic component of the chromosomal passenger complex (CPC) which plays a critical role during mitosis [141]. Almost 70% of DIPG have demonstrated overexpression of *AURKB* [142].

8.4.3.4. WEE1 kinase pathway

WEE1 kinase is an important part of G_2 checkpoint. DIPG cells, unlike normal cells, have aberrations in genes regulating the G_1 checkpoint, including *TP53*, *MDM2*, *CDKN2A*, and *ATM*

[122, 133, 143] causing a dysfunctional G_1 arrest. So, these cells rely heavily on G2 checkpoint to repair DNA damage caused by irradiation. WEE1 protein is significantly overexpressed in post-mortem DIPG samples [73]. Abrogation of the G_2 checkpoint achieved by WEE1 kinase inhibition pushes DIPG cells with unrepaired DAN damage into mitotic catastrophe resulting in cell death.

8.4.3.5. Poly (ADP-ribose) polymerase (PARP)-1 abnormalities

PARP-1 is a nuclear protein involved in the DNA damage repair processes [144]. PARP-1 activity provides an escape mechanism for cancer cells to avoid apoptosis and its overexpression may be associated with temozolomide and radiation resistance [47]. Gain of *PARP-1* is seen in DIPG tumors and provides a potentially targetable therapeutic option [47].

8.5. Chromosomal number abnormalities

Copy number abnormalities (CNAs) reported in DIPG include gain in chromosomes 1q, 2q, 8q, 9q, 7p/7q and loss in chromosomes 16q, 17p, 20p, 21q, 10q and 4q [47, 48, 122, 123, 139, 145]. The CNAs may represent the initial mutations responsible for DIPG tumorigenesis as well as the treatment effect.

8.6. Immune checkpoint abnormalities

8.6.1. B7-H3 abnormalities

B7-H3 or CD276, a member of the B7-CD28 family, is a type I transmembrane glycoprotein [146]. Many malignant neuroectodermal tumors including adult HGG over-express B7-H3. B7-H3 was found to be overexpressed in a small panel of DIPG samples obtained at autopsy [147]. A monoclonal antibody 8H9 recognizes it and binds specifically to the tumor cells [148, 149] enabling therapeutic cell selectivity. B7H3 was targeted safely in the salvage therapy of stage IV neuroblastoma using intrathecal ^{131}I-8H9 [150].

8.7. Tumor microenvironment abnormalities

Therapies targeted at intrinsic cellular pathways have yielded poor results in DIPG. Tumor microenvironment plays a vital role in tumorigenesis and progression, so studies have looked into investigating microenvironment alteration for better results.

8.7.1. Neuroligin-3 (NLGN3) role

Neuroligin-3 (NLGN3) is a synaptic adhesion molecule which is cleaved from neurons and oligodendrocyte precursor cells via the ADAM10 sheddase and released into the tumor microenvironment. This important neuronal activity promotes many types of brain cancers including DIPG, pediatric and adult HGG and anaplastic oligodendroglioma. NLGN3 release activates oncogenic pathways like focal adhesion kinase activation resulting in the downstream PI3K-mTOR pathway induction. This in turn causes upregulation of several synapse-related genes resulting in the proliferation of glioma cells [151]. HGG glioma growth in xenograft models was blocked by ADAM10 inhibitors by preventing NLGN3 release into the tumor microenvironment. Similarly, patient-derived orthotopic xenografts fail to grow in *Nlgn3* knockout mice [152].

8.7.2. Pleiotrophin (PTN) role

PTN is a growth factor secreted by neural precursor cells in the lateral ventricle subventricular zone (SVZ). It has an important role in normal neurodevelopment, plasticity and regeneration. PTN acts as a glioma chemoattractant. Through autocrine/paracrine actions, it activates Rho/Rho kinase (ROCK) signaling pathway enabling migration of DIPG cells to the SVZ [153].

9. DIPG subgroups

Proteomic, methylation and mRNA analyses have identified interesting subgroups of DIPG.

PDGFRA amplification is seen in association with H3.3 mutation and ACVR1 mutation is mainly seen in H3.1 mutant tumors [87, 115].

Upregulation of N-Myc and Hh signaling pathways [92].

Upregulation of N-Myc (H3 wild-type), silent genome and H3K27 M [115].

Mesenchymal transition with stem cell-like phenotype and oligodendroglial differentiation and PDGFRA amplification/mutation.

10. Novel therapeutic approaches

10.1. Molecularly targeted agents

10.1.1. RTK-RAS-PI3K pathway

Given DIPG tumors show aberrant activation of growth factor receptor-mediated signal transduction pathways, using drugs targeting these pathways is a rational approach. *In-vitro* studies confirmed the efficacy of tyrosine kinase inhibitors (TKI) like dasatinib in reducing tumor proliferation and inhibition of *PDGFRA* activity [154]. Phase I studies of PDGFR pathway inhibition by imatinib [155] and dasatinib [156], VEGFR2 inhibition by vandetinib [156, 157], EGFR inhibition by gefitinib [158] and erlotinib [49] revealed the safety of using these drugs in children and provided the doses for phase II studies. Temsirolimus is an mTOR inhibitor [159] and its combination with perifosine, an Akt inhibitor, was shown to be safe and feasible in a phase I study in children with recurrent/refractory solid tumors including DIPG [160]. This study tested the hypothesis of dual targeting of PI3K-Akt–mTOR pathway. Phase II studies of multi-tyrosine kinase inhibitor sunitinib [161] and farnesyl transferase inhibitor tipifarnib, which inhibits farnesylation of Ras, [162] did not show activity. BIOMEDE, a phase II study, is stratifying patients based on overexpression of EGFR and/or loss of PTEN following diagnostic biopsy. The patients are randomized or assigned to different treatment arms with erlotinib, everolimus and dasatinib [163].

10.2. Epigenetic modifying agents

Histone deacetylases (HDAC) regulate the histone acetylation in nucleosomes, which mediates changes in chromatin conformation, leading to gene expression regulation [164]. HDAC gene mutations, downregulation and altered expression are linked to tumorigenesis. Histone deacetylase (HDAC) inhibitors modify histone activity to increase expression of previously silenced genes thereby leading to cell death [165]. Panobinostat is a multi-HDAC inhibitor which increases global H3 acetylation and H3K27 M methylation and reduces oncogene expression. Panobinostat-induced polyacetylation of the H3 N-terminal tail has been shown to reverse PRC2 inhibition caused by K27 M and rescue the H3K27 hypomethylation phenotype [166]. Panobinostat has shown promising results in *in vitro* [164] and some *in vivo* [167] studies although a narrow therapeutic index causing dose limiting toxicities at the required antitumor concentrations being the likely reason for lack of efficacy [164]. Its efficacy was further enhanced by histone demethylase inhibitor GSK-J4 which increase H3K27me3 [168]. DIPG patients showed no objective responses to single agent vorinostat in a phase I clinical trial [169]. Vorinostat is currently being investigated in combination with temsirolimus and RT in DIPG in a phase I trial [170]. Pediatric Brain Tumor Consortium (PBTC) is undertaking a phase I trial of single agent Panobinostat in patients with DIPG [171].

10.3. Targeting cell cycle regulation

DIPG tumors contain cell cycle regulatory gene abnormalities like amplification of D-type cyclins and CDK4/6 or loss of Ink4a-ARF resulting in cellular proliferation [172]. Targeting the cyclin/CDK/RB pathway was investigated in a preclinical trial. PD-0332991 (PD), a CDK4/6 inhibitor, was used in a genetically engineered, PDGF-B overexpressed, Ink4a-ARF and p53 deficient brainstem glioma mouse model. PD induced cell cycle arrest both *in vitro* and *in vivo*. The survival of mice treated with PD alone or in combination with RT was significantly more than untreated or mice treated with only RT [172]. Inhibition WEE1 kinase, which is overexpressed in DIPG, was shown to increase the RT response in vitro and in vivo [73].

10.4. Immunotherapy

Interferon, IL-12 and anti-glioma monoclonal antibody have shown efficacy in mouse models of non-brainstem malignancies [173]. Recently, subcutaneous vaccinations with glioma-associated antigen epitope peptides (EphA2, IL13-Rα2 and survivin) were investigated in children with DIPG. The vaccine was tolerated well and the results were encouraging for future trials [174]. IL13-Rα2 is of particular significance as it is highly and differentially expressed in DIPG [175, 176] compared to the normal brain tissue which makes it a suitable immunotherapy target.

10.5. Human neural and mesenchymal stem cells

Neural stem cells (NSC) have been utilized as the vehicle for therapeutic agents in gene therapy for experimental malignant brain tumors [177, 178]. NSC have robust tumor tropism and this property can be used to deliver therapeutic agents to the inoperable DIPG tumors. NSC are difficult to harvest and use due to their inherent immunogenicity [179]. Mesenchymal stem cells (MSC) have been found to be a suitable alternative as they have all the properties of NSC and are more practical to use [180]. In a rat model, brainstem glioma directed migratory capacities of NSC and MSC from different sources was found to be similar *in vitro* and *in vivo*. This study showed promise as 20–30% of stem cells migrated from the site of injection in the right forebrain to the brainstem glioma cells. In addition, the group treated with genetically engineered NSC encoding cytosine deaminase (CD) suicide gene and IFNβ proinflammatory cytokine and systemic 5-fluorouracil resulted in 59% reduction in the tumor size [181].

10.6. Delivery methods to overcome blood-brain barrier (BBB)

The vast majority of brain tumors are characterized by the loss of BBB integrity due to the disordered and highly permeable tumor neovasculature [182]. In DIPG, however, the BBB integrity is normal and the drug permeability is reduced as the tumor makes use of the existing brain vasculature [183]. Traditional cytotoxic drugs have shown good efficacy against DIPG cells *in vitro* but they likely fail to penetrate the BBB which may explain the contrasting results with clinical trials [28]. To overcome the disappointing results associated with systemic therapy, methods utilizing localized and targeted drug delivery have been investigated.

10.6.1. Convection-enhanced delivery (CED)

CED is a relatively novel delivery modality which utilizes the properties of bulk flow to achieve homogeneously distributed infusions into the brain parenchyma [184]. It is a neurosurgical technique in which one to several catheters are stereotactically placed within or around the tumor mass and drug is delivered locally, bypassing the BBB and reducing systemic toxicity [185, 186]. The local concentrations achieved are significantly higher than the systemic administration and the drug distribution occurs along the patterns of the glioma cell invasion along the white matter tracts [187]. Many *in vivo* feasibility studies have confirmed that drugs can be safely delivered into the rodent brainstem [188]. CED of carmustine [74, 189], carboplatin [190, 191], temozolomide [192], small-molecule kinase inhibitors [193], cisplatin [194] and gemcitabine [190, 195] have been evaluated for safety and distribution parameters. Topotecan CED in two pediatric patients with DIPG showed initial reduction in tumor size [196]. MRI guided and robotically placed catheters were used for CED of carboplatin in DIPG patients. Three out of eight patients survived beyond 15 months and the procedure was tolerated well [197, 198]. Administration of ^{124}I-8H9, a radioactively labeled antibody and a chimeric toxin with B7-H3 specificity, is currently being explored in a phase I clinical trial for DIPG patients [199]. A patient with DIPG received CED infusion of the recombinant cytotoxin IL13-PE38QQR with GD-diethylenetriamine but the tumor progresses within a few weeks [200]. IL13-PE38QQR is a recombinant *Pseudomonas aeruginosa* toxin and some early phase clinical trials investigating its CED efficacy are being conducted or recently completed in patients with DIPG and HGG [185]. These studies have established the feasibility of CED. However, more data is required to prove safety and efficacy and CED models are undergoing rigorous investigations into the physical properties of the catheters and infusion rates [173]. CED targets the primary tumor only and not the metastatic sites. In DIPG, local and distant metastases in the brain or spine are seen in 13–17% patients. Therefore, in situations where disseminated disease is present, CED therapy alone, directed toward the primary tumor site, will be inadequate and should be complemented with therapies for the secondaries [28, 32].

10.6.2. Nanoparticle delivery

Another alternative drug delivery technique involves encapsulation of cationic substances into capsules termed micro- and nanoparticles. This reduces their tissue affinity and increases the volume of distribution [28, 201].

10.6.3. Cell-mediated delivery

Bacterial cell-derived vehicles to transport chemotherapy agents across the BBB was utilized with bi-specific antibodies recognizing cell wall and EGFR moieties [202]. Similar EGFR-targeted vehicles loaded with doxorubicin resulted in significant tumor regression in canine brain cancer models [203]. ECREST (A Study of Intravenous EEDVsMit in Children With Recurrent/Refractory Solid or CNS Tumors Expressing EGFR) is a phase I study using mitoxantrone loaded nanocells in EGFR positive relapsed/refractory solid and CNS tumors including DIPG [204].

10.6.4. BBB disruption techniques

BBB can be temporarily disrupted by ultrasound methods. This results in enhanced uptake of systemically delivered drugs [28].

11. Conclusion

DIPG remains the main cause of death in pediatric patients with brain tumors. Despite many clinical trials, minimal improvement has been achieved as compared with RT. Most of the clinical trials in the past did not have sound biological bases due to a lack of biopsy specimens. In the last few years, international collaborative research has helped to identify new molecular aberrations in DIPG. These have provided insight into the pathogenesis of DIPG and may help in identifying new targeted therapies.

Author details

Santosh Valvi* and Nicholas G. Gottardo

*Address all correspondence to: santosh.valvi@health.wa.gov.au

Perth Children's Hospital, Perth, Australia

References

[1] Scheurer ME, Bondy ML, Gurney JG. Epidemiology of childhood Cancer. In: Pizzo PA, Poplack DG, editors. Principles and Practice of Pediatric Oncology. 6th ed. Philadelphia: Lippincott Williams & Wilkins; 2011. p. 2

[2] Stiller CA, Nectoux J. International incidence of childhood brain and spinal tumours. International Journal of Epidemiology. 1994;**23**(3):458-464

[3] Ostrom QT, Gittleman H, Liao P, Vecchione-Koval T, Wolinsky Y, Kruchko C, et al. CBTRUS statistical report: Primary brain and other central nervous system tumors diagnosed in the United States in 2010-2014. Neuro-Oncology. 2017;**19**(suppl_5):v1-v88

[4] Freeman CR, Farmer JP. Pediatric brain stem gliomas: A review. International Journal of Radiation Oncology, Biology, Physics. 1998;**40**(2):265-271

[5] Warren KE. Diffuse intrinsic pontine glioma: Poised for progress. Frontiers in Oncology. 2012;**2**:205

[6] Bleyer A, O'Leary M, Barr R, Ries LAG, editors. Cancer Epidemiology in Older Adolescents and Young Adults 15 to 29 Years of Age, Including SEER Incidence and Survival: 1975-2000. NIH Pub. No. 06-5767. Bethesda, MD: National Cancer Institute; 2006

[7] Smith MA, Seibel NL, Altekruse SF, Ries LA, Melbert DL, O'Leary M, et al. Outcomes for children and adolescents with cancer: Challenges for the twenty-first century. Journal of Clinical Oncology. 2010;**28**(15):2625-2634

[8] Cohen KJ, Heideman RL, Zhou T, Holmes EJ, Lavey RS, Bouffet E, et al. Temozolomide in the treatment of children with newly diagnosed diffuse intrinsic pontine gliomas: A report from the Children's oncology group. Neuro-Oncology. 2011;**13**(4):410-416

[9] Hargrave D, Bartels U, Bouffet E. Diffuse brainstem glioma in children: Critical review of clinical trials. The Lancet Oncology. 2006;**7**(3):241-248

[10] Jansen MH, van Vuurden DG, Vandertop WP, Kaspers GJ. Diffuse intrinsic pontine gliomas: A systematic update on clinical trials and biology. Cancer Treatment Reviews. 2012;**38**(1):27-35

[11] Donaldson SS, Laningham F, Fisher PG. Advances toward an understanding of brainstem gliomas. Journal of Clinical Oncology. 2006;**24**(8):1266-1272

[12] Littman P, Jarrett P, Bilaniuk LT, Rorke LB, Zimmerman RA, Bruce DA, et al. Pediatric brain stem gliomas. Cancer. 1980;**45**(11):2787-2792

[13] Berger MS, Edwards MS, LaMasters D, Davis RL, Wilson CB. Pediatric brain stem tumors: Radiographic, pathological, and clinical correlations. Neurosurgery. 1983;**12**(3):298-302

[14] Grimm SA, Chamberlain MC. Brainstem glioma: A review. Current Neurology and Neuroscience Reports. 2013;**13**(5):346

[15] Fangusaro J. Pediatric high-grade gliomas and diffuse intrinsic pontine gliomas. Journal of Child Neurology. 2009;**24**(11):1409-1417

[16] Albright AL, Guthkelch AN, Packer RJ, Price RA, Rourke LB. Prognostic factors in pediatric brain-stem gliomas. Journal of Neurosurgery. 1986;**65**(6):751-755

[17] Fisher PG, Breiter SN, Carson BS, Wharam MD, Williams JA, Weingart JD, et al. A clinicopathologic reappraisal of brain stem tumor classification. Identification of pilocystic astrocytoma and fibrillary astrocytoma as distinct entities. Cancer. 2000;**89**(7):1569-1576

[18] Schroeder KM, Hoeman CM, Becher OJ. Children are not just little adults: Recent advances in understanding of diffuse intrinsic pontine glioma biology. Pediatric Research. 2014;**75**(1-2):205-209

[19] Fischbein NJ, Prados MD, Wara W, Russo C, Edwards MS, Barkovich AJ. Radiologic classification of brain stem tumors: Correlation of magnetic resonance imaging appearance with clinical outcome. Pediatric Neurosurgery. 1996;**24**(1):9-23

[20] Bartels U, Hawkins C, Vezina G, Kun L, Souweidane M, Bouffet E. Proceedings of the diffuse intrinsic pontine glioma (DIPG) Toronto Think Tank: Advancing basic and translational research and cooperation in DIPG. Journal of Neuro-Oncology. 2011;**105**(1):119-125

[21] Warren KE. Novel therapeutic delivery approaches in development for pediatric gliomas. CNS Oncology. 2013;**2**(5):427-435

[22] Tzika AA, Astrakas LG, Zarifi MK, Zurakowski D, Poussaint TY, Goumnerova L, et al. Spectroscopic and perfusion magnetic resonance imaging predictors of progression in pediatric brain tumors. Cancer. 2004;**100**(6):1246-1256

[23] Phillips NS, Sanford RA, Helton KJ, Boop FA, Zou P, Tekautz T, et al. Diffusion tensor imaging of intraaxial tumors at the cervicomedullary and pontomedullary junctions. Report of two cases. Journal of Neurosurgery. 2005;**103**(6 Suppl):557-562

[24] Helton KJ, Phillips NS, Khan RB, Boop FA, Sanford RA, Zou P, et al. Diffusion tensor imaging of tract involvement in children with pontine tumors. AJNR. American Journal of Neuroradiology. 2006;**27**(4):786-793

[25] Hipp SJ, Steffen-Smith E, Hammoud D, Shih JH, Bent R, Warren KE. Predicting outcome of children with diffuse intrinsic pontine gliomas using multiparametric imaging. Neuro-Oncology. 2011;**13**(8):904-909

[26] van Dongen GA, Poot AJ, Vugts DJ. PET imaging with radiolabeled antibodies and tyrosine kinase inhibitors: Immuno-PET and TKI-PET. Tumour Biology. 2012;**33**(3):607-615

[27] Jansen MH, Veldhuijzen van Zanten SEM, van Vuurden DG, Huisman MC, Vugts DJ, Hoekstra OS, et al. Molecular drug imaging: (89)Zr-Bevacizumab PET in children with diffuse intrinsic Pontine Glioma. Journal of Nuclear Medicine. 2017;**58**(5):711-716

[28] El-Khouly FE, van Vuurden DG, Stroink T, Hulleman E, Kaspers GJL, Hendrikse NH, et al. Effective drug delivery in diffuse intrinsic Pontine Glioma: A theoretical model to identify potential candidates. Frontiers in Oncology. 2017;**7**:254

[29] Mantravadi RV, Phatak R, Bellur S, Liebner EJ, Haas R. Brain stem gliomas: An autopsy study of 25 cases. Cancer. 1982;**49**(6):1294-1296

[30] Grigsby PW, Garcia DM, Ghiselli R. Analysis of autopsy findings in patients treated with irradiation for thalamic and brain stem tumors. American Journal of Clinical Oncology. 1989;**12**(3):255-258

[31] Sethi R, Allen J, Donahue B, Karajannis M, Gardner S, Wisoff J, et al. Prospective neuraxis MRI surveillance reveals a high risk of leptomeningeal dissemination in diffuse intrinsic pontine glioma. Journal of Neuro-Oncology. 2011;**102**(1):121-127

[32] Gururangan S, McLaughlin CA, Brashears J, Watral MA, Provenzale J, Coleman RE, et al. Incidence and patterns of neuraxis metastases in children with diffuse pontine glioma. Journal of Neuro-Oncology. 2006;**77**(2):207-212

[33] Donahue B, Allen J, Siffert J, Rosovsky M, Pinto R. Patterns of recurrence in brain stem gliomas: Evidence for craniospinal dissemination. International Journal of Radiation Oncology, Biology, Physics. 1998;**40**(3):677-680

[34] Maria BL, Rehder K, Eskin TA, Hamed LM, Fennell EB, Quisling RG, et al. Brainstem glioma: I. Pathology, clinical features, and therapy. Journal of Child Neurology. 1993;**8**(2):112-128

[35] Monje M, Mitra SS, Freret ME, Raveh TB, Kim J, Masek M, et al. Hedgehog-responsive candidate cell of origin for diffuse intrinsic pontine glioma. Proceedings of the National Academy of Sciences of the United States of America. 2011;**108**(11):4453-4448

[36] Schumacher M, Schulte-Monting J, Stoeter P, Warmuth-Metz M, Solymosi L. Magnetic resonance imaging compared with biopsy in the diagnosis of brainstem diseases of childhood: A multicenter review. Journal of Neurosurgery. 2007;**106**(2 Suppl):111-119

[37] Edwards MS, Wara WM, Urtasun RC, Prados M, Levin VA, Fulton D, et al. Hyperfractionated radiation therapy for brain-stem glioma: A phase I-II trial. Journal of Neurosurgery. 1989;**70**(5):691-700

[38] Laigle-Donadey F, Doz F, Delattre JY. Brainstem gliomas in children and adults. Current Opinion in Oncology. 2008;**20**(6):662-667

[39] Bugiani M, Veldhuijzen van Zanten SEM, Caretti V, Schellen P, Aronica E, Noske DP, et al. Deceptive morphologic and epigenetic heterogeneity in diffuse intrinsic pontine glioma. Oncotarget. 2017;**8**(36):60447-60452

[40] Hawkins C, Ellison DW, Sturm D. Diffuse midline glioma, H3K27M-mutant. In: Louis DN, Ohgaki H, Wiestler OD, Cavenee WK, editors. WHO Classification of Tumours of the Central Nervous System. Revised 4th ed. Lyon: International Agency for Research on Cancer (IARC); 2016. pp. 57-59

[41] Jenkin RD, Boesel C, Ertel I, Evans A, Hittle R, Ortega J, et al. Brain-stem tumors in childhood: A prospective randomized trial of irradiation with and without adjuvant CCNU, VCR, and prednisone. A report of the Childrens Cancer Study Group. Journal of Neurosurgery. 1987;**66**(2):227-233

[42] Epstein F, Wisoff JH. Intrinsic brainstem tumors in childhood: Surgical indications. Journal of Neuro-Oncology. 1988;**6**(4):309-317

[43] Albright AL, Packer RJ, Zimmerman R, Rorke LB, Boyett J, Hammond GD. Magnetic resonance scans should replace biopsies for the diagnosis of diffuse brain stem gliomas: A report from the Children's Cancer Group. Neurosurgery. 1993;**33**(6):1026-1029 discussion 9-30

[44] Cartmill M, Punt J. Diffuse brain stem glioma. A review of stereotactic biopsies. Child's Nervous System. 1999;**15**(5):235-237 discussion 8

[45] Grill J, Puget S, Andreiuolo F, Philippe C, MacConaill L, Kieran MW. Critical oncogenic mutations in newly diagnosed pediatric diffuse intrinsic pontine glioma. Pediatric Blood & Cancer. 2012;**58**(4):489-491

[46] Roujeau T, Machado G, Garnett MR, Miquel C, Puget S, Geoerger B, et al. Stereotactic biopsy of diffuse pontine lesions in children. Journal of Neurosurgery. 2007;**107**(1 Suppl):1-4

[47] Zarghooni M, Bartels U, Lee E, Buczkowicz P, Morrison A, Huang A, et al. Whole-genome profiling of pediatric diffuse intrinsic pontine gliomas highlights platelet-derived growth factor receptor alpha and poly (ADP-ribose) polymerase as potential therapeutic targets. Journal of Clinical Oncology. 2010;**28**(8):1337-1344

[48] Paugh BS, Broniscer A, Qu C, Miller CP, Zhang J, Tatevossian RG, et al. Genome-wide analyses identify recurrent amplifications of receptor tyrosine kinases and cell-cycle regulatory genes in diffuse intrinsic pontine glioma. Journal of Clinical Oncology. 2011;**29**(30):3999-4006

[49] Geoerger B, Hargrave D, Thomas F, Ndiaye A, Frappaz D, Andreiuolo F, et al. Innovative therapies for children with cancer pediatric phase I study of erlotinib in brainstem glioma and relapsing/refractory brain tumors. Neuro-Oncology. 2011;**13**(1):109-118

[50] Ogiwara H, Morota N. The efficacy of a biopsy of intrinsic brainstem lesions for decision making of the treatments. Child's Nervous System. 2013;**29**(5):833-837

[51] MacDonald TJ. Diffuse intrinsic pontine glioma (DIPG): Time to biopsy again? Pediatric Blood & Cancer. 2012;**58**(4):487-488

[52] Walker DA, Liu J, Kieran M, Jabado N, Picton S, Packer R, et al. A multi-disciplinary consensus statement concerning surgical approaches to low-grade, high-grade astrocytomas and diffuse intrinsic pontine gliomas in childhood (CPN Paris 2011) using the Delphi method. Neuro-Oncology. 2013;**15**(4):462-468

[53] Buczkowicz P, Bartels U, Bouffet E, Becher O, Hawkins C. Histopathological spectrum of paediatric diffuse intrinsic pontine glioma: Diagnostic and therapeutic implications. Acta Neuropathologica. 2014;**128**(4):573-581

[54] Hoffman LM, DeWire M, Ryall S, Buczkowicz P, Leach J, Miles L, et al. Spatial genomic heterogeneity in diffuse intrinsic pontine and midline high-grade glioma: Implications for diagnostic biopsy and targeted therapeutics. Acta Neuropathologica Communications. 2016;**4**:1

[55] Janssens GO, Gidding CE, Van Lindert EJ, Oldenburger FR, Erasmus CE, Schouten-Meeteren AY, et al. The role of hypofractionation radiotherapy for diffuse intrinsic brainstem glioma in children: A pilot study. International Journal of Radiation Oncology, Biology, Physics. 2009;**73**(3):722-726

[56] Negretti L, Bouchireb K, Levy-Piedbois C, Habrand JL, Dhermain F, Kalifa C, et al. Hypofractionated radiotherapy in the treatment of diffuse intrinsic pontine glioma in children: A single institution's experience. Journal of Neuro-Oncology. 2011;**104**(3):773-777

[57] Wolff JE, Driever PH, Erdlenbruch B, Kortmann RD, Rutkowski S, Pietsch T, et al. Intensive chemotherapy improves survival in pediatric high-grade glioma after gross total resection: Results of the HIT-GBM-C protocol. Cancer. 2010;**116**(3):705-712

[58] Massimino M, Spreafico F, Biassoni V, Simonetti F, Riva D, Trecate G, et al. Diffuse pontine gliomas in children: Changing strategies, changing results? A mono-institutional 20-year experience. Journal of Neuro-Oncology. 2008;**87**(3):355-361

[59] Wolff JE, Rytting ME, Vats TS, Zage PE, Ater JL, Woo S, et al. Treatment of recurrent diffuse intrinsic pontine glioma: The MD Anderson Cancer Center experience. Journal of Neuro-Oncology. 2012;**106**(2):391-397

[60] Frappaz D, Schell M, Thiesse P, Marec-Berard P, Mottolese C, Perol D, et al. Preradiation chemotherapy may improve survival in pediatric diffuse intrinsic brainstem gliomas: Final results of BSG 98 prospective trial. Neuro-Oncology. 2008;**10**(4):599-607

[61] Buczkowicz P, Hawkins C. Pathology, molecular genetics, and epigenetics of diffuse intrinsic pontine glioma. Frontiers in Oncology. 2015;**5**:147

[62] Jalali R, Raut N, Arora B, Gupta T, Dutta D, Munshi A, et al. Prospective evaluation of radiotherapy with concurrent and adjuvant temozolomide in children with newly diagnosed diffuse intrinsic pontine glioma. International Journal of Radiation Oncology, Biology, Physics. 2010;**77**(1):113-118

[63] Chassot A, Canale S, Varlet P, Puget S, Roujeau T, Negretti L, et al. Radiotherapy with concurrent and adjuvant temozolomide in children with newly diagnosed diffuse intrinsic pontine glioma. Journal of Neuro-Oncology. 2012;**106**(2):399-407

[64] Jakacki RI, Cohen KJ, Buxton A, Krailo MD, Burger PC, Rosenblum MK, et al. Phase 2 study of concurrent radiotherapy and temozolomide followed by temozolomide and lomustine in the treatment of children with high-grade glioma: A report of the Children's Oncology Group ACNS0423 study. Neuro-Oncology. 2016;**18**(10):1442-1450

[65] Agnihotri S, Burrell K, Buczkowicz P, Remke M, Golbourn B, Chornenkyy Y, et al. ATM regulates 3-methylpurine-DNA glycosylase and promotes therapeutic resistance to alkylating agents. Cancer Discovery. 2014;**4**(10):1198-1213

[66] Molecularly Determined Treatment of Diffuse Intrinsic Pontine Gliomas (DIPG)

[67] Bernier-Chastagner V, Grill J, Doz F, Bracard S, Gentet JC, Marie-Cardine A, et al. Topotecan as a radiosensitizer in the treatment of children with malignant diffuse brainstem gliomas: Results of a French Society of Paediatric Oncology Phase II study. Cancer. 2005;**104**(12):2792-2797

[68] Kivivuori SM, Riikonen P, Valanne L, Lonnqvist T, Saarinen-Pihkala UM. Antiangiogenic combination therapy after local radiotherapy with topotecan radiosensitizer improved quality of life for children with inoperable brainstem gliomas. Acta Paediatrica. 2011;**100**(1):134-138

[69] Bradley KA, Zhou T, McNall-Knapp RY, Jakacki RI, Levy AS, Vezina G, et al. Motexafin-gadolinium and involved field radiation therapy for intrinsic pontine glioma of

childhood: A children's oncology group phase 2 study. International Journal of Radiation Oncology, Biology, Physics. 2013;**85**(1):e55-e60

[70] Aquino-Parsons C, Hukin J, Green A. Concurrent carbogen and radiation therapy in children with high-risk brainstem gliomas. Pediatric Blood & Cancer. 2008;**50**(2):397-399

[71] Broniscer A, Baker JN, Baker SJ, Chi SN, Geyer JR, Morris EB, et al. Prospective collection of tissue samples at autopsy in children with diffuse intrinsic pontine glioma. Cancer. 2010;**116**(19):4632-4467

[72] Kambhampati M, Perez JP, Yadavilli S, Saratsis AM, Hill AD, Ho CY, et al. A standardized autopsy procurement allows for the comprehensive study of DIPG biology. Oncotarget. 2015;**6**(14):12740-12747

[73] Caretti V, Hiddingh L, Lagerweij T, Schellen P, Koken PW, Hulleman E, et al. WEE1 kinase inhibition enhances the radiation response of diffuse intrinsic pontine gliomas. Molecular Cancer Therapeutics. 2013;**12**(2):141-150

[74] Sewing AC, Caretti V, Lagerweij T, Schellen P, Jansen MH, van Vuurden DG, et al. Convection enhanced delivery of carmustine to the murine brainstem: A feasibility study. Journal of Neuroscience Methods. 2014;**238**:88-94

[75] Misuraca KL, Barton KL, Chung A, Diaz AK, Conway SJ, Corcoran DL, et al. Pax3 expression enhances PDGF-B-induced brainstem gliomagenesis and characterizes a subset of brainstem glioma. Acta Neuropathologica Communications. 2014;**2**:134

[76] Ballester LY, Wang Z, Shandilya S, Miettinen M, Burger PC, Eberhart CG, et al. Morphologic characteristics and immunohistochemical profile of diffuse intrinsic pontine gliomas. The American Journal of Surgical Pathology. 2013;**37**(9):1357-1364

[77] Jones C, Baker SJ. Unique genetic and epigenetic mechanisms driving paediatric diffuse high-grade glioma. Nature Reviews. Cancer. 2014;**14**(10):651-661

[78] Kepert JF, Toth KF, Caudron M, Mucke N, Langowski J, Rippe K. Conformation of reconstituted mononucleosomes and effect of linker histone H1 binding studied by scanning force microscopy. Biophysical Journal. 2003;**85**(6):4012-4022

[79] Marino-Ramirez L, Kann MG, Shoemaker BA, Landsman D. Histone structure and nucleosome stability. Expert Review of Proteomics. 2005;**2**(5):719-729

[80] Tagami H, Ray-Gallet D, Almouzni G, Nakatani Y. Histone H3.1 and H3.3 complexes mediate nucleosome assembly pathways dependent or independent of DNA synthesis. Cell. 2004;**116**(1):51-61

[81] Wells D, Hoffman D, Kedes L. Unusual structure, evolutionary conservation of non-coding sequences and numerous pseudogenes characterize the human H3.3 histone multigene family. Nucleic Acids Research. 1987;**15**(7):2871-2889

[82] Albig W, Bramlage B, Gruber K, Klobeck HG, Kunz J, Doenecke D. The human replacement histone H3.3B gene (H3F3B). Genomics. 1995;**30**(2):264-272

[83] Yuen BT, Knoepfler PS. Histone H3.3 mutations: A variant path to cancer. Cancer Cell. 2013;**24**(5):567-574

[84] Wu G, Diaz AK, Paugh BS, Rankin SL, Ju B, Li Y, et al. The genomic landscape of diffuse intrinsic pontine glioma and pediatric non-brainstem high-grade glioma. Nature Genetics. 2014;**46**(5):444-450

[85] Wu G, Broniscer A, McEachron TA, Lu C, Paugh BS, Becksfort J, et al. Somatic histone H3 alterations in pediatric diffuse intrinsic pontine gliomas and non-brainstem glioblastomas. Nature Genetics. 2012;**44**(3):251-253

[86] Mackay A, Burford A, Carvalho D, Izquierdo E, Fazal-Salom J, Taylor KR, et al. Integrated molecular meta-analysis of 1,000 pediatric high-grade and diffuse intrinsic pontine glioma. Cancer Cell. 2017;**32**(4):520-537 e5

[87] Castel D, Philippe C, Calmon R, Le Dret L, Truffaux N, Boddaert N, et al. Histone H3F3A and HIST1H3B K27M mutations define two subgroups of diffuse intrinsic pontine gliomas with different prognosis and phenotypes. Acta Neuropathologica. 2015;**130**(6):815-827

[88] Schwartzentruber J, Korshunov A, Liu XY, Jones DT, Pfaff E, Jacob K, et al. Driver mutations in histone H3.3 and chromatin remodelling genes in paediatric glioblastoma. Nature. 2012;**482**(7384):226-231

[89] Sturm D, Witt H, Hovestadt V, Khuong-Quang DA, Jones DT, Konermann C, et al. Hotspot mutations in H3F3A and IDH1 define distinct epigenetic and biological subgroups of glioblastoma. Cancer Cell. 2012;**22**(4):425-437

[90] Lewis PW, Muller MM, Koletsky MS, Cordero F, Lin S, Banaszynski LA, et al. Inhibition of PRC2 activity by a gain-of-function H3 mutation found in pediatric glioblastoma. Science. 2013;**340**(6134):857-861

[91] Bender S, Tang Y, Lindroth AM, Hovestadt V, Jones DT, Kool M, et al. Reduced H3K27me3 and DNA hypomethylation are major drivers of gene expression in K27M mutant pediatric high-grade gliomas. Cancer Cell. 2013;**24**(5):660-672

[92] Saratsis AM, Kambhampati M, Snyder K, Yadavilli S, Devaney JM, Harmon B, et al. Comparative multidimensional molecular analyses of pediatric diffuse intrinsic pontine glioma reveals distinct molecular subtypes. Acta Neuropathologica. 2014;**127**(6):881-895

[93] Chan KM, Fang D, Gan H, Hashizume R, Yu C, Schroeder M, et al. The histone H3.3K27M mutation in pediatric glioma reprograms H3K27 methylation and gene expression. Genes & Development. 2013;**27**(9):985-990

[94] Venneti S, Garimella MT, Sullivan LM, Martinez D, Huse JT, Heguy A, et al. Evaluation of histone 3 lysine 27 trimethylation (H3K27me3) and enhancer of Zest 2 (EZH2) in pediatric glial and glioneuronal tumors shows decreased H3K27me3 in H3F3A K27M mutant glioblastomas. Brain Pathology. 2013;**23**(5):558-564

[95] Funato K, Major T, Lewis PW, Allis CD, Tabar V. Use of human embryonic stem cells to model pediatric gliomas with H3.3K27M histone mutation. Science. 2014;**346**(6216): 1529-1533

[96] Nikbakht H, Panditharatna E, Mikael LG, Li R, Gayden T, Osmond M, et al. Spatial and temporal homogeneity of driver mutations in diffuse intrinsic pontine glioma. Nature Communications. 2016;**7**:11185

[97] Swartling FJ, Savov V, Persson AI, Chen J, Hackett CS, Northcott PA, et al. Distinct neural stem cell populations give rise to disparate brain tumors in response to N-MYC. Cancer Cell. 2012;**21**(5):601-613

[98] Bjerke L, Mackay A, Nandhabalan M, Burford A, Jury A, Popov S, et al. Histone H3.3. mutations drive pediatric glioblastoma through upregulation of MYCN. Cancer Discovery. 2013;**3**(5):512-519

[99] Khuong-Quang DA, Buczkowicz P, Rakopoulos P, Liu XY, Fontebasso AM, Bouffet E, et al. K27M mutation in histone H3.3 defines clinically and biologically distinct subgroups of pediatric diffuse intrinsic pontine gliomas. Acta Neuropathologica. 2012;**124**(3):439-447

[100] Jones DT, Hutter B, Jager N, Korshunov A, Kool M, Warnatz HJ, et al. Recurrent somatic alterations of FGFR1 and NTRK2 in pilocytic astrocytoma. Nature Genetics. 2013;**45**(8):927-932

[101] Jenuwein T, Allis CD. Translating the histone code. Science. 2001;**293**(5532):1074-1080

[102] Plass C, Pfister SM, Lindroth AM, Bogatyrova O, Claus R, Lichter P. Mutations in regulators of the epigenome and their connections to global chromatin patterns in cancer. Nature Reviews. Genetics. 2013;**14**(11):765-780

[103] Margueron R, Reinberg D. The Polycomb complex PRC2 and its mark in life. Nature. 2011;**469**(7330):343-349

[104] Eskeland R, Leeb M, Grimes GR, Kress C, Boyle S, Sproul D, et al. Ring1B compacts chromatin structure and represses gene expression independent of histone ubiquitination. Molecular Cell. 2010;**38**(3):452-464

[105] Kumar SS, Sengupta S, Lee K, Hura N, Fuller C, DeWire M, et al. BMI-1 is a potential therapeutic target in diffuse intrinsic pontine glioma. Oncotarget. 2017;**8**(38):62962-62975

[106] Louis DN, Rubio MP, Correa KM, Gusella JF, von Deimling A. Molecular genetics of pediatric brain stem gliomas. Application of PCR techniques to small and archival brain tumor specimens. Journal of Neuropathology and Experimental Neurology. 1993;**52**(5):507-515

[107] Bax DA, Mackay A, Little SE, Carvalho D, Viana-Pereira M, Tamber N, et al. A distinct spectrum of copy number aberrations in pediatric high-grade gliomas. Clinical Cancer Research. 2010;**16**(13):3368-3377

[108] Qu HQ, Jacob K, Fatet S, Ge B, Barnett D, Delattre O, et al. Genome-wide profiling using single-nucleotide polymorphism arrays identifies novel chromosomal imbalances in pediatric glioblastomas. Neuro-Oncology. 2010;**12**(2):153-163

[109] Barrow J, Adamowicz-Brice M, Cartmill M, MacArthur D, Lowe J, Robson K, et al. Homozygous loss of ADAM3A revealed by genome-wide analysis of pediatric high-grade glioma and diffuse intrinsic pontine gliomas. Neuro-Oncology. 2011;**13**(2):212-222

[110] Kyritsis AP, Bondy ML, Rao JS, Sioka C. Inherited predisposition to glioma. Neuro-Oncology. 2010;**12**(1):104-113

[111] Taylor KR, Mackay A, Truffaux N, Butterfield Y, Morozova O, Philippe C, et al. Recurrent activating ACVR1 mutations in diffuse intrinsic pontine glioma. Nature Genetics. 2014;**46**(5):457-461

[112] Fontebasso AM, Papillon-Cavanagh S, Schwartzentruber J, Nikbakht H, Gerges N, Fiset PO, et al. Recurrent somatic mutations in ACVR1 in pediatric midline high-grade astrocytoma. Nature Genetics. 2014;**46**(5):462-466

[113] Rigueur D, Brugger S, Anbarchian T, Kim JK, Lee Y, Lyons KM. The type I BMP receptor ACVR1/ALK2 is required for chondrogenesis during development. Journal of Bone and Mineral Research. 2015;**30**(4):733-741

[114] Han HJ, Jain P, Resnick AC. Shared ACVR1 mutations in FOP and DIPG: Opportunities and challenges in extending biological and clinical implications across rare diseases. Bone. 2018;**109**:91-100

[115] Buczkowicz P, Hoeman C, Rakopoulos P, Pajovic S, Letourneau L, Dzamba M, et al. Genomic analysis of diffuse intrinsic pontine gliomas identifies three molecular subgroups and recurrent activating ACVR1 mutations. Nature Genetics. 2014;**46**(5):451-456

[116] Zadeh G, Aldape K. ACVR1 mutations and the genomic landscape of pediatric diffuse glioma. Nature Genetics. 2014;**46**(5):421-422

[117] Regad T. Targeting RTK signaling pathways in Cancer. Cancers (Basel). 2015;**7**(3): 1758-1784

[118] Lemmon MA, Schlessinger J. Cell signaling by receptor tyrosine kinases. Cell. 2010; **141**(7):1117-1134

[119] Li E, Hristova K. Role of receptor tyrosine kinase transmembrane domains in cell signaling and human pathologies. Biochemistry. 2006;**45**(20):6241-6251

[120] Hubbard SR, Miller WT. Receptor tyrosine kinases: Mechanisms of activation and signaling. Current Opinion in Cell Biology. 2007;**19**(2):117-123

[121] Schlessinger J. Cell signaling by receptor tyrosine kinases. Cell. 2000;**103**(2):211-225

[122] Paugh BS, Qu C, Jones C, Liu Z, Adamowicz-Brice M, Zhang J, et al. Integrated molecular genetic profiling of pediatric high-grade gliomas reveals key differences with the adult disease. Journal of Clinical Oncology. 2010;**28**(18):3061-3068

[123] Puget S, Philippe C, Bax DA, Job B, Varlet P, Junier MP, et al. Mesenchymal transition and PDGFRA amplification/mutation are key distinct oncogenic events in pediatric diffuse intrinsic pontine gliomas. PLoS One. 2012;**7**(2):e30313

[124] Paugh BS, Zhu X, Qu C, Endersby R, Diaz AK, Zhang J, et al. Novel oncogenic PDGFRA mutations in pediatric high-grade gliomas. Cancer Research. 2013;**73**(20):6219-6629

[125] Becher OJ, Hambardzumyan D, Walker TR, Helmy K, Nazarian J, Albrecht S, et al. Preclinical evaluation of radiation and perifosine in a genetically and histologically accurate model of brainstem glioma. Cancer Research. 2010;**70**(6):2548-2557

[126] Masui K, Suzuki SO, Torisu R, Goldman JE, Canoll P, Iwaki T. Glial progenitors in the brainstem give rise to malignant gliomas by platelet-derived growth factor stimulation. Glia. 2010;**58**(9):1050-1065

[127] Corless CL, Schroeder A, Griffith D, Town A, McGreevey L, Harrell P, et al. PDGFRA mutations in gastrointestinal stromal tumors: Frequency, spectrum and in vitro sensitivity to imatinib. Journal of Clinical Oncology. 2005;**23**(23):5357-5364

[128] Guglielmi L, Cinnella C, Nardella M, Maresca G, Valentini A, Mercanti D, et al. MYCN gene expression is required for the onset of the differentiation programme in neuroblastoma cells. Cell Death & Disease. 2014;**5**:e1081

[129] Vogelstein B, Lane D, Levine AJ. Surfing the p53 network. Nature. 2000;**408**(6810):307-310

[130] Jin S, Levine AJ. The p53 functional circuit. Journal of Cell Science. 2001;**114**(Pt 23):4139-4140

[131] Harris SL, Levine AJ. The p53 pathway: Positive and negative feedback loops. Oncogene. 2005;**24**(17):2899-2908

[132] Aubrey BJ, Strasser A, Kelly GL. Tumor-suppressor functions of the TP53 pathway. Cold Spring Harbor Perspectives in Medicine. 2016;**6**(5):1-16

[133] Zhang S, Feng X, Koga H, Ichikawa T, Abe S, Kumanishi T. p53 gene mutations in pontine gliomas of juvenile onset. Biochemical and Biophysical Research Communications. 1993;**196**(2):851-857

[134] Zhang L, Chen LH, Wan H, Yang R, Wang Z, Feng J, et al. Exome sequencing identifies somatic gain-of-function PPM1D mutations in brainstem gliomas. Nature Genetics. 2014;**46**(7):726-730

[135] Richter M, Dayaram T, Gilmartin AG, Ganji G, Pemmasani SK, Van Der Key H, et al. WIP1 phosphatase as a potential therapeutic target in neuroblastoma. PLoS One. 2015;**10**(2):e0115635

[136] Zajkowicz A, Butkiewicz D, Drosik A, Giglok M, Suwinski R, Rusin M. Truncating mutations of PPM1D are found in blood DNA samples of lung cancer patients. British Journal of Cancer. 2015;**112**(6):1114-1120

[137] Kleiblova P, Shaltiel IA, Benada J, Sevcik J, Pechackova S, Pohlreich P, et al. Gain-of-function mutations of PPM1D/Wip1 impair the p53-dependent G1 checkpoint. The Journal of Cell Biology. 2013;**201**(4):511-521

[138] Duronio RJ, Xiong Y. Signaling pathways that control cell proliferation. Cold Spring Harbor Perspectives in Biology. 2013;**5**(3):a008904

[139] Warren KE, Killian K, Suuriniemi M, Wang Y, Quezado M, Meltzer PS. Genomic aberrations in pediatric diffuse intrinsic pontine gliomas. Neuro-Oncology. 2012;**14**(3):326-332

[140] Dar AA, Goff LW, Majid S, Berlin J, El-Rifai W. Aurora kinase inhibitors--rising stars in cancer therapeutics? Molecular Cancer Therapeutics. 2010;**9**(2):268-278

[141] Hauf S, Cole RW, LaTerra S, Zimmer C, Schnapp G, Walter R, et al. The small molecule Hesperadin reveals a role for aurora B in correcting kinetochore-microtubule attachment and in maintaining the spindle assembly checkpoint. The Journal of Cell Biology. 2003;**161**(2):281-294

[142] Buczkowicz P, Zarghooni M, Bartels U, Morrison A, Misuraca KL, Chan T, et al. Aurora kinase B is a potential therapeutic target in pediatric diffuse intrinsic pontine glioma. Brain Pathology. 2013;**23**(3):244-253

[143] Sung T, Miller DC, Hayes RL, Alonso M, Yee H, Newcomb EW. Preferential inactivation of the p53 tumor suppressor pathway and lack of EGFR amplification distinguish de novo high grade pediatric astrocytomas from de novo adult astrocytomas. Brain Pathology. 2000;**10**(2):249-259

[144] Ratnam K, Low JA. Current development of clinical inhibitors of poly(ADP-ribose) polymerase in oncology. Clinical Cancer Research. 2007;**13**(5):1383-1388

[145] Rickert CH, Strater R, Kaatsch P, Wassmann H, Jurgens H, Dockhorn-Dworniczak B, et al. Pediatric high-grade astrocytomas show chromosomal imbalances distinct from adult cases. The American Journal of Pathology. 2001;**158**(4):1525-1532

[146] Chapoval AI, Ni J, Lau JS, Wilcox RA, Flies DB, Liu D, et al. B7-H3: A costimulatory molecule for T cell activation and IFN-gamma production. Nature Immunology. 2001;**2**(3):269-274

[147] Zhou Z, Luther N, Ibrahim GM, Hawkins C, Vibhakar R, Handler MH, et al. B7-H3, a potential therapeutic target, is expressed in diffuse intrinsic pontine glioma. Journal of Neuro-Oncology. 2013;**111**(3):257-264

[148] Modak S, Kramer K, Gultckin SH, Guo HF, Cheung NK. Monoclonal antibody 8H9 targets a novel cell surface antigen expressed by a wide spectrum of human solid tumors. Cancer Research. 2001;**61**(10):4048-4054

[149] Xu H, Cheung IY, Guo HF, Cheung NK. MicroRNA miR-29 modulates expression of immunoinhibitory molecule B7-H3: Potential implications for immune based therapy of human solid tumors. Cancer Research. 2009;**69**(15):6275-6281

[150] Kramer K, Kushner BH, Modak S, Pandit-Taskar N, Smith-Jones P, Zanzonico P, et al. Compartmental intrathecal radioimmunotherapy: Results for treatment for metastatic CNS neuroblastoma. Journal of Neuro-Oncology. 2010;**97**(3):409-418

[151] Venkatesh HS, Johung TB, Caretti V, Noll A, Tang Y, Nagaraja S, et al. Neuronal activity promotes glioma growth through neuroligin-3 secretion. Cell. 2015;**161**(4):803-816

[152] Venkatesh HS, Tam LT, Woo PJ, Lennon J, Nagaraja S, Gillespie SM, et al. Targeting neuronal activity-regulated neuroligin-3 dependency in high-grade glioma. Nature. 2017;**549**(7673):533-537

[153] Qin EY, Cooper DD, Abbott KL, Lennon J, Nagaraja S, Mackay A, et al. Neural precursor-derived pleiotrophin mediates subventricular zone invasion by glioma. Cell. 2017;**170**(5):845-859 e19

[154] Truffaux N, Philippe C, Paulsson J, Andreiuolo F, Guerrini-Rousseau L, Cornilleau G, et al. Preclinical evaluation of dasatinib alone and in combination with cabozantinib for the treatment of diffuse intrinsic pontine glioma. Neuro-Oncology. 2015;**17**(7):953-964

[155] Pollack IF, Jakacki RI, Blaney SM, Hancock ML, Kieran MW, Phillips P, et al. Phase I trial of imatinib in children with newly diagnosed brainstem and recurrent malignant gliomas: A pediatric brain tumor consortium report. Neuro-Oncology. 2007;**9**(2):145-160

[156] Broniscer A, Baker SD, Wetmore C, Pai Panandiker AS, Huang J, Davidoff AM, et al. Phase I trial, pharmacokinetics, and pharmacodynamics of vandetanib and dasatinib in children with newly diagnosed diffuse intrinsic pontine glioma. Clinical Cancer Research. 2013;**19**(11):3050-3058

[157] Broniscer A, Baker JN, Tagen M, Onar-Thomas A, Gilbertson RJ, Davidoff AM, et al. Phase I study of vandetanib during and after radiotherapy in children with diffuse intrinsic pontine glioma. Journal of Clinical Oncology. 2010;**28**(31):4762-4768

[158] Geyer JR, Stewart CF, Kocak M, Broniscer A, Phillips P, Douglas JG, et al. A phase I and biology study of gefitinib and radiation in children with newly diagnosed brain stem gliomas or supratentorial malignant gliomas. European Journal of Cancer. 2010;**46**(18):3287-3293

[159] Holmes D. PI3K pathway inhibitors approach junction. Nature Reviews. Drug Discovery. 2011;**10**(8):563-564

[160] Becher OJ, Gilheeney SW, Khakoo Y, Lyden DC, Haque S, De Braganca, KC, et al. A phase I study of perifosine with temsirolimus for recurrent pediatric solid tumors. Pediatric Blood & Cancer. 2017;**64**:7

[161] Wetmore C, Daryani VM, Billups CA, Boyett JM, Leary S, Tanos R, et al. Phase II evaluation of sunitinib in the treatment of recurrent or refractory high-grade glioma or ependymoma in children: A children's Oncology Group Study ACNS1021. Cancer Medicine. 2016;**5**(7):1416-1424

[162] Fouladi M, Nicholson HS, Zhou T, Laningham F, Helton KJ, Holmes E, et al. A phase II study of the farnesyl transferase inhibitor, tipifarnib, in children with recurrent or progressive high-grade glioma, medulloblastoma/primitive neuroectodermal tumor, or brainstem glioma: A Children's Oncology Group study. Cancer. 2007;**110**(11):2535-2541

[163] Biological Medicine for Diffuse Intrinsic Pontine Glioma (DIPG) Eradication. Available from: https://ClinicalTrials.gov/show/NCT02233049

[164] Hennika T, Hu G, Olaciregui NG, Barton KL, Ehteda A, Chitranjan A, et al. Pre-clinical study of panobinostat in xenograft and genetically engineered murine diffuse intrinsic pontine glioma models. PLoS One. 2017;**12**(1):e0169485

[165] New M, Olzscha H, Thangue L, NB. HDAC inhibitor-based therapies: Can we interpret the code? Molecular Oncology. 2012;**6**(6):637-656

[166] Hashizume R. Epigenetic targeted therapy for diffuse intrinsic pontine glioma. Neurologia Medico-Chirurgica (Tokyo). 2017;**57**(7):331-342

[167] Anne M, Sammartino D, Barginear MF, Budman D. Profile of panobinostat and its potential for treatment in solid tumors: An update. OncoTargets and Therapy. 2013;**6**:1613-1624

[168] Grasso CS, Tang Y, Truffaux N, Berlow NE, Liu L, Debily MA, et al. Functionally defined therapeutic targets in diffuse intrinsic pontine glioma. Nature Medicine. 2015;**21**(7):827

[169] Fouladi M, Park JR, Stewart CF, Gilbertson RJ, Schaiquevich P, Sun J, et al. Pediatric phase I trial and pharmacokinetic study of vorinostat: A Children's Oncology Group phase I consortium report. Journal of Clinical Oncology. 2010;**28**(22):3623-3629

[170] Study of Suberoylanilide Hydroxamic Acid (SAHA) With Temsirolimus in Children With Diffuse Intrinsic Pontine Glioma (DIPG). Available from: https://ClinicalTrials.gov/show/NCT02420613

[171] Trial of Panobinostat in children with diffuse intrinsic Pontine Glioma. Available from: https://ClinicalTrials.gov/show/NCT02717455

[172] Barton KL, Misuraca K, Cordero F, Dobrikova E, Min HD, Gromeier M, et al. PD-0332991, a CDK4/6 inhibitor, significantly prolongs survival in a genetically engineered mouse model of brainstem glioma. PLoS One. 2013;**8**(10):e77639

[173] Goodwin CR, Xu R, Iyer R, Sankey EW, Liu A, Abu-Bonsrah N, et al. Local delivery methods of therapeutic agents in the treatment of diffuse intrinsic brainstem gliomas. Clinical Neurology and Neurosurgery. 2016;**142**:120-127

[174] Pollack IF, Jakacki RI, Butterfield LH, Hamilton RL, Panigrahy A, Potter DM, et al. Antigen-specific immune responses and clinical outcome after vaccination with glioma-associated antigen peptides and polyinosinic-polycytidylic acid stabilized by lysine and carboxymethylcellulose in children with newly diagnosed malignant brainstem and nonbrainstem gliomas. Journal of Clinical Oncology. 2014;**32**(19):2050-2058

[175] Okada H, Low KL, Kohanbash G, McDonald HA, Hamilton RL, Pollack IF. Expression of glioma-associated antigens in pediatric brain stem and non-brain stem gliomas. Journal of Neuro-Oncology. 2008;**88**(3):245-250

[176] Joshi BH, Puri RA, Leland P, Varricchio F, Gupta G, Kocak M, et al. Identification of interleukin-13 receptor alpha2 chain overexpression in situ in high-grade diffusely infiltrative pediatric brainstem glioma. Neuro-Oncology. 2008;**10**(3):265-274

[177] Benedetti S, Pirola B, Pollo B, Magrassi L, Bruzzone MG, Rigamonti D, et al. Gene therapy of experimental brain tumors using neural progenitor cells. Nature Medicine. 2000;**6**(4):447-450

[178] Kim SK, Kim SU, Park IH, Bang JH, Aboody KS, Wang KC, et al. Human neural stem cells target experimental intracranial medulloblastoma and deliver a therapeutic gene leading to tumor regression. Clinical Cancer Research. 2006;**12**(18):5550-5556

[179] Ehtesham M, Stevenson CB, Thompson RC. Stem cell therapies for malignant glioma. Neurosurgical Focus. 2005;**19**(3):E5

[180] Hamada H, Kobune M, Nakamura K, Kawano Y, Kato K, Honmou O, et al. Mesenchymal stem cells (MSC) as therapeutic cytoreagents for gene therapy. Cancer Science. 2005;**96**(3):149-156

[181] Lee DH, Ahn Y, Kim SU, Wang KC, Cho BK, Phi JH, et al. Targeting rat brainstem glioma using human neural stem cells and human mesenchymal stem cells. Clinical Cancer Research. 2009;**15**(15):4925-4934

[182] Muldoon LL, Soussain C, Jahnke K, Johanson C, Siegal T, Smith QR, et al. Chemotherapy delivery issues in central nervous system malignancy: A reality check. Journal of Clinical Oncology. 2007;**25**(16):2295-2305

[183] Subashi E, Cordero FJ, Halvorson KG, Qi Y, Nouls JC, Becher OJ, et al. Tumor location, but not H3.3K27M, significantly influences the blood-brain-barrier permeability in a genetic mouse model of pediatric high-grade glioma. Journal of Neuro-Oncology. 2016;**126**(2):243-251

[184] Bobo RH, Laske DW, Akbasak A, Morrison PF, Dedrick RL, Oldfield EH. Convection-enhanced delivery of macromolecules in the brain. Proceedings of the National Academy of Sciences of the United States of America. 1994;**91**(6):2076-2080

[185] Zhou Z, Singh R, Souweidane MM. Convection-enhanced delivery for diffuse intrinsic pontine glioma treatment. Current Neuropharmacology. 2017;**15**(1):116-128

[186] Debinski W, Tatter SB. Convection-enhanced delivery for the treatment of brain tumors. Expert Review of Neurotherapeutics. 2009;**9**(10):1519-1527

[187] Groothuis DR. The blood-brain and blood-tumor barriers: A review of strategies for increasing drug delivery. Neuro-Oncology. 2000;**2**(1):45-59

[188] Occhiogrosso G, Edgar MA, Sandberg DI, Souweidane MM. Prolonged convection-enhanced delivery into the rat brainstem. Neurosurgery. 2003;**52**(2):388-393 discussion 93-4

[189] Souweidane MM, Occhiogrosso G, Mark EB, Edgar MA, Dunkel IJ. Interstitial infusion of carmustine in the rat brain stem with systemic administration of O6-benzylguanine. Journal of Neuro-Oncology. 2004;**67**(3):319-326

[190] Degen JW, Walbridge S, Vortmeyer AO, Oldfield EH, Lonser RR. Safety and efficacy of convection-enhanced delivery of gemcitabine or carboplatin in a malignant glioma model in rats. Journal of Neurosurgery. 2003;**99**(5):893-898

[191] Wu Q, Guarnieri M, Tyler B, Clatterbuck RE, Liu Y, Carson BS. Section on tumors: Young Investigator Award: Local release of carboplatin via an Alzet mini-osmotic pump prolongs survival in a rat brainstem tumor model. Clinical Neurosurgery. 2004;**51**:332-339

[192] Yoshimura J, Siu IM, Thomale UW, Jallo GI. The effects of temozolomide delivered by prolonged intracerebral microinfusion against the rat brainstem GBM allograft model. Child's Nervous System. 2012;**28**(5):707-713

[193] Zhou Z, Ho SL, Singh R, Pisapia DJ, Souweidane MM. Toxicity evaluation of convection-enhanced delivery of small-molecule kinase inhibitors in naive mouse brainstem. Child's Nervous System. 2015;**31**(4):557-562

[194] Kroin JS, Penn RD. Intracerebral chemotherapy: Chronic microinfusion of cisplatin. Neurosurgery. 1982;**10**(3):349-354

[195] Murad GJ, Walbridge S, Morrison PF, Szerlip N, Butman JA, Oldfield EH, et al. Image-guided convection-enhanced delivery of gemcitabine to the brainstem. Journal of Neurosurgery. 2007;**106**(2):351-356

[196] Anderson RC, Kennedy B, Yanes CL, Garvin J, Needle M, Canoll P, et al. Convection-enhanced delivery of topotecan into diffuse intrinsic brainstem tumors in children. Journal of Neurosurgery. Pediatrics. 2013;**11**(3):289-295

[197] Singleton WGB, Barua NU, Morgan J, Bienemann AS, Killick-Cole CL, Asby DJ, et al. NS-21 multi-catheter intermittent convection-enhanced delivery of carboplatin as a treatment for diffuse intrinsic pontine glioma (DIPG): Pre-clinical rationale and early clinical experience. Neuro-Oncology. 2016;**18**(suppl_3):iii131-iii

[198] Barua NU, Lowis SP, Woolley M, O'Sullivan S, Harrison R, Gill SS. Robot-guided convection-enhanced delivery of carboplatin for advanced brainstem glioma. Acta Neurochirurgica. 2013;**155**(8):1459-1165

[199] Convection-Enhanced Delivery of 124I-8H9 for Patients With Non-Progressive Diffuse pontine gliomas Previously Treated With External Beam Radiation Therapy. Available from: https://ClinicalTrials.gov/show/NCT01502917

[200] Lonser RR, Warren KE, Butman JA, Quezado Z, Robison RA, Walbridge S, et al. Real-time image-guided direct convective perfusion of intrinsic brainstem lesions. Technical note. Journal of Neurosurgery. 2007;**107**(1):190-197

[201] MacKay JA, Deen DF, Szoka FC,J. Distribution in brain of liposomes after convection enhanced delivery; modulation by particle charge, particle diameter, and presence of steric coating. Brain Research. 2005;**1035**(2):139-153

[202] MacDiarmid JA, Mugridge NB, Weiss JC, Phillips L, Burn AL, Paulin RP, et al. Bacterially derived 400 nm particles for encapsulation and cancer cell targeting of chemotherapeutics. Cancer Cell. 2007;**11**(5):431-445

[203] MacDiarmid JA, Langova V, Bailey D, Pattison ST, Pattison SL, Christensen N, et al. Targeted doxorubicin delivery to brain tumors via minicells: Proof of principle using dogs with spontaneously occurring tumors as a model. PLoS One. 2016;**11**(4):e0151832

[204] A Study of Intravenous EEDVsMit in Children With Recurrent Refractory Solid or CNS Tumours Expressing EGFR. Available from: https://ClinicalTrials.gov/show/NCT02687386

3

Vestibular Schwannoma: Microsurgery or Radiosurgery

Ahmed Rizk

Abstract

A vestibular schwannoma (VS) is a benign tumor that arises from the neurilemmal sheath of the vestibular nerve. VSs make up to 6–8% of all intracranial tumors and 70–80% of all cerebellopontine angle tumors. Three therapeutic options are currently considered for VS: expectant treatment, microsurgical resection, and radiosurgery. No class I evidence exists to support one treatment over the others, and some clinical aspects are usually taken into consideration in the decision-making process. Very few comparative studies published so far have addressed the clinical aspects supporting any one treatment modality. The pathology, diagnosis and treatment of VS are discussed in this chapter. Moreover, we aim in this chapter to discuss the results of the most recent clinical studies performed on different treatment strategies for VS. In addition, the results of the comparative studies between microsurgical and radiosurgical treatments for VS are discussed.

Keywords: vestibular schwannoma, radiosurgery, microsurgery, Gamma Knife, intraoperative neurophysiological monitoring, hearing preservation, facial nerve preservation

1. Introduction

Vestibular schwannomas (VS) are benign tumors that typically occur in the internal auditory canal (IAC) and in the cerebellopontine angle (CPA). They originate from Schwann cells of the vestibular nerve. The vestibular nerves are enclosed by central glial and peripheral neurilemmal sheaths. The VS arises from the distal sheath at or close to the neuroglial-neurilemmal junction (Obersteiner-Redlich zone). The transition zone is encountered 1 cm away from the brainstem, commonly occurring at or close to the internal auditory canal (IAC) [1]. VS arises from either the inferior [2, 3] or superior [4] vestibular nerve.

The annual incidence is estimated to be between 0.5 and 1.7 per 100,000 persons, and the incidence is increasing with the widespread use of magnetic resonance imaging (MRI) [5]. VS represents 6–8% of all intracranial tumors and >80% of CPA tumor [6]. It occurs in equal frequency in adult males and females [7–9]. They typically occur between the fourth to sixth decades of life [10]. In teenagers, VSs have been rarely diagnosed [11], and in these cases, the tumor is usually associated with neurofibromatosis type II (NF2) [5]. Patients with NF2 often develop bilateral VS, which is sufficient to make the diagnosis of the disease. These tumors have different biological and clinical characteristics and must be differentiated from the unilateral spontaneous VS [12, 13].

The classical clinical presentation includes high-frequency sensorineural hearing loss, tinnitus, and vertigo. Three therapeutic options are currently considered for VS: expectant treatment, microsurgical resection, and radiosurgery. No class I evidence exists to support one treatment over the others, and some clinical aspects are usually taken into consideration in the decision-making process.

2. Diagnosis

The clinical presentation of VS may vary broadly depending upon tumor extension; whereas intrameatal tumors often present with high-frequency sensorineural hearing loss (about 90% of VS patients), tinnitus (65–75%), vestibular nerve dysfunction which includes vertigo, dizziness, and unsteadiness (in up to 61%); extrameatal tumors may also present with headache, facial hypoesthesia, facial weakness (4–8%), ataxia, lower cranial nerve damage, or hydrocephalus [14]. Another factor affecting clinical presentation is the site of origin of the tumor. Hearing is significantly better preserved in patients affected by medially arising VSs than in patients with laterally arising tumors [15]. The symptoms in VS progress slowly; however, it was noticed that sudden deterioration of symptoms may occur especially in cases of cystic tumors and usually represents intratumoral hemorrhage [16, 17].

A high degree of clinical suspicion is the best key for prompt diagnosis of VS. The clinician should be aware of VS diagnosis in patients complaining of unilateral hearing loss, tinnitus, and vertigo in any combination [7]. Patients with these complaints should undergo pure tone audiometry (PTA) and vestibular testing. Those with abnormalities on either, especially unilateral sensorineural hearing loss, should have MRI with and without contrast.

2.1. Hearing classification

Full audiometric assessment including pure tone audiometry (PTA) and speech discrimination score (SDS) should be done in cases of VS. In PTA, the mean hearing loss (in decibel "dB") at frequencies between 500 and 3000 Hz is assessed. SDS represents the percent of correct score when words are presented at a specified level above the speech recognition threshold. The Committee on Hearing and Equilibrium of the American Academy of Otolaryngology-Head Neck Surgery (AAO-HNS) published guidelines in 1995 for the evaluation of hearing in VS. Accordingly, hearing level is classified into four classes [18], in which Classes A and B represent functional/serviceable hearing, whereas hearing Classes C and D are nonfunctional/nonserviceable (**Table 1**).

2.2. Facial function

Although facial nerve weakness is a rare presentation of VS patients, transient or even permanent facial palsy may occur in VS patients after treatment. Therefore, it is important to have a systematic classification of the facial nerve function. The House-Brackmann facial nerve grading system (HBGS) [19] was introduced in 1983 and endorsed by the Facial Nerve Disorders Committee of the American Academy of Otolaryngology-Head and Neck Surgery in 1984 as the standard for reporting facial nerve function (**Table 2**).

2.3. Radiological diagnosis

MRI is now the gold standard for VS diagnosis. High-field MRI (1.5–3 T) should be done, the examination protocol should include fluid attenuated inversion recovery (FLAIR), high-resolution 2D/3D T1-weighted sequences (e.g., T1-W Spin-Echo (SE) or Turbo-Spin-Echo-S (TSE)-Sequence) with and without intravenously administered contrast agent (0.2 ml/kg body weight Gadolinium DTPA), and high-resolution 3D T2-weighted sequences (e.g., CISS = constructive interference in a steady state, FIESTA-C = fast imaging employing steady state, etc.) with a film thickness of ≤1 mm isotrope [6]. Tumors as small as 2–3 mm may be diagnosed using MRI1. VS is usually isointense on T1-weighted images, hyperintense on T2-weighted

Hearing grade	Hearing loss in PTA	SDS (%)
Class A	≤30 dB	≥70
Class B	>30 to ≤50 dB	≥50
Class C	>50 dB	≥50
Class D	Any level	<50

Table 1. AAO-HNS hearing classification system.

Grade	Description
I	Normal function in all facial muscles
II	Slight weakness noticeable only on close inspection; complete eye closure
III	Obvious but not disfiguring difference between two sides; forehead shows slight-to-moderate movement; complete eye closure with effort
IV	Disfiguring asymmetry; no forehead movement; incomplete eye closure
V	slightly perceptible motion
VI	Complete paralysis

Table 2. House-Brackmann facial nerve grading system.

images, and enhances uniformly after contrast injection. Heterogeneous contrast enhancement or cystic degeneration may be found.

VS typically produces changes in the internal auditory canal (IAC), ranging from widening to destruction of the canal. However, normal IAC has been described in up to 10% of VS [20]. We measured the IAC in bone-window CT scan of 140 cases presented with unilateral VS, and we stratified the tumors into soft and firm varieties according to the intraoperative findings, the results showed that firm tumors were associated with significantly more widening of the IAC than soft tumors [21].

2.4. Tumor grading

The grading of VS depends on both tumor size and tumor extension. Different classification systems are available in the literature. Both Koos [22] and Hannover [23] classification systems classify VS into four grades according to the degree of tumor extension, which is an indicator of tumor size. According to Hannover classification, patients are classified regarding tumor extension as follows: T1, purely intrameatal; T2, intra- and extrameatal; T3a, filling the cerebellopontine cistern; T3b, reaching the brainstem; T4a, compressing the brainstem; and T4b, severely dislocating the brainstem and compressing the fourth ventricle.

3. Treatment options

Three management options are provided for VS patients: observation, radiosurgery, and surgery. The concept behind treatment of VS has been widely changed in the last two decades. Before the widespread of radiosurgery, VS treatment was based on microsurgery (MS) with the aim of complete tumor removal to avoid recurrence. With the development of radiosurgery (RS), it could be possible to stop the growth of the tumor with minimal side effects and with a very high level of preservation of nerve functions; therefore, nowadays, preservation of function is a primary aim in VS treatment. However, it is important to remember that preservation of function is sometimes possible after surgery and at the same time, tumor could be completely removed. On the other hand, failure of tumor control (recurrence) may occur after surgery as well as after radiosurgery; also, combined treatment is not always successful. Other than preservation of function, the complaints of the patient play an important role in the treatment decision because if a patient gets a functional preservation treatment and still complaining of tinnitus or vertigo, this may be more disabling to him/her. Therefore, the choice of the treatment option for each VS patient should be based on an individualized concept [5].

3.1. Observation (wait and scan)

Before discussing the conservative strategy for treatment of VS, it is important to know the natural history of the disease. The average growth rate in VS is 2–2.5 mm/year [24]. Neurofibromatosis type II-associated vestibular schwannomas tend to be more aggressive, with an increased average growth rate of 4 mm per year [25]. Intrameatal tumors seem to have lower growth rates than extrameatal lesions, and a younger age is associated with a more rapid tumor growth.

More recently, an extensive research has been done on the natural history of VS, and it was found that there is a group of VS tumors that grows very slowly or even does not grow at all, and even hearing preservation is sometimes maintained [26]. A study was performed on the natural history of VS less than 2 cm has showed that only 17% of the intrameatal and 28.9% of the extrameatal tumors grew; it was also found that this growth exclusively occurred within 5 years of diagnosis [27]. Sughrue et al. performed a meta-analysis on conservative treatment (982 patients) and found better hearing preservation in patients with yearly tumor growth rate less than 2.5 mm (75 vs. 32%) [28].

Therefore, it is widely accepted that newly diagnosed asymptomatic VS could be considered for initial wait and scan strategy. Regular clinical and radiological examination should be performed, and active treatment is recommended in cases of significant tumor growth (more than 2 mm increase in the largest tumor diameter) [27].

3.2. Stereotactic radiosurgery

3.2.1. Techniques

Radiosurgery is a radiation procedure using converging, narrow ionizing beams, stereotactically focused on an intracranial predetermined target volume, in order to induce biological arrest or destructive effects within this volume with minimal irradiation of the surrounding tissues. The modalities currently used in stereotactic radiosurgery include either photon devices such as Gamma Knife (GK) and modified linear accelerators (LINAC) or proton and heavy-ion charged particles generated by a cyclotron or synchrotron [29].

3.2.1.1. Gamma Knife

Gamma Knife consists of a thick cast, hemispherical steel shell containing a dome-shaped core of 201 cylindrical Co-60 sources, all being radially aligned toward a common focal point situated at a distance of 40 cm [29]. During treatment, the patient's head is fixed to the stereotactic frame. Ideally, the frame is placed such that the lesion to be treated is located as close to the frame center as possible. Following frame application, imaging is performed (usually MRI), and the images are interfaced with a computer software treatment planning system. Radiosurgical dose planning is the most critical aspect of the procedure, and preservation of cochlear and facial nerve function is the main concern during planning. For moderate-sized tumors, preservation of brainstem function is also a consideration. The 50% isodose line where radiation dose is half of the central dose is usually serving as the margin isodose. With the application of recent Gamma Knife models like Leksell Gamma Knife Perfexion and Model C lead to greater improvements in precise dose planning and hence the application of lower radiation dose to the tumor periphery has been available. Currently, 13 Gy is recommended as the tumor margin dose; this dose is associated with reduced complications and yet maintains a high rate of tumor control [30].

3.2.1.2. Linear accelerator (LINAC) and CyberKnife

LINAC uses high-energy electromagnetic waves to accelerate electrons to high energy through a microwave structure. When the electron strikes a target, X-rays are produced. Like Gamma Knife, LINAC is based on using a stereotactic frame for lesion localization, treatment set-up, and patient immobilization during the treatment [29, 31]. The primary advantage of LINAC over Gamma Knife and cyclotron-based methods is the lower cost of installation. Other advantages include great flexibility in photon delivery, lack of a field size limitation, and the possibility of fractionation. Disadvantages include longer treatment times, especially for complex-shaped lesions [32].

CyberKnife has been developed using image guidance instead of an external frame. It combines a lightweight LINAC designed for radiosurgery and mounted to a robotic manipulator, which can position and point the LINAC. The advantages of CyberKnife include easier fractionation, the ability to treat young patients without general anesthesia, and the flexibility to treat lesions throughout the body [32].

3.2.1.3. *Heavy particle radiosurgery*

Heavy particles (e.g., protons, helium, carbon nuclei) involve very expensive technologies (cyclotrons and synchrocyclotrons) which are available at only few centers around the world. In contrast to the photon radiation seen with gamma and X-rays, heavy particle radiation is more conformal due to Bragg peak effect. This occurs because heavy particles deposit energy at the end of their target with little falloff of radiation to nearby structures. This phenomenon makes it easier to give efficient conformal radiation treatment to large tumors [33].

3.2.2. *Radiosurgery results*

The ultimate goals of radiosurgery for VS include control of tumor growth and, ideally, tumor shrinkage (**Figures 1** and **2**) while preserving functionality of the vestibulocochlear nerve and the surrounding cranial nerves and quality of life.

During the early period following radiosurgery, transient tumor growth may occur, usually between 6 and 24 months after radiation. In large tumors, however, compression-related symptoms may occur due to the initial expansion, and surgical treatment may be required [34]. In addition, cystic tumors may display sudden and dramatic growth; therefore, these tumors may not be eligible for radiosurgery, and primary surgery is recommended [27].

Van Eck and Horstmann introduced two entities of tumor control after Gamma Knife radiosurgery for VS: "MRI-based tumor control" was used in cases of no increase, or increase of less than 10% of the initial tumor volume at follow-up, while "clinical tumor control" was used when clinical symptoms did not progress, and no further treatment was necessary. They reported MRI-based tumor control rate of 87% and clinical control rate of 97.5% after a mean follow-up duration of 22 months [35]. Recently, the marginal radiation dose was reduced in order to avoid cranial nerve complications; therefore, more data are needed regarding long-term rates of tumor control after radiosurgery after using these new regimens. Even in cases where the tumor remained stable for 3 years after treatment, delayed tumor growth may occur [36].

Reviewing the literature on radiosurgery for VS, it is important to remember that recent studies may show better results due to advances in radiosurgery treatment with the use of high-resolution MRI and recent treatment planning software. Other factors that should be critically looked after when reviewing the literature are the definition of tumor control, the

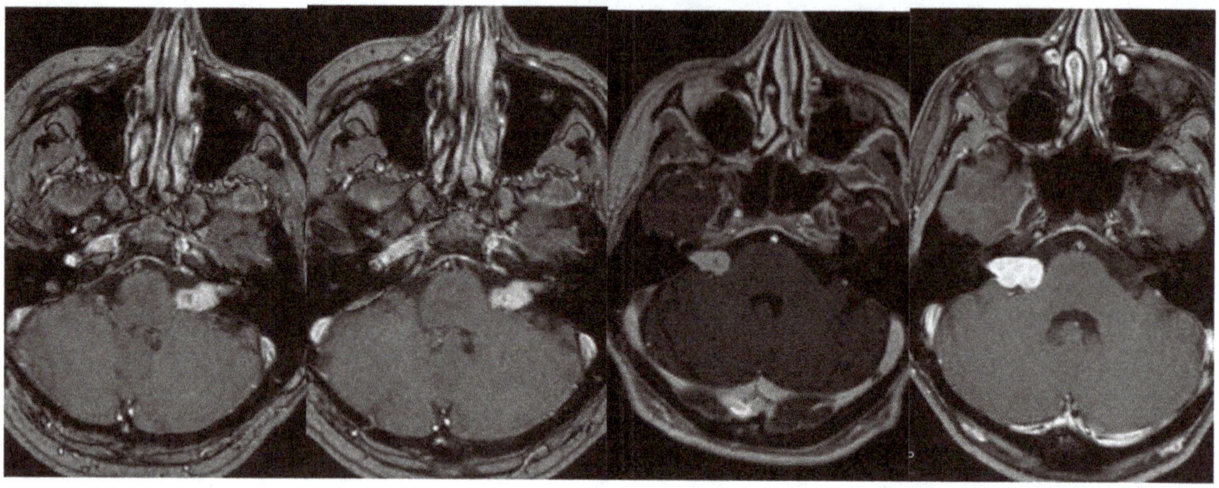

Figure 1. Axial MRI (T1-with contrast) of two cases of VS treated with Gamma Knife radiosurgery (13 Gy marginal dose) with follow-up MRI showed good tumor control after 15 months (case on the left side) and after 29 months (case on the right side).

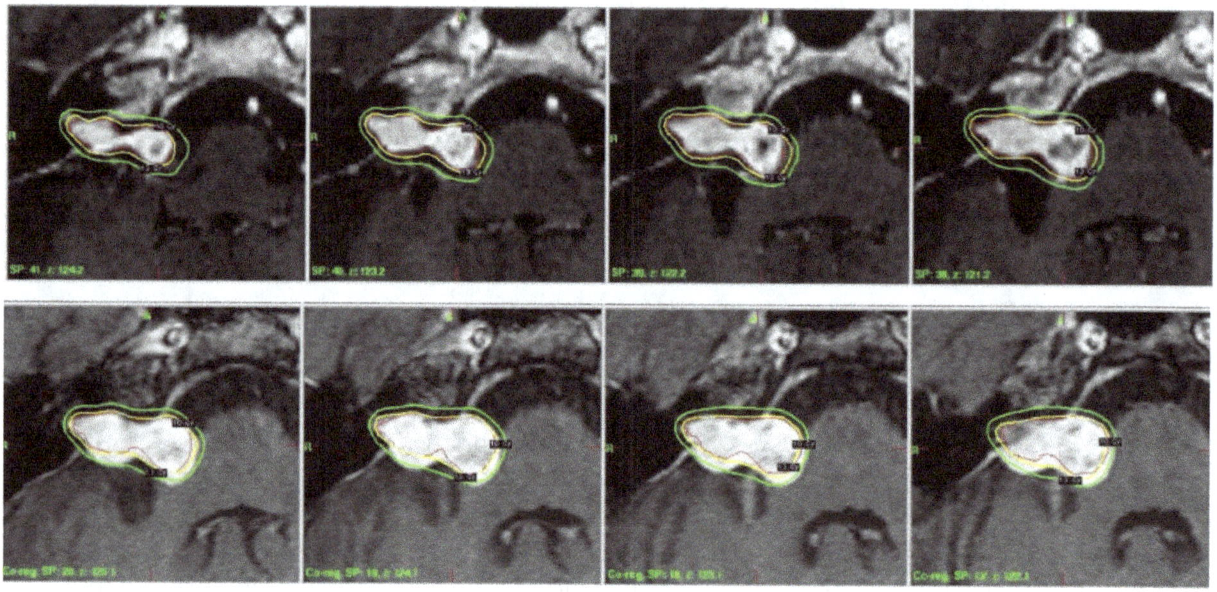

Figure 2. Axial MRI (T1-with contrast) of a VS case treated with Gamma Knife radiosurgery (13 Gy marginal dose) with follow-up MRI after 21 months (lower row) showed increase in tumor volume in comparison with the tumor volume before treatment (upper row).

duration follow-up, as well as the tumor size before treatment. In the radiosurgical literature, tumor size is usually reported in volume rather than in diameter as in the surgery literature [37].

In a meta-analysis included 3233 VS patients treated with Gamma Knife between 2007 and 2011 with an average marginal dose of 12.4 Gy and a mean follow-up of 51 months, Rykaczewski and Zabek reported tumor growth control in 92.7% and preservation of functional hearing in 66.4% of patients [30].

In another meta-analysis performed on Gamma Knife treated cases where tumors less than 4 cm were included and a mean follow-up of 2 years, the hearing preservation rate was 44% and tumor control rate was 91% [38].

The results of radiosurgery for VS are better in small tumors. A recent meta-analysis was conducted on tumors less than 2 cm treated by radiosurgery with follow-up more than 5 years and reported hearing preservation rate of 70.2% and a tumor control rate of 96.2%. They reported facial neuropathy rates using GK between 0 and 1.8% per study, while the rates of trigeminal neuropathy ranged between 0 and 3.1% per study. Interestingly, the rate of facial neuropathy in one study on LINAC was 6.9% [39].

It is important to note that a recent meta-analysis on CyberKnife for VS included 800 patients studied during 1998 and 2012 showed results similar to that of GK. The meta-analysis revealed the collective mean tumor control rate to be 96.3%. The collective hearing preservation rate was 79.1% in 427 patients with measurable hearing. The trigeminal neuropathy rate was 2.0%, facial neuropathy rate was 2.0%, and cerebellar/brainstem toxicity rate was 1.8% [26].

Maducdoc et al. performed a thorough literature review on malignant transformation of VS, they included only cases of histopathologic evidence of malignant transformation. They reported 11 cases of malignant transformation after radiosurgery, 4 cases after microsurgery, and 18 cases of either primary malignant VS or de novo transformation to malignancy without surgical intervention of any type. Therefore, it remains possible that the malignant transformation is part of the natural history of rare unfortunate event. In addition, they identified 12 cases of radiation-associated malignant tumors in the setting of NF2 and concluded that radiosurgery of NF2 tumors has been associated with a higher likelihood of malignant transformation [40]. Follow-up should be conducted for 5–20 years following radiation in order to detect any radiation-associated tumors that may develop.

3.3. Surgery

3.3.1. Surgical approaches

Three surgical approaches are available for VS removal: retrosigmoid, translabyrinthine, and middle fossa. The translabyrinthine and the retrosigmoid approaches can be used for all tumor sizes, whereas the middle fossa approach is useful only for removal of small tumors. Hearing preservation can be achieved only through the retrosigmoid or middle fossa approaches. The risk implied for patients is minimized if the surgeon and the team use the approach with which they are most familiar [23].

The middle fossa approach is suitable for intrameatal tumors and also for small tumors (less than 20 mm) with slight extrameatal extension. It is a subtemporal extradural approach that allows drilling of the roof of the internal auditory canal (IAC) and hence, removal of an intrameatal VS is possible. Retraction of the temporal lobe may be associated with the risk of seizures or sometimes temporal lobe contusion and hence neurological dysfunction [41]. When drilling into the IAC from above, the facial nerve has to be manipulated before reaching the tumor, and therefore, the facial nerve preservation results are inferior to those following other approaches [5, 42].

The translabyrinthine approach is the most widely used approach for removal of VS by neuro-otologists. This approach is hearing destructive, by definition, so it is suitable in cases of nonfunctional hearing. It is a direct approach to the IAC through drilling the mastoid air cells, and the labyrinth. It offers removal of VS of any size, as it provides wide access to the facial nerve and the contents of the CPA with minimal retraction of the cerebellum [41].

In the retrosigmoid approach, the cerebellopontine angle (CPA) is approached after retraction of the cerebellum and hence large VS extending into the CPA could be safely removed. The approach allows wide exposure of the CPA and decompression of the brainstem as well as the cranial nerves; from the trigeminal till the lower cranial nerves. Opening of the posterior wall of the IAC allows for removal of intracanalicular VS. Wide opening of the posterior wall IAC may result in violation of the posterior semicircular canal or the endolymphatic sac and therefore, may be critical for hearing preservation. Recently, endoscopic-assisted exposure of the lateral portion of the IAC allows complete removal of intracanalicular tumor through the retrosigmoid approach with less opening of the IAC [1, 43–45].

The retrosigmoid approach can be performed in supine, park-bench, or semi-sitting position. The semi-sitting position has the advantage of spontaneous drainage of cerebrospinal fluid (CSF) and blood, which provides a clean surgical field, thereby minimizing the retraction of the cerebellum and reducing the dissection time. The main risks of the setting position are brachial plexus injury and the development of venous air embolism with subsequent pulmonary embolism or even cerebral embolism in case of patent foramen oval. The complications of semi-sitting position can be avoided by the monitoring of somatosensory evoked potentials (SSEPs) during patient positioning to avoid brachial plexus injury, intraoperative monitoring of CO_2 and trans-esophageal echocardiography, as well as application of central venous catheter with the tip positioned close to the superior vena cava junction with the right atrium are important to detect the venous air embolism in the early stage, hence avoiding subsequent complications [45]. Even patients with a patent foramen oval can be operated safely in the semi-sitting position under standardized anesthesiological and neurosurgical protocols [46].

3.3.2. Intraoperative neurophysiological monitoring

Intraoperative neurophysiological monitoring in VS surgery is associated with increasing rates of hearing and facial nerve preservation. In addition, it helps to predict the postoperative functional outcome and hence helps the surgeon preoperatively counsel the patient regarding the postoperative hearing and facial nerve outcome.

Direct electrical stimulation and continuous free running electromyography (EMG) monitoring considered the gold standard for intraoperative facial nerve monitoring. However, the role of monitoring of facial nerve motor evoked potentials is still controversial [47].

Through direct electrical stimulation of the facial nerve, the EMG activity of the facial muscles is recorded. Early facial nerve identification during surgical removal of large VS is very helpful in preventing damage to the facial nerve during tumor dissection [48]. Several studies have provided parameters that can predict the postoperative facial functional outcome. The most widely accepted parameters are stimulation threshold and absolute EMG amplitude following stimulation at the root exit zone from the brainstem [49–53]. A study showed that proximal-to-distal EMG amplitude ratios (comparing the response from stimulation at the brainstem to the response at the internal auditory canal) were more predictive for initial postoperative nerve function and for functional recovery than absolute EMG potentials or stimulation thresholds [48, 54].

Continuous EMG recording from facial muscles gives important information that helps in identification of the facial nerve during tumor dissection, so it is used in conjunction with direct nerve stimulation. It has been showed that continuous sinusoidal symmetric EMG signal of high-frequency and low-amplitude known as "A" trains are predictors of poor postoperative facial nerve function [55–57].

The brainstem auditory evoked potential (BAEP) is the most widely used intraoperative electrophysiological method for auditory function monitoring because it has a high sensitivity and reliability to detect cochlear nerve damage. Classically, BAEP comprises 5–7 waves. During surgery for VS, wave III and wave V are the most relevant and should be closely monitored. The surgeon is alerted when the change in latency of Wave V exceeds 0.5 ms or if any wave is significantly changed or disappeared [47].

Direct cochlear nerve action potential monitoring has been used in multiple centers, and it represents a near-field technique in which electrodes are placed close to the cochlear nerve. Therefore, larger amplitude signals are produced and acquisition takes only 2–3 s (in contrast to minutes with BAEP), thus allowing near real-time feedback to the surgeon [47].

3.3.3. Surgery results

Total removal of VS is possible by dissecting the neurovascular structures from the false capsule of the tumor [58]. Although total tumor removal should be the aim in VS surgery, near-total removal is also accepted when a thin layer of tumor is intentionally left attached to one or more nerves in an attempt to preserve the neurological function. The results of long-term rates of tumor control do not differ significantly between cases of gross total resection and cases in which a small amount of tumor is left behind [59]. Recurrent tumors should be treated by radiosurgery whenever possible, as repeat surgery is more difficult; however, in case of large recurrent tumors or radiosurgery failure, repeat surgery will be needed [59] (**Figures 3** and **4**).

It has been reported that anatomical preservation of the facial nerve is achieved in 93–99% of VS surgeries [23, 58, 60–64]. Although transient deterioration of facial nerve function usually occurs after surgery, gradual recovery usually follows during the first 3–6 months postoperatively. The main predictor of facial nerve preservation after surgery is tumor size [65–68].

The rate of hearing preservation following surgery for VS varies widely in the literature. The most significant factors predicting hearing preservation are tumor size and extension, and preoperative hearing level. Some authors have suggested that hearing preservation surgery should be undertaken only for small- or medium-sized VSs [25, 65, 69–71]. However, hearing preservation may be possible even with large VS. Hearing preservation rates of 9.1–50% have been reported for tumors >3 cm [72–78] and 22.2–56.3% for tumors >2 cm [58, 62, 79, 80]. Therefore, patients with functional preoperative hearing should be offered hearing preservation surgery with intraoperative monitoring of hearing function.

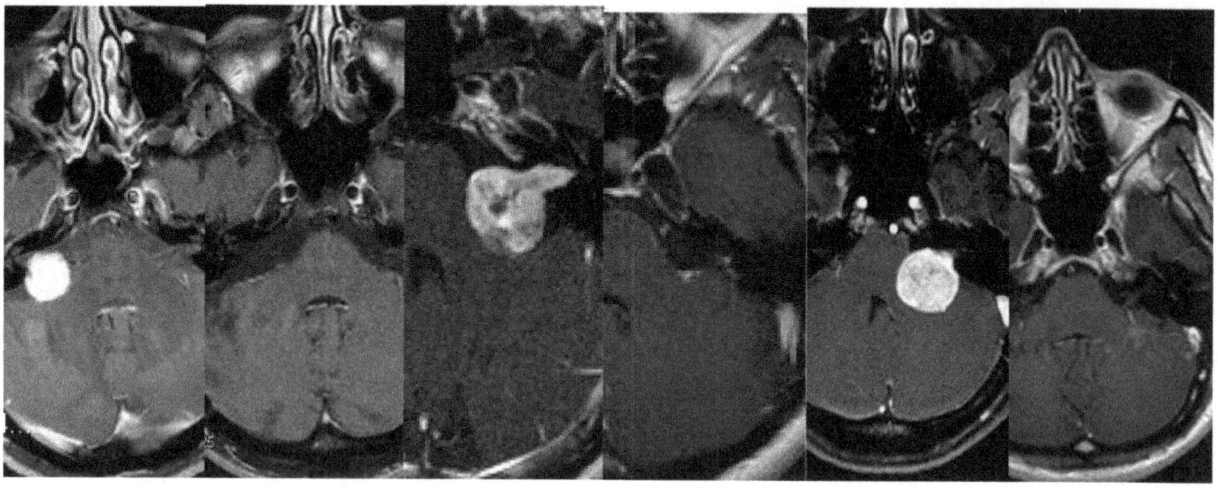

Figure 3. Axial MRI (T1-with contrast) of three operated cases (complete removal-retrosigmoid approach) with follow-up MRI after 31 months (case on the left side), after 29 months (case on the middle), and after 17 months (case on the right side) showing no tumor rest or recurrence.

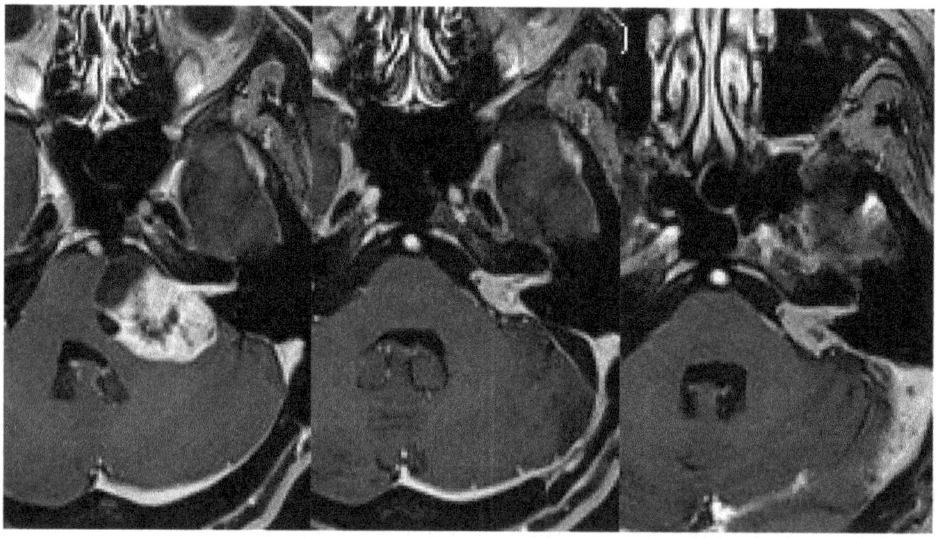

Figure 4. Axial MRI (T1-with contrast) of a case of partially cystic VS (T4a), subtotal removal-retrosigmoid approach. Follow-up MRI after 18 months (image in the middle) showed residual tumor, after 31 months (image on the right) showed progress in size of the residual tumor, so that radiosurgery was indicated.

The results of a large systematic review evaluating the use of microsurgery in more than 5000 patients with VS with a mean follow-up of 66 months, revealed tumor control rate of 98.2%, hearing preservation outcome of 36%, facial neuropathy in 13%, CSF-leak in 6%, and mortality rate of 0.6%. In a cohort of about 1000 patients with tumors smaller than 3 cm in diameter, they reported hearing preservation outcome of 49% and facial neuropathy in 10% [81].

In their meta-analysis on small VS cases (size less than 2 cm in diameter) with follow-up more than 5 years, Maniakas and Saliba included 153 operated cases. They reported tumor control rate of 98.7% and the overall hearing preservation outcome of 50.3%, while facial neuropathy rate was ranged from 0 to 5.3% per study and trigeminal neuropathy in 0% [39].

Ahsan et al. performed a systematic review and meta-analysis on long-term hearing preservation after resection of VS, and they reported immediate postoperative hearing preservation rate of 50–70%; in addition, the hearing durability at 5 years was found to be 70% [82].

Possible complications of surgery include CSF leakage in 3–13% [72, 83], postoperative hemorrhage in 2.2% [84], meningitis in 0.8–2.5% [85, 86], lower cranial nerve deficit in 0.5–5.5%, and hydrocephalus in 1–3% [84]. The possible complications associated with microsurgery may result in death; however, mortality rates are very low; a 3-month mortality rate of 0.5% was recently reported in a hospital-based study that included 2643 VS surgeries in 265 US Hospitals [87].

3.4. Studies comparing microsurgery and radiosurgery

To the best of our knowledge, currently, there is no class 1 evidence to support one treatment modality for vestibular schwannoma (VS). There are six studies that compared microsurgery (MS) and radiosurgery (RS) for treatment of VS, two of which are prospective controlled studies with predefined inclusion criteria [88, 89]. The other four studies are retrospective cohort studies with a matched control group, all comparing microsurgery with radiosurgery [90–93]. The results of these studies are summarized in **Table 3**. The relatively small patient groups, short follow-up periods, and heterogeneity in the comparison groups are potential weaknesses of some of these comparison studies [94].

3.5. Summary of the literature review

Until additional prospective comparisons or randomized trials can be accomplished, systematic meta-analysis of the available literature offers the most powerful guidance for clinical

Authors and publication year	**Pollock 2006**	**Myrseth 2009**	**Pollock 1995**	**Myrseth 2005**	**Regis 2002**	**Kaprinos 2000**
Follow-up (mean in months)	42	24	36	69	36	MS 24 RS 48
Tumor control	Not included	Not included	Not included	94.2% (MS) 89.2% (RS)	Retreatment MS (9%) RS (3%)	100% (MS) 91%(RS)
Hearing preservation (%)						
MS	5	0	14	5	36	40
RS	63	68	75	32	50	44
Facial preservation (%)						
MS	83	82	78	80	67	64.7
RS	98	100	91	95	100	93.9

Table 3. Cohort studies comparing microsurgery (MS) and radiosurgery (RS) for solitary VS.

decisions. We have performed analysis of the available meta-analyses in the literature that reported the results of MS and RS for treatment of VS. The results of tumor control rate ranged between 98.2 and 98.7 in MS [39, 81], and between 91 and 96.2% in RS [26, 30, 38, 39]. The results of hearing were found to be higher in small tumors both after MS as well as after RS, with rates of hearing preservation 39–70% after MS [39, 81, 82] and 44–79.1% after RS [26, 30, 38, 39]. The results of facial neuropathy following Gamma Knife and CyberKnife RS ranged between 0 and 2% [26, 39]; however, LINAC was associated with 6.9% risk of facial neuropathy [39]. The rate of facial neuropathy following MS is highly dependent on tumor size and experience of the surgery team as well as the use of intraoperative neuromonitoring, and the results ranged widely between 0 and 13% in the reviewed meta-analyses [39, 81].

Author details

Ahmed Rizk[1,2*]

*Address all correspondence to: arizkrizk@gmail.com

1 Benha University Hospital, Benha, Egypt

2 Barmherzigen Brüder Hospital, Trier, Germany

References

[1] Tatagiba M, Acioly MA. Vestibular schwannoma: Current state of the art. In: Ramina R, Aguiar P, Tatagiba M, editors. Samii's Essentials in Neurosurgery. Heidelberg: Springer-Verlag Berlin; 2008. pp. 175-189

[2] Jacob A, Robinson LL Jr, Bortman JS, et al. Nerve of origin, tumor size, hearing preservation, and facial nerve outcomes in 359 vestibular schwannoma resections at a tertiary care academic center. The Laryngoscope. 2007;**117**:2087-2092

[3] Khrais T, Romano G, Sanna M. Nerve origin of vestibular schwannoma: A prospective study. The Journal of Laryngology and Otology. 2008;**122**:128-131

[4] Clemis JD, Ballad WJ, Baggot PJ, et al. Relative frequency of inferior vestibular schwannoma. Archives of Otolaryngology—Head & Neck Surgery. 1986;**112**:190-194

[5] Myrseth E, Pedersen PH, Møller P, et al. Treatment of vestibular schwannomas. Why, when and how? Acta Neurochirurgica. 2007;**149**:647-660

[6] Rosahl S, Bohr C, Lell H, et al. Diagnosis and management of vestibular schwannomas—An inter-disciplinary challenge. Laryngo-Rhino-Otologie. 2017;**96**:S152-S182

[7] Sampath P, Long DM. Acoustic neuroma. In: Winn HR, editor. Youmans Neurological Surgery. Philadelphia: Saunders; 2004. pp. 1147-1168

[8] Matthies C, Samii M. Management of 1000 vestibular schwannomas (acoustic neuromas): Clinical presentation. Neurosurgery. 1997;**40**:1-9

[9] Stangerup SE, Tos M, Thomsen J, et al. True incidence of vestibular schwannoma? Neurosurgery. 2010;**67**:1335-1340

[10] Brown CM, Ahmad ZK, Ryan AF, et al. Estrogen receptor expression in sporadic vestibular schwannomas. Otology & Neurotology. 2011;**32**:158-162

[11] Mirzayan MJ, Gerganov VM, Lüdemann W, et al. Management of vestibular schwannomas in young patients—Comparison of clinical features and outcome with adult patients. Child's Nervous System. 2007;**23**:891-895

[12] Ojemann RG. Acoustic neuroma. In: Winn HR, editor. Youmans Neurological Surgery. Philadelaphia: Saunders; 1996. pp. 2841-2846

[13] Lawson McLean A, Rosahl SK. Growth dynamics of intracranial tumors in patients with neurofibromatosis type 2. World Neurosurgery. 2017;**98**:152-161

[14] Moffat DA, Golledge J, Baguley DM, et al. Clinical correlates of acoustic neuroma morphology. The Journal of Laryngology and Otology. 1993;**107**:290-294

[15] Berrettini S, Ravecca F, Sellari-Franceschini S, et al. Acoustic neuroma: Correlations between morphology and otoneurological manifestations. Journal of the Neurological Sciences. 1996;**144**:24-33

[16] Ganslandt O, Fahrig A, Strauss C. Hemorrhage into cystic vestibular schwannoma following stereotactic radiation therapy. Zentralblatt für Neurochirurgie. 2008;**69**:204-206

[17] Metwali H, Samii M, Samii A, et al. The peculiar cystic vestibular schwannoma: A single-center experience. World Neurosurgery. 2014;**82**:1271-1275

[18] Committee on Hearing and Equilibrium guidelines for the evaluation of hearing preservation in acoustic neuroma (vestibular schwannoma): American Academy of Otolaryngology–Head Neck Surgery Foundation, Inc. Otolaryngology and Head and Neck Surgery. 1995;**113**:179-180

[19] House JW. Facial nerve grading system. The Laryngoscope. 1983;**93**:1056-1069

[20] Yamakami I, Uchino Y, Kobayashi E, et al. Prognostic significance of changes in the internal acoustic meatus caused by vestibular schwannoma. Neurologia Medico-Chirurgica (Tokyo). 2002;**42**:465-470

[21] Rizk AR, Adam A, Gugel I, et al. Implications of vestibular schwannoma consistency: Analysis of 140 cases regarding radiologic and clinical features. World Neurosurgery. 2016;**99**:159-163

[22] Koos WT, Spetzler RF, Böck FW, et al. Microsurgery of cerebellopontine angle tumors. In: Koos WT, Böck FW, Spetzler RF, editors. Clinical Microneurosurgery. Stuttgart: Thieme; 1976. pp. 91-112

[23] Samii M, Matthies C. Management of 1000 vestibular schwannomas (acoustic neuromas): Hearing function in 1000 tumor resections. Neurosurgery. 1997;**40**:248-260

[24] Thakur JD, Banerjee AD, Khan IS, et al. An update on unilateral sporadic small vestibular schwannoma. Neurosurgical Focus. 2012;**33**:E1

[25] Slattery WH 3rd, Brackmann DE, Hitselberger W. Middle fossa approach for hearing preservation with acoustic neuromas. The American Journal of Otology. 1997;**18**:596-601

[26] Mahboubi H, Sahyouni R, Moshtaghi O, et al. CyperKnife for treatment of vestibular schwannoma: A meta-analysis. Otolaryngology and Head and Neck Surgery. 2016;**157**:7-15

[27] Stangerup SE, Caye´-Thomasen P, Tos M, et al. The natural history of vestibular schwannoma. Otology & Neurotology. 2006;**27**:547-552

[28] Sughrue ME, Yang I, Aranda D, et al. The natural history of untreated sporadic vestibular schwannomas: A comprehensive review of hearing outcomes. Journal of Neurosurgery. 2010;**112**:163-167

[29] Pellet W, Regis J, Roche PH, et al. Relative indications for radiosurgery and microsurgery for acoustic schwannoma. Advances and Technical Standards in Neurosurgery. 2003;**28**: 227-282

[30] Rykaczewski B, Zabek M. A meta-analysis of treatment of vestibular schwannoma using Gamma Knife radiosurgery. Contemporary Oncology (Poznań, Poland). 2014;**18**:60-66

[31] Suh JH, Macklis RM. Principles of radiotherapy. In: Winn HR, editor. Youmans Neurological Surgery. Philadelphia: Saunders; 2004. pp. 4005-4015

[32] Chang S, Adler J, Steinberg G. General and historical considerations of radiotherapy and radiosurgery. In: Winn HR, editor. Youmans Neurological Surgery. Philadelphia: Saunders; 2004. pp. 3991-3999

[33] Conley GS, Hirsch BE. Stereotactic radiation treatment of vestibular schwannoma indications, limitations, and outcomes. Current Opinion in Otolaryngology & Head and Neck Surgery. 2010;**18**:351-356

[34] Fukuokaa S, Takanashi M, Hojyoa A, et al. Gamma Knife radiosurgery for vestibular schwannomas. In: Yamamoto M, editor. Japanese Experience with Gamma Knife Radiosurgery. Prog Neurol Surg: Basel, Karger; 2009. pp. 45-62

[35] van Eck AT, Horstmann GA. Increased preservation of functional hearing after gamma knife surgery for vestibular schwannoma. Journal of Neurosurgery. 2005;**102**:204-206

[36] Roche PH, Khalil M, Thomassin JM, et al. Surgical removal of vestibular schwannoma after failed gamma knife radiosurgery. Basel, Karger: Prog Neurol Surg; 2008. pp. 152-157

[37] Arthurs BJ, Fairbanks RK, Demakas JJ, et al. A review of treatment modalities for vestibular schwannoma. Neurosurgical Review. 2011;**34**:265-277

[38] Kaylie DM, Horgan MJ, Delashaw JB, et al. A meta-analysis comparing outcomes of microsurgery and gamma knife radiosurgery. The Laryngoscope. 2000;**110**:1850-1856

[39] Maniakas A, Saliba I. Microsurgery versus stereotactic radiation for small vestibular schwannomas: A meta-analysis of patients with more than 5 years' follow-up. Otology & Neurotology. 2012;**33**:1611-1620

[40] Maducdoc MM, Ghavami Y, Linskey ME, et al. Evaluation of reported malignant transformation of vestibular schwannoma: De novo and after stereotactic radiosurgery or surgery. Otology & Neurotology. 2015;**36**:1301-1308

[41] Doherty JK, Friedman RA. Controversies in building a management algorithm for vestibular schwannomas. Current Opinion in Otolaryngology & Head and Neck Surgery. 2006; **14**:305-313

[42] Wilkinson EP, Roberts DS, Cassis A, et al. Hearing outcomes after middle fossa or retrosigmoid craniotomy for vestibular schwannoma tumors. Journal of Neurological Surgery Part B: Skull Base. 2016;**77**:333-340

[43] Roland PS, Meyerhoff WL, Wright CG, et al. Anatomic considerations in the posterior approach to the internal auditory canal. The Annals of Otology, Rhinology, and Laryngology. 1988;**97**:621-625

[44] Kumon Y, Kohno S, Ohue S, et al. Usefulness of endoscope-assisted microsurgery for removal of vestibular schwannomas. Journal of Neurological Surgery Part B: Skull Base. 2012;**73**:42-47

[45] Porter JM, Pidgeon C, Cunningham AJ. The sitting position in neurosurgery: A critical appraisal. British Journal of Anaesthesia. 1999;**82**:117-128

[46] Feigl GC, Decker K, Wurms M, et al. Neurosugical procedures in semi-sitting position: An evaluation of the risk of a paradoxical venous air embolism for patients with a patent foramen ovale. World Neurosurgery. 2014;**81**:149-164

[47] Youssef AS, Downes AE. Intraoperative neurophysiological monitoring in vestibular schwannoma surgery: Advances and clinical implications. Neurosurgical Focus. 2009;**27**(4):E9

[48] Sobottka SB, Schackert G, May SA, et al. Intraoperative facial nerve monitoring (IFNM) predicts facial nerve outcome after resection of vestibular schwannoma. Acta Neurochirurgica. 1998;**140**:235-243

[49] Kirkpatrick PJ, Watters G, Strong AJ, et al. Prediction of facial nerve function after surgery for cerebellopontine angle tumors. Use of facial nerve stimulator and monitor. Skull Base Surgery. 1991;**1**:171-176

[50] Lalwani AK, Butt FY, Jackler RK, et al. Facial nerve outcome after acoustic neuroma surgery: A study from the era of cranial nerve monitoring. Otolaryngology and Head and Neck Surgery. 1994;**111**:561-570

[51] Nissen AJ, Sikand A, Curto FS, et al. Value of intraoperative threshold stimulus in predicting postoperative facial nerve function after acoustic tumor resection. The American Journal of Otology. 1997;**18**:249-251

[52] Prasad S, Hirsch BE, Kamerer DB, et al. Facial nerve function following cerebellopontine angle surgery: Prognostic value of intraoperative thresholds. The American Journal of Otology. 1993;**14**:330-333

[53] Selesnick SH, Carew JF, Victor JD. Predictive value of facial nerve electrophysiologic stimulation thresholds in cerebellopontine-angle surgery. The Laryngoscope. 1996;**106**: 633-638

[54] Taha JM, Tew JM, Keith RW. Proximal-to-distal facial amplitude ratios as predictors of facial nerve function after acoustic neuroma excision. Journal of Neurosurgery. 1995;**83**: 994-998

[55] Neff BA, Ting J, Dickinson SL, et al. Facial nerve monitoring parameters as a predictor of postoperative facial nerve outcomes after vestibular schwannoma resection. Otology & Neurotology. 2005;**26**:728-732

[56] Romstock J, Strauss C, Fahlbusch R. Continuous electromyography monitoring of motor cranial nerves during cerebellopontine angle surgery. Journal of Neurosurgery. 2000;**93**: 586-593

[57] Prell J, Rampp S, Romstöck J, et al. Train time as a quantitative electromyographic parameter for facial nerve function in patients undergoing surgery for vestibular schwannoma. Journal of Neurosurgery. 2007;**106**:826-832

[58] Samii M, Gerganov V, Samii A. Improved preservation of hearing and facial nerve function in vestibular schwannoma surgery via the retrosigmoid approach in a series of 200 patients. Journal of Neurosurgery. 2006;**105**:527-535

[59] Sughrue ME, Kaur R, Rutkowski MJ, et al. Extent of resection and the long-term durability of vestibular schwannoma surgery. Journal of Neurosurgery. 2011;**114**:1218-1223

[60] Ojemann RG. Management of acoustic neuromas (vestibular schwannomas) (honored guest presentation). Clinical Neurosurgery. 1993;**40**:498-535

[61] Sekhar LN, Gormley WB, Wright DC. The best treatment for vestibular schwannoma (acoustic neuroma): Microsurgery or radiosurgery? The American Journal of Otology. 1996;**17**:676-682

[62] Gormley WB, Sekhar LN, Wright DC, et al. Acoustic neuromas: Results of current surgical management. Neurosurgery. 1997;**41**:50-58

[63] Sampath P, Holliday MJ, Brem H, et al. Facial nerve injury in acoustic neuroma (vestibular schwannoma) surgery: Etiology and prevention. Journal of Neurosurgery. 1997;**87**: 60-66

[64] Lanman TH, Brackmann DE, Hitselberger WE, et al. Report of 190 consecutive cases of large acoustic tumors (vestibular schwannoma) removed via the translabyrinthine approach. Journal of Neurosurgery. 1999;**90**:617-623

[65] Briggs RJ, Fabinyi G, Kaye AH. Current management of acoustic neuromas: Review of surgical approaches and outcomes. Journal of Clinical Neuroscience. 2000;**7**:521-526

[66] Jung S, Kang SS, Kim TS, et al. Current surgical results of retrosigmoid approach in extralarge vestibular schwannomas. Surgical Neurology. 2000;**53**:370-377

[67] Staecker H, Nadol JB Jr, Ojeman R, et al. Hearing preservation in acoustic neuroma surgery: Middle fossa versus retrosigmoid approach. The American Journal of Otology. 2000;**21**:399-404

[68] Wiet RJ, Mamikoglu B, Odom L, et al. Long-term results of the first 500 cases of acoustic neuroma surgery. Otolaryngology and Head and Neck Surgery. 2001;**124**:645-651

[69] Brackmann DE, Owens RM, Friedman RA, et al. Prognostic factors for hearing preservation in vestibular schwannoma surgery. The American Journal of Otology. 2000;**21**:417-424

[70] Holsinger FC, Coker NJ, Jenkins HA. Hearing preservation in conservation surgery for vestibular schwannoma. The American Journal of Otology. 2000;**21**:695-700

[71] Yates PD, Jackler RK, Satar B, et al. Is it worthwhile to attempt hearing preservation in larger acoustic neuromas? Otology & Neurotology. 2003;**24**:460-464

[72] Fischer G, Fischer C, Remond J. Hearing preservation in acoustic neurinoma surgery. Journal of Neurosurgery. 1992;**76**:910-917

[73] Yokoh A, Kobayashi S, Tanaka Y, et al. Preservation of cochlear nerve function in acoustic neurinoma surgery. Acta Neurochirurgica. 1993;**123**:8-13

[74] Cohen NL. Retrosigmoid approach for acoustic tumor removal. Otolaryngologic Clinics of North America. 1992;**25**:295-310

[75] Fahlbusch R, Neu M, Strauss C. Preservation of hearing in large acoustic neu-rinomas following removal via suboccipito-lateral approach. Acta Neurochirurgica. 1998;**140**:771-777

[76] Iwai Y, Yamanaka K, Ishiguro T. Surgery combined with radiosurgery of large acoustic neuromas. Surgical Neurology. 2003;**59**:283-289

[77] Yamakami I, Uchino Y, Kobayashi E, et al. Removal of large acoustic neurinomas (vestibular schwannomas) by the retrosigmoid approach with no mortality and minimal morbidity. Journal of Neurology, Neurosurgery, and Psychiatry. 2004;**75**:453-458

[78] Raftopoulos C, Abu Serieh B, Duprez T, et al. Microsurgical results with large vestibular schwannomas with preservation of facial and cochlear nerve function as the primary aim. Acta Neurochirurgica. 2005;**147**:697-706

[79] Frerebeau P, Benezech J, Uziel A, et al. Hearing preservation after acoustic neurinoma operation. Neurosurgery. 1987;**21**:197-200

[80] Wanibuchi M, Fukushima T, McElveen JT Jr, et al. Hearing preservation in surgery for large vestibular schwannomas. Journal of Neurosurgery. 2009;**111**:845-854

[81] Yamakami I, Uchino Y, Kobayashi E, et al. Conservative management, gamma-knife radiosurgery, and microsurgery for acoustic neurinomas: A systematic review of outcome and risk of three therapeutic options. Neurological Research. 2003;**25**:682-690

[82] Ahsan S, Huq F, Seidman M, et al. Long-term hearing preservation after resection of vestibular schwannoma: A systematic review and meta-analysis. Otology & Neurotology. 2017;**38**:1505-1511

[83] Glasscock ME III, McKennan KX, Levine SC. Acoustic neuroma surgery: The results of hearing conservation surgery. The Laryngoscope. 1987;**97**:785-789

[84] Samii M, Matthies C. Management of 1000 vestibular schwannomas (acoustic neuromas): Surgical management and results with an emphasis on complications & how to avoid them. Neurosurgery. 1997;**40**:11-23

[85] Ebersold MJ, Harner SG, Beatty CW, et al. Current results of the retrosigmoid approach to acoustic neuroma. Journal of Neurosurgery. 1992;**76**:901-909

[86] Wiegand DA, Fickel V. Acoustic neuroma-the patient's perspective: Subjective assessment of symptoms, diagnosis, therapy, and outcome in 541 patients. The Laryngoscope. 1989; **99**:179-187

[87] Barker FG 2nd, Carter BS, Ojemann RG, et al. Surgical excision of acoustic neuroma: Patient outcome and provider caseload. The Laryngoscope. 2003;**113**:1332-1343

[88] Pollock BE, Driscoll CL, Foote RL, et al. Patient outcomes after vestibular schwannoma management: A prospective comparison of microsurgical resection and stereotactic radiosurgery. Neurosurgery. 2006;**59**:77-85

[89] Myrseth E, Moller P, Pedersen PH, et al. Vestibular schwannoma: Surgery or gamma knife radiosurgery? A prospective, nonrandomized study. Neurosurgery. 2009;**64**:654-661

[90] Pollock B, Lunsford L, Kondziolka D, et al. Outcome analysis of acoustic neuroma management: A comparison of microsurgery and stereotactic radiosurgery. Neurosurgery. 1995;**36**:215-224

[91] Karpinos M, Teh B, Kawaguchi T, et al. Treatment of acoustic neuroma: Stereotactic radiosurgery vs. microsurgery. International Journal of Radiation Oncology, Biology, Physics. 2002;**54**:1410-1421

[92] Régis J, Pellet W, Delsanti C, et al. Functional outcome after gamma knife surgery or microsurgery for vestibular schwannomas. Journal of Neurosurgery. 2002;**97**:1091-1100

[93] Myrseth E, Møller P, Pedersen PH, et al. Vestibular schwannomas: Clinical results and quality of life after microsurgery or gamma knife radiosurgery. Neurosurgery. 2005;**5**: 927-935

[94] Wolbers JG, Dallenga AH, Romero AM, et al. What intervention is best practice for vestibular schwannomas? A systematic review of controlled studies. BMJ Open. 2013;**22**:2

4

Current Trends in Glioblastoma Treatment

Ligia Gabriela Tataranu, Vasile Ciubotaru,
Tabita Larisa Cazac, Oana Alexandru,
Oana Stefana Purcaru, Daniela Elise Tache,
Stefan Alexandru Artene and Anica Dricu

Abstract

Glioblastoma (also called glioblastoma multiforme – GBM) is a primary brain neoplasm, representing about 55% of all gliomas. It is a very aggressive and infiltrative tumor. Glioblastoma is usually highly malignant, with more than 90% 5-year mortality and a median survival of about 14.6 months. Compared to other cancers, the survival rate has not greatly changed over time and no current treatment is curative for this disease. Because the tumor has a heterogeneous cell population containing several types of cells, the treatment for GBM is one of the most challenging in clinical oncology. This chapter will discuss the current approaches in glioblastoma treatment, including resection techniques, chemotherapy and radiation therapy.

Keywords: glioblastoma, surgical resection, intraoperative guidance, radiation therapy, chemotherapy, intratumoral therapies, targeted therapy

1. Introduction

Glioblastoma is the most common primary brain malignancy in adults. It is the most aggressive of the gliomas, largely resistant to conventional therapies, having a very poor prognosis. The global incidence is 2–3 newly diagnosed cases per 100,000 people per year in the United States and Europe. According to Central Brain Tumor Registry of the United States, GBM accounts for 14.9% of all primary brain tumors and 55.4% of all gliomas. It represents the highest number of cases of all malignant tumors, with an estimated 12,390 new cases predicted in 2017. Currently, the standard of care (SoC) for patients with GBM consists of maximal safe surgical resection, followed by concurrent chemoradiotherapy and adjuvant chemotherapy with temozolomide (TMZ). New discoveries are being made in basic and translational research, novel therapeutic approaches have been tried and tested, some of them finding their way into clinical practice. Despite the synergistic multimodal strategies and individualized therapies, the available treatment is of limited utility, and patients have a poor prognosis, with a progression-free survival (PFS) of 7–8 months, a median survival of 14–16 months and 5-year overall survival (OS) of 9.8% [1]. This review focuses on the current treatment strategies and perspectives in the management of GBM.

2. Histology and classification

The cellular origin of GBM is unknown. Astrocyte, oligodendrocyte precursor cell and neural stem cell can all serve as the cell of origin for this type of brain tumor. For this reason, in the recent version of the 2016 World Health Organization (WHO) Classification of Tumors of the Central Nervous System (CNS), which is the current international standard for the nomenclature and diagnosis, GBM is incorporated into the category of "diffuse astrocytic and oligodendroglial tumors", being considered a grade IV tumor.

There are **some properties of the tumor cells that render GBM incurable**. First, the diffuse infiltrative nature of the cells makes complete tumor resection impossible, despite the advances in neurosurgical techniques. Glioma cells have the ability to migrate away from the main tumor mass, through the brain. Typical migration routes include white matter tracts, along the basal lamina of the blood vessels, perineuronal and in between the glia limitans and the pia mater. Tumor cells are still detectable at a distance greater than 4 cm away from macroscopic and radiologic margin of the tumor [2]. Second, there is a resistance of the glioma cells to conventional radiation therapy, chemotherapy and other therapies, as they are spared from eradication. This resistance is correlated with the heterogeneous character of the tumor itself, with its "multiforme" appearance [3]. GBM is multiforme macroscopically, featuring multifocal hemorrhage, necrosis and cystic areas. It is multiforme microscopically, demonstrating pleomorphic cell population, hypercellularity with mitotic activity, nuclear atypia, pseudopalisading necrosis and microvascular proliferation. And it is multiforme genetically, with various genetic abnormalities and heterogeneous subclones within the tumor cell population.

The histological diagnosis of GBM should be undertaken by a neuropathologist by standard histopathology methods and should include tumor type and tumor grade according to WHO Classification of Tumors of the CNS.

Progress has been made in knowledge of the GBM biology in relation to its microenvironment. Patterns of **molecular genetic alterations** have been associated with specific types of GBMs. Recent medical advances have indicated the importance of molecular typing in determining the prognosis and personalized treatment strategies for the patient. For this reason, in the recent version of the 2016 WHO Classification of Tumors of the CNS, molecular parameters are used in addition to histology to define diagnostic entities. This adds a level of objectivity to diagnostic and should lead to improvements in determination of prognosis and treatment response. So, GBMs are further defined by the presence or absence of **isocitrate dehydrogenase (IDH) gene mutations**. IDH is an enzyme encoded by the IDH gene, whose mutations occur in gliomas. These mutations are oncogenic and they lead to a hypermethylation phenotype, as well as changes in cellular metabolism and response to hypoxic and oxidative stress [4, 5]. Mutated IDH can now be detected by immunohistochemistry and magnetic resonance spectroscopy (MRS). IDH mutation is identified as a genetic marker of secondary GBM. It can indicate a favorable prognosis and a relatively good response to radiation and/or alkylating chemotherapy.

GBMs are divided into: GBM, IDH-wildtype; GBM, IDH-mutant and GBM, NOS [6]. IDH-wildtype GBM corresponds with clinically described primary or de novo GBM. It represents about 90% of GBMs. It arises without clinical, radiologic or histologic evidence of a pre-existing less malignant lesions, in elderly patients (median age of 62 years), usually supratentorial. The mean length of clinical history is 4 months and the median overall survival after conventional surgery, radiotherapy and chemotherapy is 15 months, the prognosis being poor [6, 7]. IDH-mutant GBM corresponds with secondary GBM (approximately 10% of GBMs). It typically develops from lower grade diffuse glioma. It occurs in younger patients (median age of 45 years), preferentially in the frontal lobe. The mean duration of the clinical history of secondary GBM is 15 months and the median overall survival after multimodal treatment (including surgical resection, radiotherapy and chemotherapy) is 31 months, a significantly better prognosis than primary GBM [6, 7]. Primary and secondary GBMs carry distinct genetic abnormalities. Other common genetic alterations in secondary GBMs include TP53 mutations (~65%), ATRX mutations (~65%) and loss of heterozygosity (LOH) on chromosome 19q (~50%). In primary GBMs, there is a high frequency of EGFR amplification (~35%), phosphatase and tensin homolog (PTEN) mutation (~25%) and LOH on chromosome 10 (LOH 10p ~50%, LOH 10q ~70%) [7, 8]. There is now increasing evidence that primary and secondary GBMs are in fact different tumor entities that develop from distinct cells of origin [7]. Despite the differences in their phenotypic and genotypic profiles, these two subtypes of GBM are histopathologically indistinguishable, except that extensive necrosis is more frequent in primary GBM and oligodendroglioma components are more frequent in secondary GBM [7]. Recent findings in pediatric GBMs regarding mutations in the histone H3F3A gene suggest that these tumors may represent a third major category of GBMs, separate from adult primary and secondary GBMs [9]. The terminology NOS (i.e., not otherwise specified) is used for GBM when molecular information is insufficient, either because testing cannot be fully performed or the results do not fit within a defined category.

In the 2016 update of the WHO Classification of Tumors of the CNS, there are **three variants of IDH-wildtype GBMs**: giant cell GBM, gliosarcoma and epithelioid GBM. It is to be noted that variants are subtypes of accepted entities that are sufficiently well characterized pathologically and have potential clinical utility [6]. There are also **different patterns in GBMs**, including small cell GBMs, granular cell GBM and GBM with primitive neuronal component (previously referred as GBM with primitive neuroectodermal tumor (PNET)-like component). Patterns are histological features that are readily recognizable, but usually do not have clear clinicopathological significance [6].

3. Patient evaluation

GBMs are typically large tumors at diagnosis. They occur most commonly in the supratentorial compartment and are less common in the posterior fossa and brainstem. Lesions usually start within the deep white matter, but often infiltrate into cortex (**Figure 1**), deep nuclei or through commissural pathways into the contralateral hemisphere.

When a GBM spreads across the corpus callosum, there is a characteristic appearance of bihemispheric involvement, resulting in the classic "butterfly" pattern on imaging (**Figure 2**).

The vast majority of GBMs are solitary lesions, but cases of multiple GBMs were observed in 0.5–1% of cases. Multiple gliomas can be categorized as multifocal or multicentric. Multifocal disease consists of multiple tumors which result from dissemination along an established route of CNS, spreading through white matter tracts, cerebrospinal fluid pathways or through local extension by satellite formations. They can be separated by abnormal white matter tracts within the same hemisphere (demonstrated by contiguous areas of modified T2-weighted signal on cerebral MRI (**Figure 3**).

On the other hand, multicentric disease represents multiple tumors with normal intervening brain, so widely separated masses in different lobes or hemispheres (**Figure 4**).

Although GBM is an invasive tumor, dissemination remains limited to the central nervous system and extracranial metastases are very rare (0.4–2%). GBMs usually appear like a mass with thick, irregular margins and a central necrotic core, sometimes with a hemorrhagic component. Tumors are surrounded by a vasogenic edema, characterized by extensive infiltration of tumor cells. This edema causes additional mass effect and leads to neurological disturbances.

The diagnosis of brain tumors must be evoked in any adult with symptoms of raised intracranial pressure, seizures or focal neurological deficit, the onset being usually weeks to months before. The **clinical presentation** is nonspecific and can vary widely, depending on the tumor localization and the rate of growth. Rarely, an intratumoral hemorrhage occurs and patient may present with sudden stroke-like symptoms. GBMs may occur at any age, but 70% of cases are seen between 45 and 70 years of age, with a mean age at the time of diagnosis being 53 years [10]. Men are more frequently involved (there is a sex ratio of 3:2).

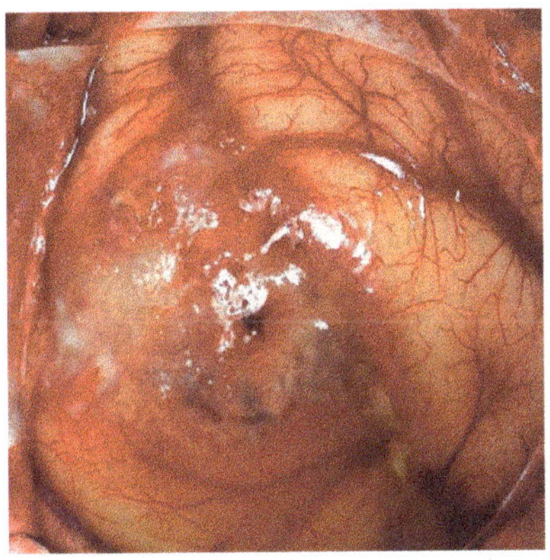

Figure 1. Corticalized glioblastoma – Macroscopic appearance.

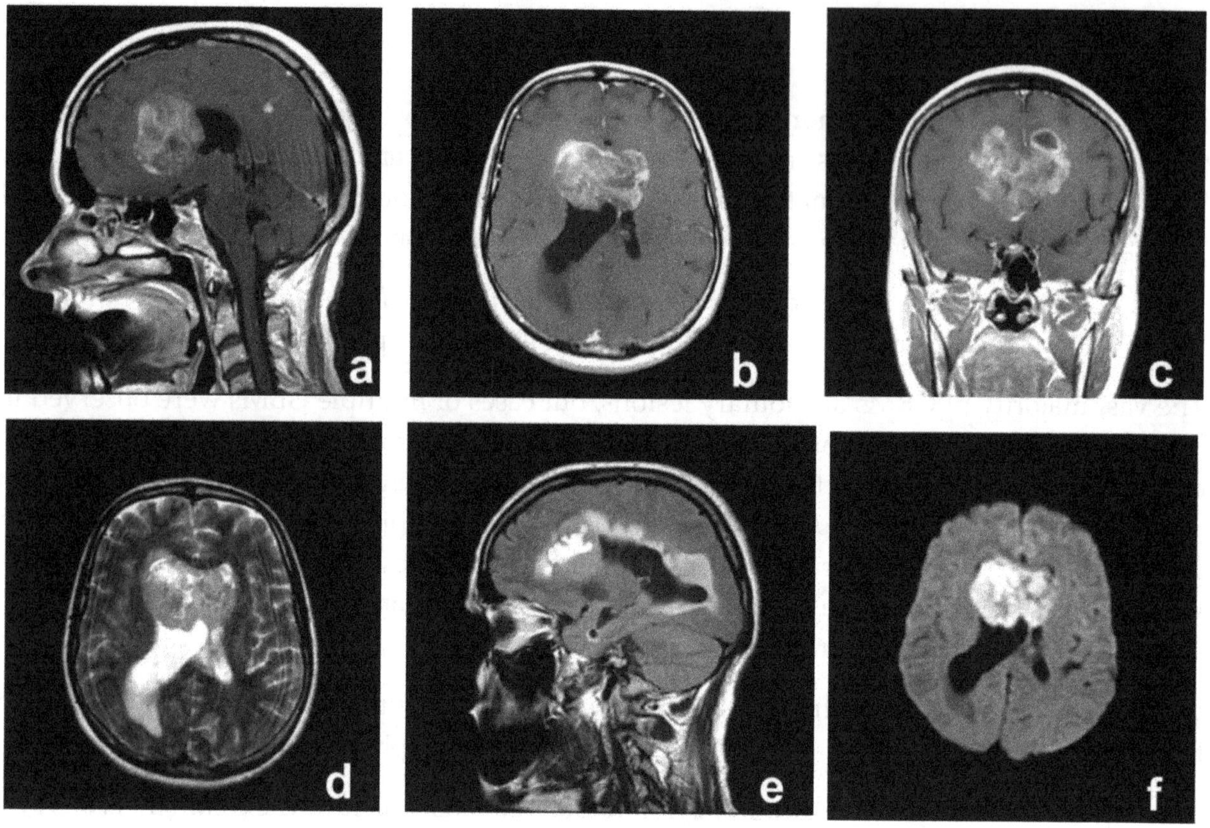

Figure 2. Butterfly glioblastoma – MRI features. Tumor involves both cerebral hemispheres by crossing the corpus callosum – Bifrontal localization. (a) Sagittal T1-weighted image with contrast; (b) axial T1-weighted image with contrast; (c) coronal T1-weighted image with contrast; (d) axial T2-weighted image; (e) sagittal fluid-attenuated inversion recovery (FLAIR) sequence; (f) axial diffusion-weighted image (DWI).

All patients, who are presented with symptoms that could be caused by an intracranial mass, require **neuroimaging** to establish the cause of these symptoms. **CT scan** is often the first examination, because it is widely available, fast and inexpensive. Typical findings for GBM on CT scan are a heterogeneous mass lesion, with an isodense to slightly hyperdense irregular thick ring and a hypodense core representing necrosis. There is an intense, irregular and heterogeneous contrast enhancement of the tumor mass (**Figure 5**). Images highlight a significant surrounding cerebral edema and a marked mass effect. CT scan is helpful in demonstrating the presence of intratumoral hemorrhage or calcification, which is thought to be related to a pre-existing oligodendroglial lesion.

While CT scan provides initial data, **contrast-enhanced MRI** is the imaging modality of choice for GBMs, because of his greater accuracy and multi-planar imaging capabilities. All patients with a suspected brain tumor should have an MRI evaluation, unless it would be unsafe for them. It will confirm the diagnosis, will refine the diagnosis and will provide additional data needed for treatment planning. On T1-weighted images, GBMs typically appear as a hypo to isointense mass with central heterogeneous signal (necrosis, intratumoral hemorrhage and cysts), thick, irregular or poorly defined margins and peritumoral edema. After the administration of contrast medium, a heterogeneous or irregular ring-like enhancement is almost always present. T2-weighted and fluid-attenuated inversion recovery (FLAIR) images reveal a heterogeneous, hyperintense mass with adjacent tumor infiltration/vasogenic edema.

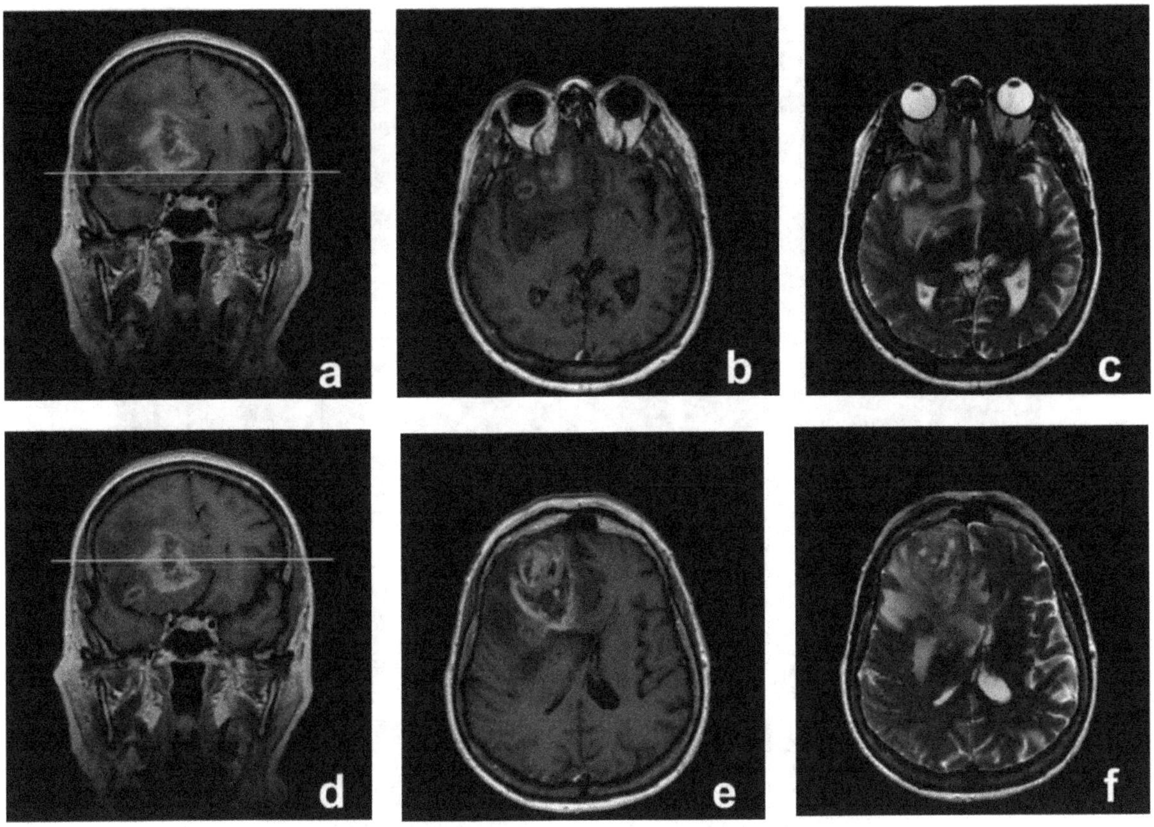

Figure 3. Multifocal glioblastoma – MRI features. There are two separate tumor foci in the right frontal lobe: A smaller one in the basal frontal region and a bigger one in the anterior frontal region. The presence of connecting signal alteration in T2-weighted images defines multifocal lesions. (a) Coronal T1-weighted image with contrast, with section line at the level of smaller tumor; (b) axial T1-weighted image with contrast – Section level is indicated in (a); (c) axial T2-weighted image – Section level is indicated in (a); (d) coronal T1-weighted image with contrast, with section line at the level of bigger tumor; (e) axial T1-weighted image with contrast – Section level is indicated in (d); (f) axial T2-weighted image – Section level is indicated in (d).

Surrounding infiltrative edema (which is a combination of increased interstitial water and neoplastic cells) is better appreciated in T2-weighted images as compared with T1-weighted images (**Figures 5** and **6**).

Advanced imaging technologies have been developed, including diffusion-weighted imaging (DWI), diffusion tensor imaging (DTI), perfusion-weighted imaging (PWI) and MR spectroscopy (MRS). Diffusion-weighted imaging (DWI) allows the calculation of the apparent diffusion coefficient (ADC) that is correlated with tumor cellularity and tumor grade. Diffusion tensor imaging (DTI) offers the possibility to identify and to characterize the white matter tracts. Perfusion-weighted imaging (PWI) provides useful information about the cerebral microcirculation and allows the development of cerebral blood volume maps. MR spectroscopy (MRS) allows in vivo measurements of certain tissue metabolites. These techniques focus on pathophysiological changes in disease and offer potential indications on differential diagnosis and individual anatomy. Post-therapeutic MRI examinations are used to monitor treatment response and to differentiate radionecrosis from residual or recurrent tumor.

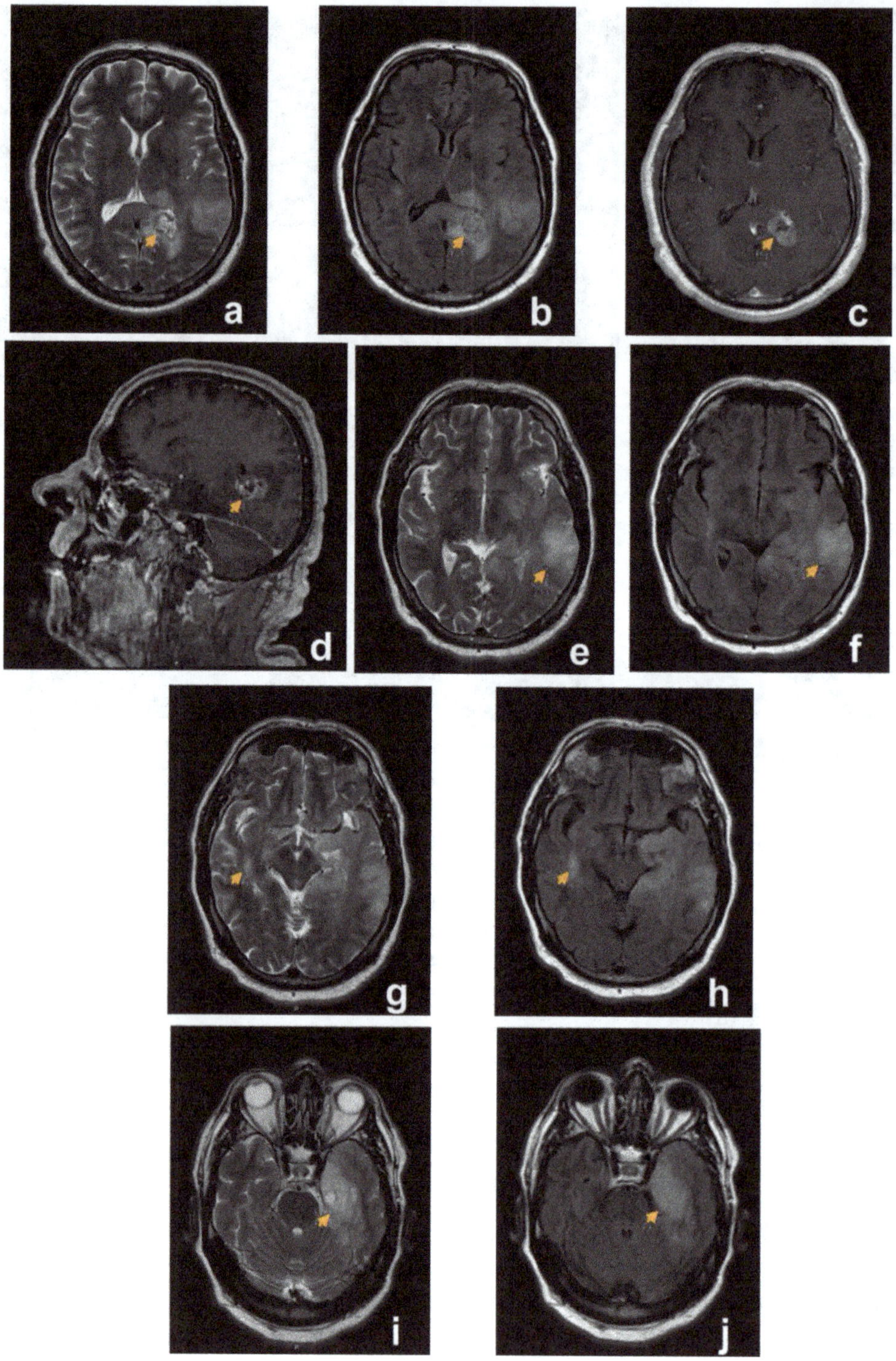

Figure 4. Multicentric synchronous glioblastoma – MRI features. There are widely separated lesions, occurring in different lobes or hemispheres, with no connection between foci. They were already present at the time of initial radiological investigation. The figures (a), (b), (c) and (d) demonstrate a left paraventricular occipital tumor: (a) axial T2-weighted image; (b) axial FLAIR sequence; (c) axial T1-weighted image with contrast; (d) sagittal T1-weighted image with contrast. The figures (e) and (f) illustrate a left posterior temporal lesion: (e) axial T2-weighted image; (f) axial FLAIR sequence. The figures (g) and (h) present a right deep temporal lesion: (g) axial T2-weighted image; (h) axial FLAIR sequence.The figures (i) and (j) reveals a left temporomesial lesion: (i) axial T2-weighted image; (j) axial FLAIR sequence.

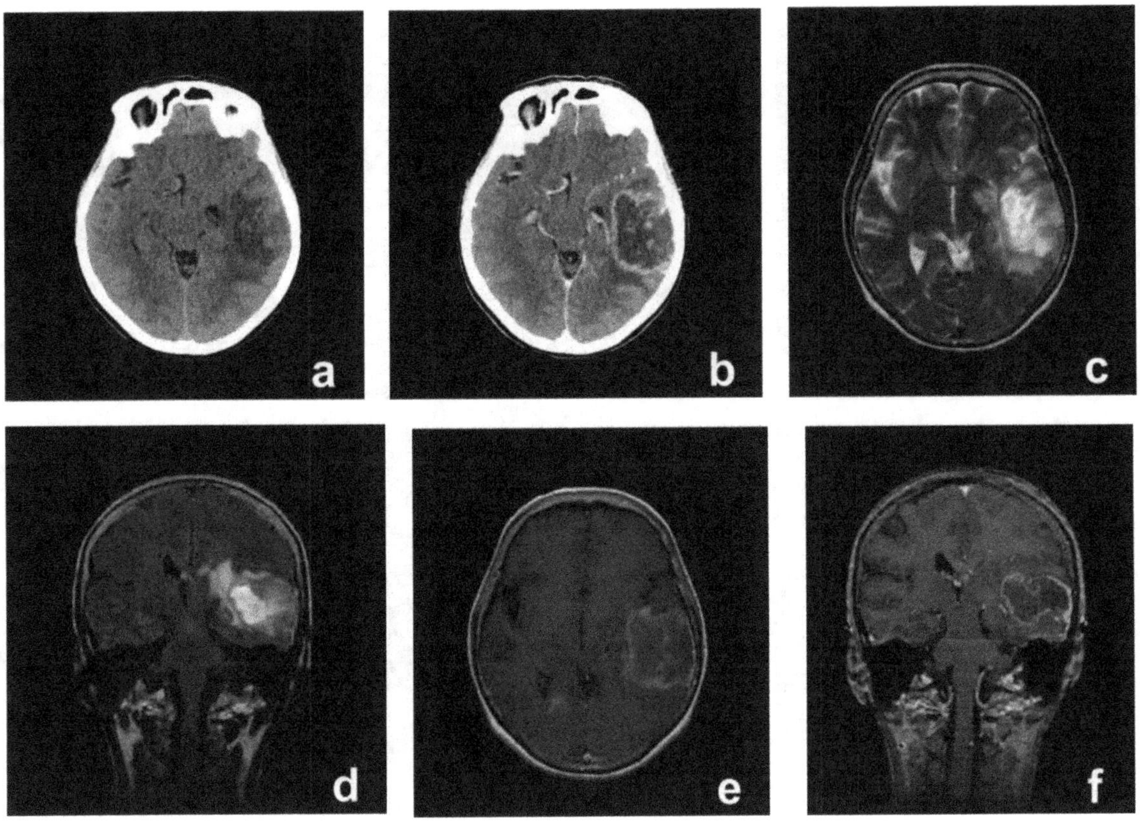

Figure 5. Left temporal glioblastoma. (a) CT scan without contrast; (b) CT scan with contrast; (c) MRI – Axial T2-weighted image; (d) MRI – Coronal FLAIR sequence; (e) MRI – Axial T1-weighted image with contrast; (f) MRI – Coronal T1-weighted image with contrast.

Positron emission tomography (PET) can be used to provide additional metabolic information of the tumor. This technique is based on the detection of radioactivity emitted by biochemically active molecules labeled with radiotracers. Different molecular processes can be investigated including glucose consumption, expression of amino acid transporters, proliferation rate, membrane biosynthesis and hypoxia. The glucose analog ^{18}F-fluorodeoxyglucose (^{18}F FDG) is the most commonly used radiotracer for PET to measure the local metabolic rate of glucose. Increased glucose metabolism is a feature of high-grade glioma (HGG) and a positive correlation between glycolysis rate and malignancy was demonstrated. Radiolabeled amino acids (like ^{11}C Methionine—^{11}C MET) have been introduced as suitable tracers in brain tumors, because amino acid transport as well as protein synthesis were both demonstrated to be enhanced in HGG. Even more, ^{11}C MET has increased specificity and sensitivity, highlighting areas of cellular proliferation correlating well with the Ki-67 labeling index of proliferation and with microvascular density. PET can help distinguish GBMs from other brain lesions pre-operatively, can reveal malignant transformation in low-grade gliomas (LGG), and can evaluate the tumor extension for an appropriate site for biopsy, for surgery planning or for radiation therapy planning. PET is also important in assessment of treatment response, being beneficial for differentiation of tumor tissue from post-therapeutic changes.

In patients with a suspected diagnosis of GBMs, **initial management** is intended to control symptoms and prepare the patients for surgery. Corticosteroid therapy reduces peritumoral edema and alleviates symptoms of raised intracranial pressure and neurologic

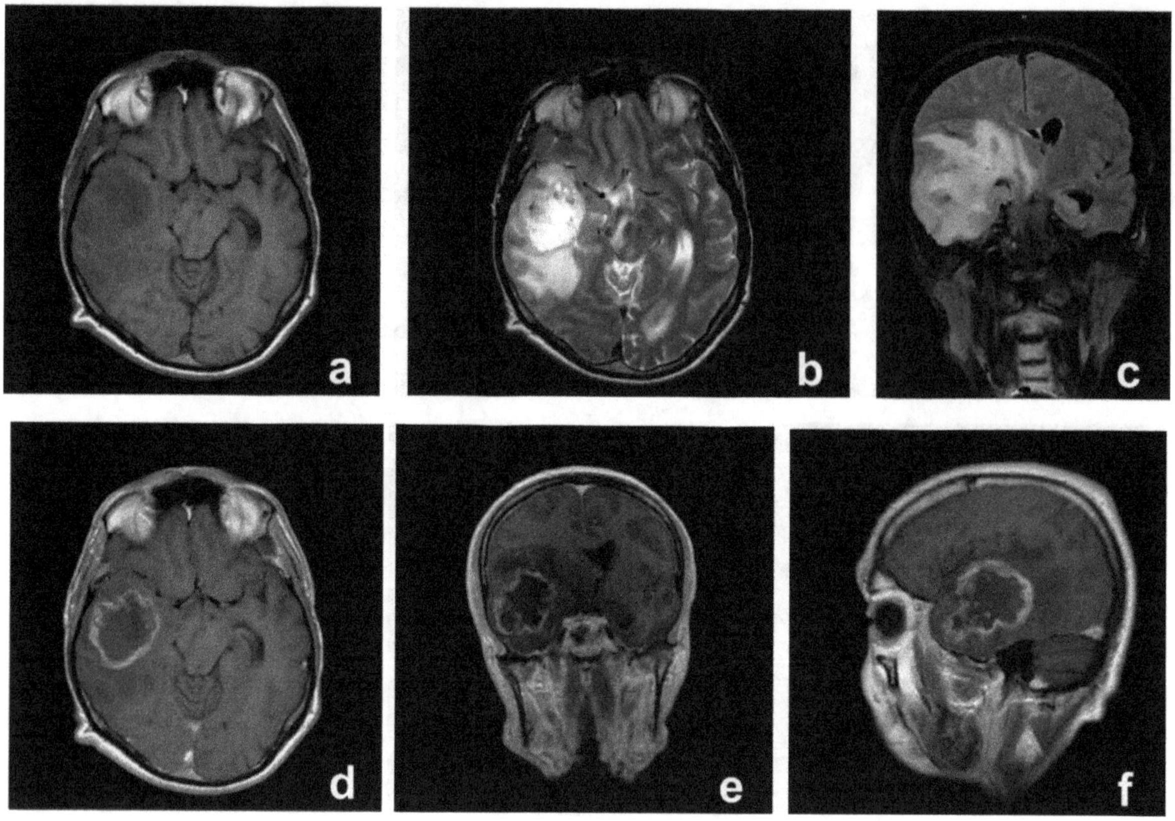

Figure 6. Right temporal glioblastoma – MRI features. (a) Axial T1-weighted image; (b) axial T2-weighted image; (c) coronal FLAIR sequence; (d) axial T1-weighted image with contrast; (e) coronal T1-weighted image with contrast; (f) sagittal T1-weighted image with contrast.

symptoms, making surgery safer. Anticonvulsants are necessary when a history of seizures exists. However, prophylactic use of antiepileptic drugs outside the perioperative phase is controversial.

Ideally, all patients with GBMs should be managed by a multidisciplinary team in a centralized neurosciences center. The neuro-oncology group should include specialists from neuroradiology, neurology, neurosurgery, neuropathology, intensive care, medical and radiation oncology, neurorehabilitation, etc.

4. Surgical management

Neuroimaging modalities provide a lot of data about mass lesion, but cannot reliably predict the diagnosis of tumor type and grade. Histological assessment is required. Thus, **a representative tissue sample should be obtained by biopsy or resection** to have a correct diagnosis before specific adjunctive therapies have been initiated. The neurosurgeon is involved in decision-making regarding the appropriate surgical procedure for patients with GBM. Based on preoperative evaluation, he must indicate either an open surgical resection for both diagnosis and treatment or only a biopsy for diagnosis. Special consideration should be given to some important factors, including age of the patient, location and size of the tumor, neurological status, functional impairment (quantified by Karnofsky Performance Status (KPS) Scale), significant comorbidity and patient and family preferences. Patients with GBM should have **surgery for maximal tumor removal** whenever safe, because this could prolong their survival when compared with biopsy, subtotal or partial resection. **Biopsy** is only indicated in cases of "inoperability" of the tumor, because of the associated risks are minimal. The image-guided stereotactic techniques are preferred over open biopsy.

4.1. Stereotactic biopsy

Stereotactic biopsy enables safe retrieval of sufficient material to allow pathologic diagnosis from precise targets in GBMs with the help of MRI or CT scan. Framed or frameless stereotactic biopsy can be performed. The main indications are inaccessible tumor location (deep-seated lesion), multiple or bilateral disease, potential unacceptable surgical morbidity because of eloquent adjacent brain areas, poor performance status (KPS < 60), lesion in a surgically poor candidate because of significant medical problems. When the diagnosis of GBM versus other space-occupying lesions is in doubt, biopsy may be a better initial step. Stereotactic biopsy is a minimally invasive technique, with low risk and good diagnostic accuracy, which can provide valuable information, guiding further treatment. However, an average morbidity rate of 4.1% (range, 0.7–7%) and a mortality rate of 0.9% (range, 0.2–2.3%) have been demonstrated [11]. Owing to histological heterogeneity, it leads to an inaccurate or imprecise diagnosis in about 10% of cases. There are approximately 15–20% of patients who undergo only biopsy as a surgical procedure [12].

4.2. Open surgical resection

To date, surgery for resection remains **the first and the most important treatment modality** in GBMs. **The goal of surgery** should be to remove as much of the tumor as possible, while minimizing damage to surrounding healthy brain. Unfortunately, surgery is not curative. Because of the highly aggressive and invasive nature of the GBM, a complete resection is not possible. Despite the relative lack of appropriately designed trials, experience strongly supports the fact that gross-total resection (GTR) of the entire area of gadolinium-enhancement tumor is associated with improved outcome. Therefore, the current trend is to perform maximal tumor removal whenever possible, while minimizing the risk for unacceptable neurological deficit, aimed to both improve the quality of life and prolong survival.

There are **some reasons for surgery** on lesions thought to be GBMs. The first indication is to obtain a histological diagnosis. Owing to glioma histological heterogeneity, multiple biological samples from separate places of the tumor should be taken and examined. Open resection can provide a larger tissue specimen as compared to biopsy. Provision of tumor for research and scientific analysis also could be beneficial for the patient. The second indication is to perform a surgical decompression that can relieve intracranial hypertension, can improve neurologic functions and can prevent death due to brain herniation. The third indication is to reduce the tumor mass as much as possible. Reduction of the tumor burden provides a rapid drop in the global tumoral cell population, removes resistant cells and prolongs survival. Extensive resection of the tumor may potentiate or facilitate radiation therapy, chemotherapy, immunotherapy or other modalities of treatment. The fourth indication is to deliver adjuvant therapies, including intratumoral chemotherapy, intracavitary brachytherapy, gene therapy, immunotherapy, photodynamic therapy, etc. Radical surgery to the extent feasible should be recommended whenever is possible, regardless of age. Relative contraindications include inaccessible or eloquent location, poor performance status and important comorbidities. Typically, tumors located in the basal ganglia, thalamus, corpus callosum, brain stem or multiple tumors are biopsied only.

Proper patient selection and preoperative planning are very important for the success of the surgical intervention. The decision to undergo radical surgery needs to be reasonable and the surgical approach must be individualized for each patient. Careful assessment of the preoperative MRI imaging studies is essential for preoperative planning. The tumor location determines the type of approach to be used and the optimal trajectory to the lesion. The neurosurgeon should measure the tumor dimensions in all three axes on the contrast-enhanced MRI and compare them with on-site measurements for a good estimation of the extent of resection (EOR). If there is concern regarding proximity of the tumor to eloquent areas, a functional MRI can help to highlight the location of critical brain regions. Consequently, the surgeon can plan the operative technique and can take the decision to perform intraoperative mapping (sometimes an awake craniotomy is needed). The blood oxygenation level-dependent functional MRI (BOLDfMRI) is used in the clinical practice for presurgical mapping of motor areas and language areas (lateralization and localization). It works by recording subtle changes in blood oxygenation and flow that occur in response to a particular neural activity. It produces activation maps.

Maximal safe tumor resection represents the mainstay in GBM treatment. **Tumor removal** involves standard neurosurgical techniques. A good knowledge of surgical anatomy and a meticulous microsurgical technique, while preserving brain functions are essential. To increase the precision and the safety of the surgery, the specialist can use various technologies which allow intraoperative guidance. Neurosurgery for patients with GBM should be conducted in accredited facilities, that have the appropriate neurosurgical equipment and trained staff and where there is a specific multidisciplinary team.

Ideally, **the extent of resection (EOR)** should be assessed after surgery. This must be carried out by a contrast-enhanced MRI within 24–48 hours postoperatively, in order to distinguish between residual GBM, postoperative reactive changes and parenchymal damage as a result of surgery. Postoperative contrast-enhancing tumor mass is typically used to delineate residual GBM and completeness of removal. It is better to use volumetric analysis of the preoperative and postoperative tumor to accurately measure EOR and residual volume (RV). Reactive postoperative changes can be seen as early as 18 hours on MRI, but usually does not appear in the first 3–4 days. The EOR was identified as a strong prognostic factor for survival in GBM, together with patient's age and patient's functional status. Surgical removal has a critical role in GBM management because the only potentially modifiable risk factor associated with survival is EOR. The gross-total resection is not always possible. Thus, several studies have been conducted to evaluate EOR threshold which may serve as minimum surgical goal to achieve. Other studies demonstrated that EOR is not an ideal indicator to the success of the surgery, because it is a percentage value, reported to initial volume of the tumor, which can vary widely. Contrast-enhancing RV is considered a more clinically relevant measure and a stronger predictor of survival than EOR, representing the tumor mass existing prior to starting medical therapy. Chaichana et al. in 2014 evaluated newly diagnosed GBM patients who underwent surgery and found that the minimum EOR of 70% and the maximal RV of 5 cm^3 showed statistical significance for prolonged survival and delayed recurrence [13]. Grabowsky et al. in 2014 reported that RV of 2 cm^3 or less confers survival benefit to the patient [14]. There are models that argue for a continuous relationship between EOR and median survival, suggesting that there is a survival advantage associated with any degree of resection [15]. This is evident for the practice of maximal safe resection for GBM.

Surgery is associated with some **risk**. Complications encountered in open surgery for GBM are those of craniotomy in general. There are reported morbidity rates ranging from 5 to 15% and mortality rates from 1 to 5% [8].

4.3. Intraoperative neurosurgical guidance

The key issue for glioma surgery is to accurately delineate the tumor into the operative field, which can be a challenge for the neurosurgeon. Many useful tools have been created to help the surgeon differentiate between tumor and normal tissue. It is important to adapt modern technologies to successfully guide maximal surgical resection without postoperative neurological deficit. Multiple studies suggest that extensive resection is beneficial for the patient. But an excessive excision should be avoided, since it can induce permanent neurological dysfunction. At the same time, an incomplete resection can be therapeutically ineffective. The ideal goal of neurosurgery is to maximize the resection of the tumor mass safely, without impairing eloquent functions and quality of life. For higher efficacy and lower risk, the current concept of neurosurgery is an "information-guided surgery", using multimodal intraoperative information to identify the positions of the eloquent brain areas accurately and in real-time [16, 17]. Anatomical information from navigation, ultrasonography and intraoperative MRI, functional information from mapping and monitoring and histopathological data must all be considered to prevent unexpected deficits and promote extensive resection.

4.3.1. Image-based navigation

MRI neuronavigation (frameless stereotactic navigation) is based on preoperative MR-imaging data, taken with fiducial markers that are left in place on the scalp. This data is projected into the operative field for better anatomical orientation. It is useful for surgical planning and image guidance, particularly when the tumor cannot be seen on the cortical surface of the brain. However, it is rendered unreliable when variations in brain volume or shifts of the intracranial content appear during the surgery, because this technology is based on a preoperative set of images, without updating during surgery.

Intraoperative ultrasonography is helpful when the tumor is not isoechoic with the brain or the density difference is greater (when there is a hematoma or a cystic component into the mass lesion). It is a dynamic imaging modality that can guide the neurosurgeon in real-time during resection. It has the advantage that brain shift and brain relaxation that occur during the excision of the lesion do not influence the accuracy of the procedure. Three-dimensional sonography with navigation software solves any orientation problems.

Intraoperative MRI systems are available, but the equipment is expensive and therefore the access is somewhat restricted for many neurosurgeons and patients alike. It has the advantage to avoid potential errors caused by brain shift. It provides information about the completeness of tumor resection during surgery and allows the surgeon to perform an additional tumor excision, if needed. However, it has a limited ability to delineate between residual glioma and adjacent normal brain. The system has been shown to improve the extent of tumor removal.

4.3.2. Intraoperative functional mapping and monitoring

Intraoperative functional mapping and monitoring are essential for safe excision of GBM localized near eloquent cortex. It can accurately identify individual eloquent brain areas, including somatosensory cortex, motor cortex and language cortex, enabling the neurosurgeon to avoid these regions during tumor resection and thereby minimizing the risk of neurological morbidity. One of the most important advantages of this method over the imaging techniques is allowing assessment of the cortical and subcortical function in real-time. In addition, continuous monitoring of the patient's neurological findings during surgery is very useful for intraoperative feedback to the surgeon. Using these functional methods, the edge of resection can exceed the anatomical borders of the tumor (contrast-enhancing regions) to reach the functional border of the tumor (placed in the peritumoral tissues, invaded by the tumoral cells) [18].

Localization of the primary somatosensory cortex can be achieved by somatosensory evoked potentials (SSEPs) mapping, performed under general anesthesia or in awake patient. Techniques are similar to those used for routine diagnostic studies. Evoked potentials are recorded by stimulating peripheral afferent nerves (median nerve, posterior tibial nerve, etc.), usually electrically. Recording electrodes are placed on the cortical surface (typically proximal to the lesion). When recording SSEPs, the primary sensory cortex and primary motor cortex generate potentials that are mirror images of each other. This "phase reversal" across the central sulcus aids in the localization of the primary motor cortex. Localization of the primary somatosensory cortex can also be performed by direct cortical electrical stimulation of the postcentral region. The awake patient communicates the presence or absence of the sensory symptoms triggered by stimulation.

Localization of the primary motor cortex can be accomplished using the SSEPs "phase reversal" technique or by direct cortical electrical stimulation (with patient under general anesthesia). It is recommended to use both techniques, starting with central sulcus identification and continuing with cortical stimulation of precentral regions and recording the muscle motor evoked potentials (mMEPs) from the corresponding muscles or observing clinical movements [19]. The former technique is preferred, because the stimulation threshold for obtaining mMEPs is smaller than that for obtaining clinical movements [8, 17, 19]. Thus, the risk of eliciting local or generalized seizure activity is decreased. During the cortical stimulation, simultaneous electrocorticogram (EcoG) recording is required for the safety of the patient. It is used to identify spontaneous or stimulation-induced epileptic discharges (after discharges), marking a subclinical seizure activity. It is important to have an adequate serum anticonvulsant level pre-operatively and, if necessary, additional intravenous boluses of antiepileptic drugs may be considered [8]. It is of paramount importance to distinguish primary from supplementary motor areas as it is known that damage of the motor strip will cause a permanent postoperative motor deficit, while damage of the supplementary and premotor areas will result in a temporary postoperative deficit. Once the motor strip was identified, direct cortical stimulation or subcortical stimulation can be used for continuous evaluation of the functional integrity of the motor pathways during glioma resection.

Localization of the language cortex is performed under awake craniotomy (AC), by cortical and subcortical direct electrical stimulation (DES). A "positive mapping" strategy can be used: a large craniotomy exposes the brain a good distance from the tumor and makes it possible to identify "positive" language sites (areas where a cortical stimulation induces a language function) prior to excision. Lately, a "negative mapping" strategy emerged as preferable. It supposes to identify "negative" language sites, meaning regions where a cortical stimulation blocks a language function. This technique allows a smaller, tailored craniotomy, with a minimal cortical exposure around the tumor (up to 2 cm of surrounding brain) and a less extensive mapping. It is a more time-efficient neurosurgical procedure [17, 20, 21].

It is important to emphasize that stimulation mapping is used to identify essential language cortex, whose injury will lead to permanent deficit. But there are also multiple nonessential speech areas. The essential language cortex is obviously different from involved language cortex identified by functional imaging techniques, such as functional MRI (fMRI) and positron emission tomography (PET). Although these imaging techniques have advanced considerably, they have some limitations and cannot replace intraoperative mapping. Patients who speak multiple languages have separate language sites for each of their different languages [8]. Different language tasks performed by a patient may lead to delineate distinct language sites. There is significant individual variability in the location of the language areas, sometimes the Broca area or the Wernicke area having a location beyond the classic anatomical boundaries or more than two essential speech areas being identified. Quinones-Hinojosa et al. found a variability of more than 4 cm in the location of speech arrest when using classical neuroanatomic landmarks [22, 23]. Furthermore, cerebral topography is distorted by the tumor mass effect and brain plasticity can induce a functional reassignment [17, 20, 23]. Thus, intraoperative identification of the language areas is essential for extensively and safely removing GBMs located near these eloquent regions in the dominant-hemisphere. It is best to continuously monitor the patient's ability to speak, especially during the part of the excision which is close to the identified language sites (within 2 cm). If the distance between resection border and the nearest language area is more than 1 cm, significantly fewer permanent language deficits occur [20, 24]. A subcortical stimulation can be used into the resection cavity to guide the removal technique (when stimulation block the language function, the location is very close to the subcortical language pathways – 5 mm or less) [17, 25].

A new intraoperative method to assess integrity of functional interconnections between language areas during surgery was proposed by Yamao et al. [17, 26, 27]. The authors monitored the integrity of the dorsal language pathway (arcuate fasciculus) using cortico-cortical evoked potentials (CCEPs). The technique is based on the electrical stimulation of the anterior perisylvian language area while recording the average response from posterior perisylvian language area. It is clinically useful for evaluating the integrity of the language network and have the advantages that is task-free, do not require the cooperation of the patient and therefore can be performed also under general anesthesia [27, 28].

4.3.3. Enhanced visual tumor demarcation

The ideal technique for sharper intraoperative delineation between tumor and the surrounding cerebral tissue should provide real-time information during resection, without concern about changes into the operative field and still be affordable.

Intraoperative tumoral tissue fluorescence due to specific enhancing agents provides a real-time GBM discrimination in situ. The differences are visualized using specially designed microscopes, equipped with appropriate filters to detect fluorescent light emission. Fluorescence is the emission of light with a short wavelength by a substance that has absorbed light of a longer wavelength. Fluorochrome is a fluorescent dye, used to stain biological material before microscopic examination. In neurosurgery of the gliomas, a specific fluorochrome is associated with glioma tissue (selectively if possible) and then illuminated by light. Fluorescent dye will emit light, which will be perceived by the surgeon using special filters. There are four types of approaches to intraoperative fluorescence: (1) tissue fluorescence induced by specific metabolic activity; (2) tissue fluorescence-based on passive permeability; (3) tissue fluorescence due to targeted fluorescent probes accumulated into the tumor tissue; and (4) autofluorescence [29].

Tissue fluorescence induced by specific metabolic activity is the basis to use of 5-aminolevulinic acid (5-ALA) in fluorescence-guided surgery. 5-ALA is an endogenous amino acid, the first compound in the porphyrin synthesis pathway. It is finally converted to protoporphyrin IX (PPIX), which chelates with iron in presence of enzyme ferrochelatase to produce heme (component of hemoproteins). GBM cells lack or have reduced ferrochelatase activity and this results in accumulation of protoporphyrin IX into the tumor tissue after oral administration of 5-ALA. Protoporphyrin IX is clearly visualized by its red fluorescence under blue-violet light conditions, enabling differentiation of viable tumor from normal adjacent brain. 5-ALA is the only agent that has been approved in fluorescence-guided neurosurgery in Europe, Canada and Japan, and is commonly used in surgery of GBMs. It induces GBM tissue fluorescence, having high sensitivity, specificity, and positive predictive values for identifying malignant glioma tumor tissue [30, 31]. In recurrent malignant gliomas, fluorescence is observed in anaplastic foci, in regions of gliosis or invaded by inflammatory cells, but not in normal brain. Prior alternative treatment such as radiotherapy or chemotherapy does not invalidate 5-ALA-induced fluorescence [32]. Fluorescence can discriminate malignant glioma cells down to a tumor cell density of approximately 10% [29, 33]. It is now demonstrated that visible fluorescence clearly extends beyond the border of preoperative MRI contrast-enhancement, PPIX accumulation being more sensitive than gadolinium enhancement [33, 34]. Thus, an extensive glioma resection beyond radiologically evident tumor can be performed. 5-ALA-guided resection of GBM was found to be beneficial, enabling surgeons to achieve a double rate of complete resections of malignant gliomas in comparison with conventional techniques [31, 35]. A randomized controlled multicenter phase III trial conducted by Stummer et al. involving 270 patients in 17 centers has examined a group undergoing 5-ALA fluorescence-guided surgery and a group undergoing conventional white light-guided surgery. The authors reported that gross-total resection evaluated on postoperative imaging was 65% in cases undergoing fluorescence guidance compared with 36% in the white light group ($p < 0.001$), and progression-free survival was 41 versus 21.1% ($p < 0.003$) [35].

Tissue fluorescence based on passive permeability uses fluorescein or indocyanine green, which has not been approved for intracranial use. Fluorescein is a typical marker of compromised blood-brain barrier (BBB), rather than a selective tumor marker, therefore its presence is highly nonspecific. It displays a yellow-green fluorescence visualized by the naked eye. Given its limited specificity, there is a great risk to remove normal, functional brain tissue, and given its sensitivity concerns, there is a risk of leaving residual tumor [36]. Recently, a dual-labeling approach has been proposed, using both PPIX and fluorescein fluorescence simultaneously. The advantage is that PPIX provides a reliable tumor detection and fluorescein gives a better background visualization, as it would be expected to accelerate surgery, while maintaining safety and efficacy [37]. Indocyanine green enables evaluation of tumoral and peritumoral blood flow and vascularization. It has the advantage of emitting light in the near-infrared region of the spectrum, therefore the fluorochrome can be visualized deeper in the tumoral tissue. However, the visualization requires special technologies.

Tissue fluorescence due to targeted fluorescent probes accumulated into the malignant tumor tissue is an ongoing subject of research. There are some fluorescent agents targeted or being retained by brain tumor cells undergoing clinical testing. Their effective application in clinical settings requires development of detection instrumentation and additional studies. Agents that show promise for intraoperative discrimination of GBM include Tumor Paint (chlorotoxin linked to a fluorophore), Angiopep-2 targeting agents, epidermal growth factor receptor (EGFR)-targeted agents, PTPμ-targeted SBK agents, the fluorescently labeled poly (ADP-ribose) polymerase 1 (PARP-1) inhibitor (CLR1502) and $\alpha v\beta 3$ integrin-targeted agents [38, 39].

Microspectrofluorometry can be used to measure the autofluorescence spectrum of biological tissues both *ex vivo* on resected samples and *in vivo*, during surgery, by means of fiber optic probe. It is a dye-free method, based on the intrinsic autofluorescence properties of a tissue. In glioma, the autofluorescence profile is distinct from normal brain, due to changes of biochemical composition and histological organization. There are differences in both spectral shape and signal amplitude relative to normal cortex and white matter. These differences allow the use of autofluorescence in situ as a parameter for distinguishing neoplastic from normal condition and so to better delineate GBM resection margins [40–42].

Confocal microscopy (laser scanning confocal microscopy – LSCM) may provide *in vivo* images by optical sectioning, characterized by higher resolution and contrast, with magnification up to 1000x. These images enable intraoperative visualization of tumor histopathological features and cell morphology in real-time, in three dimensions, without the need for extensive traditional tissue processing [36]. Intraoperative confocal imaging correlates with histopathological analysis, the diagnostic accuracy being of up to 93% [43]. The major application of confocal microscopy is for imaging tissues labeled with fluorescent probes. In GBM surgery, confocal microscopy combined with tissue fluorescence provides a reliable identification of tumor cells and tumor-brain interfaces.

4.3.4. Intraoperative sampling

The diagnostic of GBM is usually confirmed by standard postoperative histopathological examination of tissue sections with results only available several days after the surgery has finished. But the maximal removal of the glioma is the key component in the specific treatment, a smaller volume of postoperative residual tumor being associated with an improved prognosis. One of the difficulties of achieving an optimal excision is failure to delineate the resection margins. Nevertheless, histopathological assessment is also available during the surgery, providing important diagnostic information. Even if such information is less reliable compared with that of postoperative approaches, sometimes **intraoperative sampling** is the sole source of diagnostic arguments for deciding the extent of resection. Precision increases with the number of tissue sections. Traditional histopathological techniques made intraoperative include frozen section and imprint cytology. They are time-consuming (requiring nearly 30 mins), laborious and subjective. It is desirable that they are performed by a skilled pathologist.

Mass spectrometry-based molecular analysis can rapidly provide detailed molecular information about tumor and adjacent brain tissue, allowing an intraoperative diagnosis and guidance in detection of the boundaries between glioma and normal brain. The desorption electrospray ionization mass spectrometry (DESI-MS) is a mass spectrometric imaging technique for characterizing lipid profile within tumor specimens. Because DESI-MS can be performed rapidly (minutes) and routinely, in the ambient conditions, with minimal pretreatment of biological samples, it can be used during surgery. It quickly provides a valuable diagnosis of tumor type based on lipid pattern [44]. It can also detect oncometabolites: 2-hydroxyglutarate and N-acetylaspartate. 2-hydroxyglutarate is present in small amounts in normal brain tissue, but its concentrations are extremely high in gliomas with mutations in IDH1 and IDH2 [45–47]. It could be used as a biomarker and serve as an important prognostic indicator. Detection of 2-hydroxyglutarate in operative field with precise spatial distribution could also help define surgical margins. DESI-MS provide valuable information that is unattainable by traditional histopathological techniques.

4.4. Intratumoral therapies

Given that GBM is typically a solitary tumor, with local recurrence and very rare metastases, the disease is a proper candidate for local treatment. On the other hand, availability of drugs which can cross the BBB has severely limited the effective therapies against GBM. Strategies to bypass this barrier have been developed. Localized drug delivery into a postoperative tumor bed is an attractive option for administration of therapeutics while avoiding systemic side effects. Furthermore, this way provides a means for administration of new, tumor-selective molecules that are often largely excluded by brain.

Controlled-release polymer systems, like carmustine wafers (Gliadel wafers) can be implanted in the resection cavity. Another local approach is catheter-based convection-enhanced delivery (CED) of conventional or novel agents through continuous low-positive-pressure bulk flow. Intracavitary delivery of highly localized doses of irradiation is feasible through GliaSite system brachytherapy.

4.5. Recurrence

Standard therapy in newly diagnosed GBM involves maximal safe surgical resection followed by radiotherapy (RT) with concurrent and adjuvant TMZ. Despite this first-line treatment, recurrence inevitably occurs, most patients experiencing it after 7–8 months of primary treatment. There are no well-defined management protocols for recurrent GBM. Options for second-line treatment are limited and include repeat surgery, re-irradiation, chemotherapy, novel therapies, supportive care or, better, a combination of these.

The standard neuroimaging modality for the follow-up of GBM is contrast-enhanced MRI, which is performed every 2–3 months while the patient is on therapy. Criteria to assess treatment response and progression have been established by the Response Assessment in Neuro-Oncology (RANO) Working Group [48]. Progression is defined as at least 25% increase in the contrast-enhancing MRI lesion (the product of the maximal cross-sectional enhancing diameters of tumor area). Diagnosing a true progressive tumor growth after chemoradiation by MRI alone remains a challenge, because it is very difficult to distinguish between post-treatment radiation effects (such as pseudoprogression or radiation necrosis) and tumor recurrence. Post-treatment radiation effects can be divided into pseudoprogression and radiation necrosis. Pseudoprogression appears several weeks up to 3 months after RT (5.5–31%), whereas radiation necrosis occurs 3 months to years after irradiation (3–24%) [49]. Radiation necrosis is a space-occupying necrotic lesion, with mass effect and neurological dysfunction. It is irreversible and progressive. Its features on MRI are often identical to that of recurrent GBM. The differentiation is very important, because the management is different. Advanced MRI techniques such as DWI, DTI and PWI provide additional information. Metabolic imaging techniques like PET, single-photon emission computed tomography (SPECT) and MR spectroscopy (MRS) are helpful in differentiating between tumor recurrence and therapy-related changes. Tumor recurrence appears as a lesion metabolically active, while radiation necrosis appears metabolically inactive. However, no imaging modality has sufficient specificity and tissue biopsy remains the gold standard to obtain a definitive diagnosis.

GBMs typically recur focally and in many cases surgery is possible. **Repeat surgery** is performed in approximately 25% of cases. Although a repeat surgery is associated with a higher complication rates than the initial surgery, this increase is rather small and clearly acceptable [50, 51]. However, its efficacy is debated. Many recent studies reported a survival benefit and an improvement of quality of life resulting from repeat resections in selected patients. Performing an overview of the current literature on second surgery for recurrent GBM, Montemurro et al. found the median overall survival from diagnosis being 18.5 months and the median survival from second surgery being 9.7 months [51]. Extent of resection at reoperation has been demonstrated to improve overall survival, thus a maximum safe excision should be the surgical goal. The decision of a second surgery should be individualized and should involve a multidisciplinary team approach. The age and the preoperative performance status are the most important predictors of a prolonged survival. A more favorable prognosis following surgery for recurrence is associated with a younger age (< 60 years) and a good preoperative performance status (KPS ≥ 70) [51]. Reoperation is not recommended for patients with involvement of eloquent brain regions.

Thus, patients with recurrent GBM may benefit from resection of tumor whenever safely possible. Repeat surgery can help in providing symptom relief and differentiating tumor recurrence from pseudoprogression, radiation necrosis, respectively. But surgery should be followed by adjuvant therapies.

5. Radiation therapy

The SoC for newly diagnosed GBM consists of maximal safe surgical resection followed by radiotherapy (RT) plus concomitant and adjuvant TMZ.

Following gross-tumor removal, the final histological diagnosis is established, and RT should start. **The optimal time to initiate** radiation is controversial. There are studies showing worse outcomes and even decreased survival when radiation is delayed [52, 53]. Irwin et al. found that a 6 weeks delay (from 2 weeks postoperative to 8 weeks) reduces median survival by 11 weeks for a "typical" patient [52]. But there also studies showing no association between timing of radiation initiation and outcomes [54, 55] and studies suggesting a possible benefit of delay (however, up to a reference range of time) [56, 57]. Blumenthal et al. analyzed the relationship between the delay of RT and the outcome on a large cohort of more than 2800 patients. They observed no obvious reduction in survival with increasing delay (within relatively narrow temporal limits—6 weeks). Indeed, median survival time was unexpectedly greater in the group with the longest interval (>4 weeks) than in those with the shortest delay (≤2 weeks), respectively, 12.5 months versus 9.2 months ($P < 0.0001$). The authors do not exclude the possibility that an adjuvant treatment initiated beyond 6 weeks postoperatively may be detrimental [56]. In other studies, Han et al. found a narrow range of time (from 30 to 34 days after surgery) where there is prolonged overall survival and prolonged progression-free survival compared with early initiation of concurrent chemoradiation [57, 58]. In common practice, the patient commonly waits about 4 weeks before adjuvant therapies. It is generally agreed that a postoperative delay of 6 weeks may not be critical.

Concomitant TMZ and RT (known as the Stupp regimen) have been shown to be more effective than radiation alone with minimal additional toxicity. **After the end of radiation, an adjuvant treatment with TMZ is indicated.** Patients who received RT and concurrent TMZ presented a median survival of 14.6 months versus 12.1 months with RT alone [59]. Furthermore, the two-year survival rate was 26.5% with RT plus TMZ versus 10.4% with RT alone. This is the current SoC for patients with newly diagnosed GBM up to age 70, with a good performance status (Karnofsky Performance Status (KPS) ≥ 60).

RT using three-dimensional conformal beam or intensity-modulated RT is used now. The typical total dose delivered is 60 Gy in 2 Gy fractions, administered 5 days per week for 6 weeks and there is no evidence that higher doses improve outcome [60, 61]. The RT involved fields should include the tumor bed with a 2–3 cm margin, based on the observation that GBM commonly recurs within 2 cm of the original tumor location in 80–90% of cases.

The optimal management of **elderly patients** is controversial. In practice, for patients >70 years old or for patients <70 years old with a poor performance status (KPS < 60), an alternative hypofractionated regimen can be considered. For elderly not suitable for radiation, chemotherapy alone may be an option.

Despite maximal multimodal treatment, GBM invariably recur, disease progression occurring within the first year in about 70% of cases. In selected cases of **recurrences**, a second course of radiation may be possible, but tolerance of local brain tissue to radiation is limited and there is an increased risk of radiation necrosis. This may lead to neurological dysfunction, edema and mass effect. Radiation necrosis is very difficult to distinguish from progressive disease solely by imaging techniques. Histology remains the gold standard for diagnosis. Combs et al. investigated the role of re-irradiation using the fractionated stereotactic approach and demonstrated a median survival of 8 months and a progression-free survival of 5 months for patients with GBM [62].

Stereotactic radiosurgery offers the potential of providing a "boost" radiation to a portion of the radiation field in newly diagnosed patients or treating a small recurrence, being an alternative to open surgery [63]. However, its applicability remains very limited in absence of studies which could demonstrate a statistically significant benefit.

Intracavitary brachytherapy using the GliaSite system can be used in selected newly diagnosed patients or in recurrent disease, intending to deliver an additional radiation to the surgical cavity wall. It is a medical device, composed of a balloon that will contain a radioactive solution with ^{125}I during the period of irradiation, connected through a catheter to an infusion port. The balloon is placed in the resection cavity during surgery and the radioactive solution is injected later. Re-irradiation of recurrent GBM with GliaSite Radiation Therapy System after resection seems to provide a median survival of approximately 9 months [64, 65].

6. Chemotherapy

For the time being, **TMZ** is considered the first-line chemotherapy drug in GBM. It is an oral systemic drug with a good penetration of the BBB and limited side effects. The mechanism of action is based on its ability to alkylate/methylate DNA. This alkylation damages the DNA and triggers the death of tumor cells. *MGMT* (O^6-methylguanine-DNA methyltransferase) is a DNA-repair enzyme that rescues glioma cells from damages induced by alkylating agents like TMZ or carmustine. High activity of MGMT in tumor cells creates resistance to chemotherapy with alkylating agents and may determine treatment failure. Epigenetic silencing of the MGMT gene by promoter methylation is associated with decrease of DNA-repair activity and thus tumor cells will be more responsive to TMZ. In other words, the methylation status of MGMT promoter is associated with a benefit from alkylating agent-based chemotherapy in GBM. Numerous studies have confirmed that carriers of the methylated form of MGMT promoter with GBM treated with TMZ and RT have a prolonged overall survival [66–68]. Hegi et al. found that their median survival was 21.7 months as compared with 15.3 months among those who were assigned to only RT [69]. Furthermore, assessing MGMT methylation status in a cohort of patients with GBM who underwent radiation treatment but did not receive chemotherapy, Rivera et al. have demonstrated an 50% reduction in the rate of tumor progression during RT in methylated tumors versus those that were unmethylated. These data suggest that MGMT promoter methylation may predict a better response to any form of therapy, including RT [70]. Consequently, MGMT promoter methylation status has been established as an important prognostic biomarker, helping in performing a risk stratification of cases. National Comprehensive Cancer Network (NCCN) guidelines consider MGMT promoter methylation status in clinical management of the patients with GBM.

For newly diagnosed GBM, TMZ is typically given following surgical resection, concurrent and adjuvant, in addition to RT. It is administered daily at a dose of 75 mg/m^2 for 6 weeks during irradiation, followed by a rest period of about 1 month after RT is completed (concurrent treatment). When restarted, TMZ is dosed at 150 mg/m^2 daily for 5 days every 4 weeks for 6 cycles (adjuvant treatment). If tolerated, the dose of the adjuvant treatment can be escalated up to 200 mg/m^2 daily. This is the well-known Stupp regimen. In common practice, some medical centers have attempted to prolong TMZ administration for 12–18 months. Some evidence suggests that long-term therapy with TMZ in selected patients is superior to Stupp regimen [71–73], but there is no definitive data to prove this.

The use of standard or hypofractionated RT plus concomitant and/or adjuvant TMZ has been extended to **elderly** (> 70 years old) with a good performance status (KPS ≥ 60). For patients >70 years old with a poor performance status (KPS < 60), TMZ alone can be an option.

At the time of **recurrence**, reoperation should be proposed if the tumor is resectable and if prognostic factors suggest a benefit. Local chemotherapy can be administered during surgery by implantation of Gliadel wafers. Second-line chemotherapy is indicated based on MGMT promoter methylation, time to disease recurrence and toxicity profile. The nitrosourea-based regimen is the preferred choice. Restarting therapy with TMZ may be an option in MGMT-methylated patients. Other agents, such as carboplatin, etoposide, irinotecan may be tried as single agents or in regimens.

Gliadel wafers are composed of a biodegradable polymer impregnated with carmustine (BCNU), an alkylating agent of the nitrosourea family. During the surgery, after removal of the tumor, up to 8 wafers (containing a maximum of 61.6 mg BCNU) are deposited along the wall of the resection cavity and left in situ. BCNU will be release over a period of 2–3 weeks, the tumor cells being directly and efficiently exposed to high levels of drug starting immediately after surgery. Gliadel has received FDA (USA) approval for use in both newly diagnosed GBM and recurrences. Studies have consistently reported an increase of median survival by about 2 months [74–76]. Local delivery of carmustine reduces systemic adverse events, but sometimes induces complications: cerebral edema, seizure, poor wound healing, cerebrospinal fluid (CSF) leak, infection, headache, hemiparesis, hydrocephalus, particularly in patients with recurrent GBM. Combining local and systemic chemotherapy offers advantages that may explain the prolonged survival. First, systemic TMZ is most effective in regions of the tumor that are most vascular, whereas local release of BCNU allows direct access to relatively avascular areas of walls of the surgical cavity. Second, following the Stupp protocol, between surgery and chemoradiotherapy there is a period without treatment. Gliadel allows treatment of residual tumor cells within this period. Therefore, the combination of different treatment modalities allows continuous therapy up to 9 months, beginning immediately following surgery [77].

7. Other therapies

Optune (formerly NovoTTF-100A) is a device that delivers tumor-treating fields (TTFields), meaning low-intensity, intermediate-frequency, alternating electric fields that have antiproliferative properties with minimal toxicity. It has been approved (FDA 2015) as an alternative treatment for adult patients having a newly diagnosed supratentorial GBM following debulking surgery and completion of RT, with concomitant SoC chemotherapy. It has also been approved (FDA, 2011) for the treatment of adult patients with supratentorial confirmed recurrences of GBM, to be used as a monotherapy, as an alternative to standard medical therapy after surgical and radiation options have been exhausted (Novocure, 2017). Current evidence supports the use of TTFs as a therapeutic option. Stupp et al. analyzed 315 patients with GBM who had completed standard chemoradiation therapy, adding TTFields to maintenance TMZ chemotherapy and found a significantly prolonged progression-free survival and overall survival. Median progression-free survival was 7.1 months in the TTFields plus TMZ group and 4 months in the TMZ alone group. Median overall survival was 20.5 months in the TTFields plus TMZ group and 15.6 months in the TMZ-alone group [78].

8. Emergent treatments strategies

As the field of neuro-oncology continues to progress, numerous novel therapies have been tried and tested. Results from preclinical and clinical studies applying new treatments alone or in combination with conventional methods are promising.

GBM has abnormalities in **cellular signal transduction pathways**. All these pathways include receptor tyrosine kinases (RTKs) like vascular endothelial growth factor (VEGF), epidermal growth factor (EGF), platelet-derived growth factor (PDGF), etc., and share common mechanisms of activation and intracellular signaling, meaning RAS or phosphoinositol-3-kinase (PI3K) pathways. Genetic alterations of RTK/RAS/PI3K occur in about 88% of primary GBMs; the pathways are overactivated, allowing uncontrolled cellular proliferation, survival and invasion [79, 80]. Targeted molecular drugs have been developed to inhibit aberrantly activated signaling pathways in the clinical setting.

Increased epidermal growth factor receptor (EGFR) signaling has been reported in approximately 45% of GBM [79, 80]. It results in tumor cell proliferation, invasiveness, migration, angiogenesis and inhibition of apoptosis. Moreover, in the clinical setting, EGFR overexpression is associated with resistance to RT while EGFR inhibitions increased sensibility to RT [81]. Inhibitors of EGFR have been developed to block-specific pathways, but the results are disappointing. These include: monoclonal antibodies (cetuximab and nimotuzumab), small molecule tyrosine kinases inhibitors TKIs (gefitinib and erlotinib), a dual EGFR and ErbB-2 inhibitor (lapatinib), a pan-ErbB inhibitor (canertinib), a dual EGFR and vascular endothelial growth factor receptor (VEGFR) inhibitor (vandetanib), irreversible EGFR inhibitors (BIBW 2992 and PF-00299804), etc. It is to be noted that the ErbB family of proteins contains four receptor tyrosine kinases, structurally related to EGFR, marked as ErbB-1 to ErbB-4. ErbB-1 and ErbB-2 are found in many human cancers.

Overexpression of alpha subtype of PDGF receptor (PDGFR) occurs in about 13% of GBM [79]. Imatinib mesylate and tandutinib are inhibitors of PDGFR and other molecules involved in intracellular signaling pathways.

VEGF is a key factor implicated in tumor neoangiogenesis. GBM is a highly vascular tumor, that depends on vascular proliferation for growth. Recent evidence suggests vasculogenic mimicry in GBM, meaning formation of vessel-like network by tumor cells, allowing a blood supply for tumor growth. This process differs from angiogenesis, it is happening without the presence of endothelial cells. Angiogenesis is driven primarily by tumor-secreting VEGF-A (one member of the VEGF family), but there are many secreted proangiogenic factors [82]. The level of VEGF in HGG is greater than 10-fold compared with LGG [83]. Thus, drugs have been developed to interfere with angiogenesis by directly blocking ligand (VEGF) or receptor (VEGFR) or by targeting proangiogenic molecules that function by alternative mechanisms [84]. Of all targeted biological agents, only **bevacizumab** (Avastin) has demonstrated efficacy. It is a humanized monoclonal antibody that selectively blocks VEGF and so the BBB becomes more stable, with a resultant decrease in vascular permeability and edema, such that the corticosteroid doses can be reduced or suspended. Bevacizumab may be useful during and after RT, because of reduction of peritumoral edema, sometimes refractory to corticosteroid drugs and because of reduction of radiation necrosis rate following improving oxygenation. It has been approved by FDA (2009) as a single agent in the treatment of recurrent GBM following prior therapy, based on improvement in progression-free survival (that however did not translate into an improvement in overall survival) and a modest toxicity profile. Patients treated with bevacizumab inevitably relapse and sometimes an aggressive, invasive "gliomatosis" pattern of recurrence, unresponsive to subsequent therapy is observed. In addition to bevacizumab, there are many inhibitors of VEGF/VEGFR and other relevant targets under investigation, including: vatalanib, cediranib, sunitinib, sorafenib, vandetanib, VEGF trap, ramucirumab, pazopanib, etc. Dually targeted VEGFR/PDGFR inhibitors may prove useful, because of role of PDGFR in pericyte recruitment.

Other antiangiogenic approach targets **the integrins $\alpha v\beta 3$ and $\alpha v\beta 5$** that are overexpressed by tumor endothelial cells. They are transmembrane receptors that interact with extracellular matrix proteins to facilitate angiogenesis and invasion. Cilengitide inhibits these integrins.

There are clinical studies focused on **substances that inhibit intracellular signaling molecules**. Overactivation of the PI3K/Akt/mTOR signaling in GBM has been observed, because of receptor tyrosine kinase overactivity, mutated oncogenic PI3K subunits, and/or loss of PTEN tumor suppressor activity. Several mTOR inhibitors are currently tested, including sirolimus, temsirolimus, everolimus, and ridaforolimus. Enzastaurin is an inhibitor of protein kinase C-β2 that suppresses PI3K/Akt pathway. Overactivation of RAS/RAF/mitogen-activated protein kinase pathway in malignant glioma has provided the rationale to study farnesyl transferase inhibitors (farnesylation is a critical step in activation of RAS). Tipifarnib, lonafarnib and sorafenib may inhibit farnesyltransferase. Histone deacetylase inhibitors (vorinostat, romidepsin, valproic acid, etc.) prevent gene transcription, resulting in cell cycle arrest, differentiation, and/or apoptosis of tumor cells. Clinical trials are in progress.

Immunotherapy has become a promising cancer treatment, which allows for synergistic multimodal strategies. There are different immunotherapeutic approaches in GBM, including active immunotherapy (tumor vaccination therapy) and passive immunotherapy (antibody-based immunotherapy, adoptive cell therapy and other immune-modulatory therapy). **Tumor**

vaccination therapy uses administration of the antigens to activate an antitumor immune response. There is a vaccine targeting the mutant of epidermal growth factor receptor EGFRvIII (only expressed in GBM cells in about 20–25% of cases) – rindopepimut. Vaccination with dendritic cells is based on their ability to absorb all kinds of antigens and to secrete interleukin-2, thus activating T lymphocytes and initiating an efficient and specific immune response [85]. The application of tumor-derived heat shock proteins as tumor antigen carrier may be effective in boosting immune response. **Antibody-based immunotherapy** refers to the use of specific interaction between antibodies and antigens to block negative immune regulatory molecules that would have been preventing activated T cells from attacking the cancer cells. The most promising class of drugs that emerged is based on immune checkpoint inhibitors. Nivolumab and pembrolizumab are antibodies targeting the receptor programmed cell death-1 (PD-1) receptor of lymphocytes. Ipilimumab is an antibody that binds cytotoxic T lymphocyte-associated antigen 4 (CTLA-4), which would have inhibiting cytotoxic T lymphocyte to destroy cancer cells. **Adoptive cell therapy** is based on infusion of activated immune effector cells into cancer patients with the goal to enhance antitumor immunity. Immune effector cells include lymphokine-activated killer (LAK) cells, natural killer (NK) cells, T cells, tumor-infiltrating lymphocytes (TILs), cytotoxic T lymphocyte (CTLs), tumor antigen-specific TCR-transgenic T cells and chimeric antigen receptors-modified T cells (CAR T) [86]. This approach would be beneficial to non-responsive patients and non-immunogenic tumors.

Gene therapy is designed for delivery of genetic material, usually transgenes or viruses, into cells for therapeutic purposes. There are four types of gene therapy proposed for the treatment of GBM: suicide gene therapy, immunomodulatory gene therapy, tumor-suppressor gene therapy, and oncolytic virotherapy. **Suicide gene therapy** uses genes that encode enzymes able to convert a non-toxic drug into an active cytotoxic compound. The herpes simplex virus (HSV) type 1 thymidine kinase (tk) gene has been used as a "suicide gene", allowing to tumor cells to produce high levels of tk. Ganciclovir is the systemically injected prodrug, that will be converted by tk into a toxic metabolite. This compound is incorporated into DNA of actively proliferating tumor cells, and consequently blocks DNA replication and inhibits cell division. Apoptosis underlies the mechanism of cytotoxicity [87]. Another "suicide gene" is cytosine deaminase (CD), an enzyme capable to convert an antifungal drug, 5-fluorocytosine (5-FC), into the highly toxic compound 5-fluorouracil (5-FU). This is again converted into molecules which interfere with RNA processing and DNA synthesis and apoptosis invariably occurs. **Immunomodulatory gene therapy** induces or augments an enhanced specific antitumoral immune response, overcoming the tumor-induced immunosuppression. **Tumor-suppressor gene therapy** aims to restore the function of a tumor-suppressor gene lost or functionally inactivated in cancer cells. They play a critical role in maintaining genome integrity and in regulating cell proliferation, differentiation, and apoptosis. In GBM, there is at least one tumor-suppressor gene mutated or deleted in all cases; in 91% of patients, 2 or more of these tumor-suppressor genes are inactivated [88]. Correcting the genetic abnormalities in the glioma cells has been demonstrated to suppress tumor growth via induction of apoptosis and cell cycle arrest. Genes encoding p53, p16, or phosphatase and tensin homolog (PTEN) can be candidates for this type of therapy. **Oncolytic virotherapy** employs replication-competent viruses with natural or engineered tropism and activity against tumors. They specifically infect and replicate in target tumor cells. During progeny particle release, tumor host cells are destroyed, and tumor-associated antigens are released, while progeny virions infect neighboring tumor cells. Finally, a complete destruction of the tumor can be achieved, multiple mechanisms being involved together with direct oncolysis, meaning induction of an effective antitumor immune response, cancer cell starvation by destruction of tumor vasculature, and sometimes the activity of virally encoded therapeutic transgenes. The two most studied oncolytic virus types are adenoviruses and herpes simplex viruses. **Another strategy of gene therapy targets genes that may modulate the tumor microenvironment**, to create unfavorable conditions for tumor growth or enhance the efficacy of therapy. Although there is a limited evidence of a therapeutic benefit of gene therapy to date, it is important to note that these therapies appear to be safe.

9. Conclusions

Effective treatment in GBM remains one of the most formidable challenge in neuro-oncology. Treatment is multimodal and despite significant advances in diagnostic technology, surgical technique, radiation, chemotherapy and targeted therapy, the prognosis remains poor. Large-scale research efforts are required to understand the molecular biology of brain tumors and to discover novel therapies. Synergistic multimodal strategies and individualized treatments are likely to be the best approach of these complex tumors to finally improve survival and quality of life of the patients.

Author details

Ligia Gabriela Tataranu[1,2], Vasile Ciubotaru[2], Tabita Larisa Cazac[2], Oana Alexandru[3], Oana Stefana Purcaru[4], Daniela Elise Tache[4], Stefan Alexandru Artene[4] and Anica Dricu[4*]

*Address all correspondence to: anica.dricu@live.co.uk

1 University of Medicine and Pharmacy "Carol Davila", Bucharest, Romania

2 Department of Neurosurgery,"Bagdasar-Arseni" Emergency Clinical Hospital, Bucharest, Romania

3 Department of Neurology, University of Medicine and Pharmacy of Craiova, Romania

4 Department of Biochemistry, University of Medicine and Pharmacy of Craiova, Romania

References

[1] Stupp R et al. Effects of radiotherapy with concomitant and adjuvant temozolomide versus radiotherapy alone on survival in glioblastoma in a randomised phase III study: 5-year analysis of the EORTC-NCIC trial. The Lancet Oncology. 2009;**10**(5):459-466

[2] Silbergeld DL, Chicoine MR. Isolation and characterization of human malignant glioma cells from histologically normal brain. Journal of Neurosurgery. 1997;**86**(3):525-531

[3] Holland EC. Glioblastoma multiforme: The terminator. Proceedings of the National Academy of Sciences of the United States of America. 2000;**97**(12):6242-6244

[4] Cohen AL, Holmen SL, Colman H. IDH1 and IDH2 mutations in gliomas. Current Neurology and Neuroscience Reports. 2013;**13**(5):345

[5] Dang L, Yen K, Attar EC. IDH mutations in cancer and progress toward development of targeted therapeutics. Annals of Oncology. 2016;**27**(4):599-608

[6] Louis DN et al. The 2016 World Health Organization classification of Tumors of the central nervous system: A summary. Acta Neuropathologica. 2016;**131**(6):803-820

[7] Ohgaki H, Kleihues P. The definition of primary and secondary glioblastoma. Clinical Cancer Research. 2013;**19**(4):764-772

[8] Rostomily RC, Spence AM, Silbergeld DL. Neurosurgical management of high-grade gliomas. In: Moore AJ, Newell DW, editors. Neurosurgery: Principles and Practice. London: Springer-Verlag; 2005. pp. 167-186

[9] Aldape K et al. Glioblastoma: Pathology, molecular mechanisms and markers. Acta Neuropathologica. 2015;**129**(6):829-848

[10] Ohgaki H, Kleihues P. Population-based studies on incidence, survival rates, and genetic alterations in astrocytic and oligodendroglial gliomas. Journal of Neuropathology and Experimental Neurology. 2005;**64**(6):479-489

[11] Jackson RJ et al. Limitations of stereotactic biopsy in the initial management of gliomas. Neuro-Oncology. 2001;**3**(3):193-200

[12] Kole AJ et al. Concurrent chemoradiotherapy versus radiotherapy alone for "biopsy-only" glioblastoma multiforme. Cancer. 2016;**122**(15):2364-2370

[13] Chaichana KL et al. Establishing percent resection and residual volume thresholds affecting survival and recurrence for patients with newly diagnosed intracranial glioblastoma. Neuro-Oncology. 2014;**16**(1):113-122

[14] Grabowski MM et al. Residual tumor volume versus extent of resection: Predictors of survival after surgery for glioblastoma. Journal of Neurosurgery. 2014;**121**(5):1115-1123

[15] Marko NF et al. Extent of resection of glioblastoma revisited: Personalized survival modeling facilitates more accurate survival prediction and supports a maximum-safe-resection approach to surgery. Journal of Clinical Oncology. 2014;**32**(8):774-782

[16] Tamura M et al. Strategy of surgical resection for glioma based on intraoperative functional mapping and monitoring. Neurologia Medico-Chirurgica (Tokyo). 2015;**55**(5):383-398

[17] Saito T et al. Intraoperative functional mapping and monitoring during glioma surgery. Neurologia Medico-Chirurgica (Tokyo). 2015;**55**(Suppl 1):1-13

[18] Li T et al. Glioma localization and excision using direct electrical stimulation for language mapping during awake surgery. Experimental and Therapeutic Medicine. 2015; **9**(5):1962-1966

[19] Simon MV. Intraoperative neurophysiologic sensorimotor mapping-a review. Journal of Neurology & Neurophysiology. 2011:S3

[20] Sanai N, Berger MS. Intraoperative stimulation techniques for functional pathway preservation and glioma resection. Neurosurgical Focus. 2010;**28**(2):E1

[21] Sanai N, Berger MS. Operative techniques for gliomas and the value of extent of resection. Neurotherapeutics. 2009;**6**(3):478-486

[22] Quinones-Hinojosa A et al. Preoperative correlation of intraoperative cortical mapping with magnetic resonance imaging landmarks to predict localization of the Broca area. Journal of Neurosurgery. 2003;**99**(2):311-318

[23] Garrett MC, Pouratian N, Liau ML. Use of language mapping to aid in resection of gliomas in eloquent brain regions. Neurosurgery Clinics of North America. 2012;**23**(3):497-506

[24] Haglund MM et al. Cortical localization of temporal lobe language sites in patients with gliomas. Neurosurgery. 1994;**34**(4):567-576; discussion 576

[25] Ozawa N et al. Identification of the pyramidal tract by neuronavigation based on intraoperative diffusion-weighted imaging combined with subcortical stimulation. Stereotactic and Functional Neurosurgery. 2009;**87**(1):18-24

[26] Yamao Y et al. Intraoperative dorsal language network mapping by using single-pulse electrical stimulation. Human Brain Mapping. 2014;**35**(9):4345-4361

[27] Yamao Y et al. Clinical impact of intraoperative CCEP monitoring in evaluating the dorsal language white matter pathway. Human Brain Mapping. 2017;**38**(4):1977-1991

[28] Matsumoto R et al. Functional connectivity in the human language system: A cortico-cortical evoked potential study. Brain. 2004;**127**(Pt 10):2316-2330

[29] Stummer W, Suero Molina E. Fluorescence imaging/agents in tumor resection. Neurosurgery Clinics of North America. 2017;**28**(4):569-583

[30] Hadjipanayis CG, Widhalm G, Stummer W. What is the surgical benefit of utilizing 5-aminolevulinic acid for fluorescence-guided surgery of malignant gliomas? Neurosurgery. 2015;**77**(5):663-673

[31] Zhao S et al. Intraoperative fluorescence-guided resection of high-grade malignant gliomas using 5-aminolevulinic acid-induced porphyrins: A systematic review and meta-analysis of prospective studies. PLoS One. 2013;**8**(5):e63682

[32] Nabavi A et al. Five-aminolevulinic acid for fluorescence-guided resection of recurrent malignant gliomas: A phase ii study. Neurosurgery. 2009;**65**(6):1070-1076; discussion 1076-7

[33] Stummer W et al. 5-Aminolevulinic acid-derived tumor fluorescence: The diagnostic accuracy of visible fluorescence qualities as corroborated by spectrometry and histology and postoperative imaging. Neurosurgery. 2014;**74**(3):310-319; discussion 319-20

[34] Schucht P et al. 5-ALA complete resections go beyond MR contrast enhancement: Shift corrected volumetric analysis of the extent of resection in surgery for glioblastoma. Acta Neurochirurgica. 2014;**156**(2):305-12; discussion 312

[35] Stummer W et al. Fluorescence-guided surgery with 5-aminolevulinic acid for resection of malignant glioma: A randomised controlled multicentre phase III trial. The Lancet Oncology. 2006;**7**(5):392-401

[36] Valdes PA et al. Optical technologies for intraoperative neurosurgical guidance. Neurosurgical Focus. 2016;**40**(3):E8

[37] Suero Molina E et al. Dual-labeling with 5-aminolevulinic acid and fluorescein for fluorescence-guided resection of high-grade gliomas: Technical note. Journal of Neurosurgery. 2017:1-7

[38] Senders JT et al. Agents for fluorescence-guided glioma surgery: A systematic review of preclinical and clinical results. Acta Neurochirurgica. 2017;**159**(1):151-167

[39] Craig SEL et al. Fluorescent-guided surgical resection of Glioma with targeted molecular imaging agents: A literature review. World Neurosurgery. 2016;**90**:154-163

[40] Zhang ZZ et al. The art of intraoperative glioma identification. Frontiers in Oncology. 2015;**5**:175

[41] Croce AC et al. Diagnostic potential of autofluorescence for an assisted intraoperative delineation of glioblastoma resection margins. Photochemistry and Photobiology. 2003;**77**(3):309-318

[42] Bottiroli G et al. Brain tissue autofluorescence: An aid for intraoperative delineation of tumor resection margins. Cancer Detection and Prevention. 1998;**22**(4):330-339

[43] Eschbacher J et al. In vivo intraoperative confocal microscopy for real-time histopathological imaging of brain tumors. Journal of Neurosurgery. 2012;**116**(4):854-860

[44] St John ER et al. Intraoperative tissue identification by mass spectrometric technologies. Trends in Analytical Chemistry. 2016;**85**:2-9

[45] Santagata S et al. Intraoperative mass spectrometry mapping of an onco-metabolite to guide brain tumor surgery. Proceedings of the National Academy of Sciences of the United States of America. 2014;**111**(30):11121-11126

[46] Jarmusch AK et al. Lipid and metabolite profiles of human brain tumors by desorption electrospray ionization-MS. Proceedings of the National Academy of Sciences of the United States of America. 2016;**113**(6):1486-1491

[47] Eberlin LS et al. Ambient mass spectrometry for the intraoperative molecular diagnosis of human brain tumors. Proceedings of the National Academy of Sciences of the United States of America. 2013;**110**(5):1611-1616

[48] Wen PY et al. Updated response assessment criteria for high-grade gliomas: Response assessment in neuro-oncology working group. Journal of Clinical Oncology. 2010; **28**(11):1963-1972

[49] Parvez K, Parvez A, Zadeh G. The diagnosis and treatment of pseudoprogression, radiation necrosis and brain tumor recurrence. International Journal of Molecular Sciences. 2014;**15**(7):11832-11846

[50] Ringel F et al. Clinical benefit from resection of recurrent glioblastomas: Results of a multicenter study including 503 patients with recurrent glioblastomas undergoing surgical resection. Neuro-Oncology. 2016;**18**(1):96-104

[51] Montemurro N et al. Second surgery for recurrent glioblastoma: A concise overview of the current literature. Clinical Neurology and Neurosurgery. 2016;**142**:60-64

[52] Irwin C et al. Delay in radiotherapy shortens survival in patients with high grade glioma. Journal of Neuro-Oncology. 2007;**85**(3):339-343

[53] Valduvieco I et al. Impact of radiotherapy delay on survival in glioblastoma. Clinical & Translational Oncology. 2013;**15**(4):278-282

[54] Randolph DM 2nd et al. Impact of timing of radiotherapy in patients with newly diagnosed glioblastoma. Clinical Neurology and Neurosurgery. 2016;**151**:73-78

[55] Seidlitz A et al. Impact of waiting time after surgery and overall time of postoperative radiochemotherapy on treatment outcome in glioblastoma multiforme. Radiation Oncology. 2015;**10**:172

[56] Blumenthal DT et al. Short delay in initiation of radiotherapy may not affect outcome of patients with glioblastoma: A secondary analysis from the radiation therapy oncology group database. Journal of Clinical Oncology. 2009;**27**(5):733-739

[57] Han SJ et al. The effect of timing of concurrent chemoradiation in patients with newly diagnosed glioblastoma. Neurosurgery. 2015;**77**(2):248-53; discussion 253

[58] Han SJ et al. Impact of timing of concurrent chemoradiation for newly diagnosed glioblastoma: A critical review of current evidence. Neurosurgery. 2015;**62**(Suppl 1):160-165

[59] Stupp R et al. Radiotherapy plus concomitant and adjuvant temozolomide for glioblastoma. The New England Journal of Medicine. 2005;**352**(10):987-996

[60] Davis ME. Glioblastoma: Overview of disease and treatment. Clinical Journal of Oncology Nursing. 2016;**20**(5):S2-S8

[61] Hau E et al. The evolving roles and controversies of radiotherapy in the treatment of glioblastoma. Journal of Medical Radiation Sciences. 2016;**63**(2):114-123

[62] Combs SE et al. Efficacy of fractionated stereotactic reirradiation in recurrent gliomas: Long-term results in 172 patients treated in a single institution. Journal of Clinical Oncology. 2005;**23**(34):8863-8869

[63] Skeie BS et al. Gamma knife surgery versus reoperation for recurrent glioblastoma multiforme. World Neurosurgery. 2012;**78**(6):658-669

[64] Gabayan AJ et al. GliaSite brachytherapy for treatment of recurrent malignant gliomas: A retrospective multi-institutional analysis. Neurosurgery. 2006;**58**(4):701-709; discussion 701-9

[65] Chan TA et al. Treatment of recurrent glioblastoma multiforme with GliaSite brachytherapy. International Journal of Radiation Oncology, Biology, Physics. 2005;**62**(4):1133-1139

[66] Thon N, Kreth S, Kreth FW. Personalized treatment strategies in glioblastoma: MGMT promoter methylation status. OncoTargets and Therapy. 2013;**6**:1363-1372

[67] Shen D et al. MGMT promoter methylation correlates with an overall survival benefit in Chinese high-grade glioblastoma patients treated with radiotherapy and alkylating agent-based chemotherapy: A single-institution study. PLoS One. 2014;**9**(9):e107558

[68] Zhao H et al. The prognostic value of MGMT promoter status by pyrosequencing assay for glioblastoma patients' survival: A meta-analysis. World Journal of Surgical Oncology. 2016;**14**(1):261

[69] Hegi ME et al. MGMT gene silencing and benefit from temozolomide in glioblastoma. The New England Journal of Medicine. 2005;**352**(10):997-1003

[70] Rivera AL et al. MGMT promoter methylation is predictive of response to radiotherapy and prognostic in the absence of adjuvant alkylating chemotherapy for glioblastoma. Neuro-Oncology. 2010;**12**(2):116-121

[71] Bhandari M et al. Comparative study of adjuvant temozolomide six cycles versus extended 12 cycles in newly diagnosed glioblastoma multiforme. Journal of Clinical and Diagnostic Research. 2017;**11**(5):XC04-XC08

[72] Barbagallo GM et al. Long-term therapy with temozolomide is a feasible option for newly diagnosed glioblastoma: A single-institution experience with as many as 101 temozolomide cycles. Neurosurgical Focus. 2014;**37**(6):E4

[73] Xu W et al. Efficacy and safety of long-term therapy for high-grade glioma with temozolomide: A meta-analysis. Oncotarget. 2017;**8**(31):51758-51765

[74] Ashby LS, Smith KA, Stea B. Gliadel wafer implantation combined with standard radiotherapy and concurrent followed by adjuvant temozolomide for treatment of newly diagnosed high-grade glioma: A systematic literature review. World Journal of Surgical Oncology. 2016;**14**(1):225

[75] Xing WK et al. The role of gliadel wafers in the treatment of newly diagnosed GBM: A meta-analysis. Drug Design, Development and Therapy. 2015;**9**:3341-3348

[76] Chowdhary SA, Ryken T, Newton HB. Survival outcomes and safety of carmustine wafers in the treatment of high-grade gliomas: A meta-analysis. Journal of Neuro-Oncology. 2015;**122**(2):367-382

[77] McGirt MJ et al. Gliadel (BCNU) wafer plus concomitant temozolomide therapy after primary resection of glioblastoma multiforme. Journal of Neurosurgery. 2009;**110**(3):583-588

[78] Stupp R et al. Maintenance therapy with tumor-treating fields plus temozolomide vs temozolomide alone for glioblastoma: A randomized clinical trial. JAMA. 2015;**314**(23): 2535-2543

[79] Van Meir EG et al. Exciting new advances in neuro-oncology: The avenue to a cure for malignant glioma. CA: a Cancer Journal for Clinicians. 2010;**60**(3):166-193

[80] Grimm SA, Chamberlain MC. State of the art and perspectives in the treatment of glioblastoma. CNS Oncology. 2012;**1**(1):49-70

[81] Alexandru O et al. The influence of EGFR inactivation on the radiation response in high grade glioma. International Journal of Molecular Sciences. 2018;**19**(1)

[82] Serban F et al. Epidermal growth factor, latrophilin, and seven transmembrane domain-containing protein 1 marker, a novel angiogenesis marker. OncoTargets and Therapy. 2015;**8**:3767-3774

[83] Schmidt NO et al. Levels of vascular endothelial growth factor, hepatocyte growth factor/scatter factor and basic fibroblast growth factor in human gliomas and their relation to angiogenesis. International Journal of Cancer. 1999;**84**(1):10-18

[84] Serban F et al. Silencing of epidermal growth factor, latrophilin and seven transmembrane domain-containing protein 1 (ELTD1) via siRNA-induced cell death in glioblastoma. Journal of Immunoassay & Immunochemistry. 2017;**38**(1):21-33

[85] Artene SA et al. Dendritic cell immunotherapy versus bevacizumab plus irinotecan in recurrent malignant glioma patients: A survival gain analysis. OncoTargets and Therapy. 2016;**9**:6669-6677

[86] Zhou Q, Wang Y, Ma W. The progress of immunotherapy for glioblastoma. Human Vaccines & Immunotherapeutics. 2015;**11**(11):2654-2658

[87] Okura H, Smith CA, Rutka JT. Gene therapy for malignant glioma. Molecular and Cellular Therapies. 2014;**2**:21

[88] Kane JR et al. Sui generis: Gene therapy and delivery systems for the treatment of glioblastoma. Neuro-Oncology. 2015;**17**(Suppl 2):ii24-ii36

5

Primary Brain Tumors in Childhood

Romana Richterová and Branislav Kolarovszki

Abstract

This chapter offers literary review of most frequently observed brain tumors in childhood. It offers basics of epidemiology, clinical presentation and diagnostics of most often occurring types of tumors according to new WHO classification of brain tumors from 2016 and emphasizes molecular biological characteristics and role of altered genes and genetic pathways in brain tumor etiology, classification and treatment. This review not only concentrates on gliomas, medulloblastomas and ependymomas, but also offers characterization of other less frequently observed lesions. Each tumor characteristics also contains basics of therapeutical possibilities of these lesions with focus on targeted and individually designed therapy according to molecular and genetic alterations found in tumor tissue sample.

Keywords: brain tumors, childhood, glioma

1. Introduction

Brain tumors are the second most common group of tumors (following hematological malignancies) as well as the most frequent solid tumors in childhood [1] in age category up to 1 year and between 5 and 19 years of age, even the most common childhood malignancy [2], as well as the most frequent death cause from all oncological diagnoses [3]. Despite the significant progress in imaging and neurosurgical techniques, molecular genetic diagnostics and therapeutic protocols as well as the introduction of concomitant chemoradiotherapy, cure and survival rates of these children did not significantly change – except for medulloblastoma [4].

2. Epidemiology of brain tumors in children

The incidence of pediatric CNS tumors varies worldwide with an average of 4 cases per 100,000 children with the highest occurrence is in the United States [3]. By age groups, the highest incidence is in adolescents (15–19 years, 6.38/100,000), followed by a group of children under 1 year (6.2/100,000). Subsequently, it is slightly declining, with 5.5/100,000 children aged between 1 and 4 years; in 5–14 years, the incidence is 5.1/100,000 [2, 5]. About 25–30% are in supratentorial localization, followed by the cerebellum (15–20%), the brain stem (10–12%), the pituitary and suprasellar region (10–15%), cranial nerves (6–7%), brain ventricles (5–6.4%), spinal cord (4.3–4.6%) and 2.6–2.9% are tumors of meninges [2, 6], as shown in **Figure 1**. Also a typical localization and histological type occur in certain age group. By 1 year of age, tumors most often occur at multiple locations in the brain and in ventricles. At the age of 1–4 years, the most common site is the cerebellum, cerebral hemispheres and brain stem. In the age range from 5 to 9 years, tumors occur frequently in the cerebellum, brain stem and cerebral hemispheres. At the age from birth to 9 years, the most common tumors are gliomas and embryonal tumors (up to 1 year is the most common embryonic atypical teratoma/rhabdoid tumor (AT/RT), in the older children it is medulloblastoma (MB)). In 10–14 year age group, the most typical site is cerebral hemisphere and most frequently occurring are gliomas, tumors of the pituitary region and embryonal tumors. Adolescents (aged 15–19 years) most often have pituitary tumors, then astrocytomas and neoplastic tumors, but the incidence of meningiomas also increases. Typical localizations in this age group are the pituitary and suprasellar regions, followed by cerebral hemispheres and cerebellum. In general, brain tumors are more common in boys [2, 5].

There are many risk factors for brain tumor development, but to date only some hereditary syndromes (type 1 and 2 neurofibromatosis, tuberous sclerosis, Li-Fraumeni syndrome, Gorlin syndrome, Turcot syndrome, Cowden syndrome, Rubinstein-Taybi syndrome and hereditary retinoblastoma) and ionizing radiation have been verified. Other possible risk factors include: a personal history of previous cancer treatment, a family history of the CNS tumor, the parent age at the time of conception, the later contact of the child with common childhood infectious

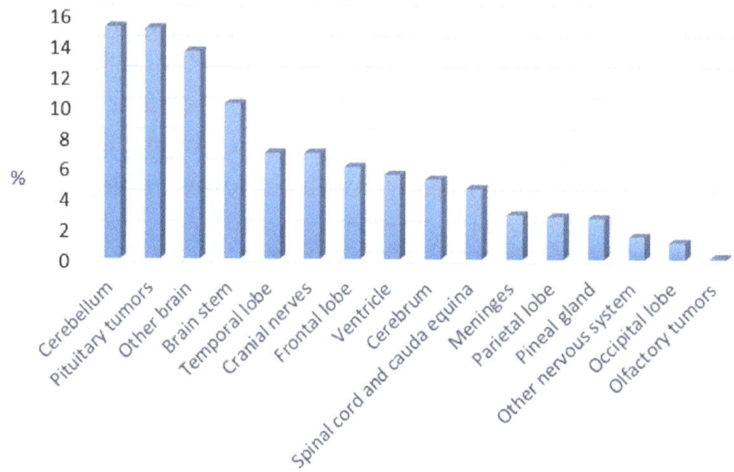

Figure 1. Localization of CNS tumors in pediatric population [5].

diseases [7], congenital anomalies [8], higher birth weight and larger head circumference [9]. Interestingly, the results of studies suggest lower incidence of CNS tumors in children with allergies and asthma [10, 11].

3. Classification of brain tumors in children

The new WHO classification of CNS tumors from 2016 for the first time uses molecular genetic characteristics for tumor classification in some cases. In this new edition, some new tumor entities appeared, some have been merged while others were excluded. Changes involving childhood tumors include: inclusion of epithelial glioblastoma, removal of the term brain gliomatosis, reclassification of the diffuse intrinsic pontine glioma to diffuse midline glioma, *H3 K27*–mutant, inclusion of the ependymoma, *RELA* fusion–positive as a separate unit and inclusion of the diffuse leptomeningeal glioneuronal tumor. The change also affected the classification of medulloblastomas, where genetically defined classification was added. The term primitive neuroectodermal tumors (CNS PNET) was eliminated while an embryonal tumor with multilayered rosettes, *C19MC*–altered was included [12].

Childhood brain tumors are also classified according to their localization into: infratentorial, supratentorial tumors and tumors of parasellar region. Most frequently observed histological types of pediatric CNS tumors are shown in **Figure 2**.

Infratentorial localization is typical for cerebellar astrocytoma (pilocytic astrocytoma – PA, but also diffuse less frequently anaplastic astrocytoma and glioblastoma), medulloblastomas, ependymomas, brain stem gliomas (most commonly diffuse midline glioma, *H3 K27*–mutant, PA), AT/RT and choroid plexus tumors.

Supratentorial localization are common: low-grade glioma—LGG (PA, diffuse astrocytoma, oligodendroglioma, mixed oligoastrocytoma, subependymal giant cell astrocytoma—SEGA, pleomorphic xanthoastrocytoma—PXA), high-grade glioma—HGG (anaplastic astrocytoma, anaplastic oligodendroglioma and glioblastoma), neuronal and mixed neuronal-glial

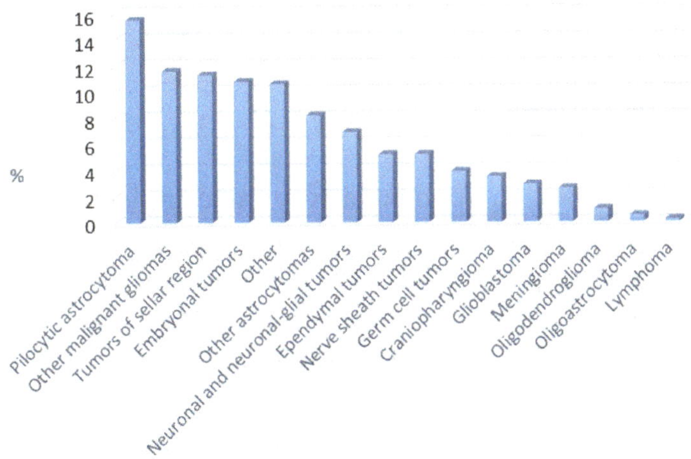

Figure 2. Most frequent histological types of CNS tumors in children [5].

tumors (ganglioglioma—GG, desmoplastic infantile astrocytoma—DIA, ganglioglioma—DIGG, dysembryoplastic neuroepithelial tumor—DNET and papillary glioneuronal tumor), embryonal tumors (embryonal tumor with multilayered rosettes, *C19MC*-altered—ETMR, medulloepithelioma, CNS neuroblastoma, CNS ganglioneuroblastoma, CNS embryonal tumor and CNS embryonal tumor with rhabdoid features), AT/RT, ependymomas, meningiomas, choroid plexus tumors, pineal tumors (pineocytomas, pineal parenchymal tumor of intermediate differentiation and papillary tumors of the pineal region) and rarely metastases of extra-neural malignant tumors.

Tumors occurring in **parasellar** region usually are: craniopharyngiomas, adenomas, LGG astrocytomas (tumors of central regions, chiasma, hypothalamus, thalamus, PA or diffuse astrocytomas) as well as germ cell tumors.

4. Brain tumors symptoms in children

Symptoms of brain tumors can develop gradually and worsen over time, or they may manifest suddenly and dramatically. Symptoms may be general or specific, resulting from tumor localization. **General symptoms** are manifestation of intracranial hypertension that is caused either by tumor growth, brain swelling or onset of hydrocephalus or a combination of these factors. Symptoms of intracranial hypertension include: headache (especially in the morning after awakening), nausea or vomiting, diplopia and strabismus, disturbances of balance, personality changes, epileptic seizures or loss of consciousness. Infants may experience irritability, loss of appetite, delay or regression of psychomotor development. There is also bulging of the fontanelle and the disproportionate enlargement of the head circumference. Children of school age may suffer from increased fatigue, psychological changes, impairment of school performance, disturbances of memory and impaired concentration. Regarding the localization of the tumor, other locally **specific neurological symptoms** may also occur: visual disturbances, narrowing and outages of visual field, abnormal bulb movements, nystagmus, hearing or speech disorders, paresis or hemiparesis, muscle weakness, loss of sensitivity or coordination, ataxia, posture disorder, walking instability, tingling of body parts, cranial nerves palsy as well as hormonal disorders.

5. Brain tumors diagnostics

Diagnosis of brain tumor is based on a patient history and complete neurological examination. Imaging examination is performed when a brain tumor is suspected. Basic imaging examination is **magnetic resonance imaging (MRI).** It is the most spectacular imaging for intracranial structures that is currently available in medicine. In brain tumor diagnostics the use of contrast media—gadolinium—is essential. **MR-angiography** displays brain vessels alongside with pathological tumor vasculature, what is important for planning of the surgical treatment. **MR-spectroscopy** is a metabolic examination of the brain. The **perfusion MRI** monitors blood flow in the investigated area. Tumors are metabolically active and require greater blood supply. **Functional MRI** and **MR-tractography** are used for planning of surgical approach.

Preoperatively, the navigational MRI is performed for the needs of intraoperative navigation. Among the disadvantages of MRI is relatively longer duration, which in smaller children requires general anesthesia. However, a huge advantage is the absence of radiation [13].

Computer tomography (CT) is mostly used for the display of bones and their lesions, which do not appear in detail in MRI. Another indication may be **CT-angiography.** Due to the high dose of radiation; however, CT is reserved for cases of sudden changes in the neurological condition when rapid imaging is necessary.

Positron emission tomography (PET) uses radioactive fluorodeoxyglucose for visualization of tumor tissue that is metabolically more active. The radioactive load is very low and is excluded in 1 day. It can be used preoperatively for diagnostics as well as for postoperative distinguishing between residues, recurrences and postoperative changes in unclear cases [14].

Angiography (mostly DSA) uses vessel imaging after contrast agent administration to assess tumor vascular supply. It is also associated with radiation and though is currently replaced by MR- or CT-angiography. However, it remains reserved for preoperative embolization of the tumor, which is carried out by DSA [13].

Specimen of CSF obtained from **lumbar puncture** is used for cytological examination to detect the presence of tumor cells that occur in CSF in tumor dissemination or in leukemia tumors. It is also used to detect the presence of tumor markers, in particular bHCG and AFP in germ cell tumors. It also serves to verify the presence of infection, especially in the postoperative period [13].

Biopsy of brain tumor is essential for definitive diagnosis. In most cases, tissue sample is obtained during surgery. However, there are also cases of inoperable tumors according to their localization or extent. If a tumor resection cannot be performed, a stereotactic biopsy can be useful. In some cases, however, the biopsy is too risky, and therefore the diagnosis is determined only by MRI (e.g., diffuse pontine gliomas).

Also **other examinations** could be useful, such as: EEG, evoked potentials, evaluation of neurocognitive functions, ophthalmological examination (papilledema of optic nerve and perimeter), evaluation of hearing disorder and hormone levels and function [13].

6. Treatment of brain tumors

Treatment consists of surgical intervention, followed by oncological and symptomatic treatment and requires multidisciplinary approach.

Surgical treatment is the basis of treatment and, in some tumors, it is the only sufficient form of therapy. Also histologically, benign tumors can be a surgical challenge by their localization. An essential part of brain tumor surgery is the use of microscope and micro instruments. Nowadays, it belongs to the usual equipment of surgical department, as well as ultrasonic aspirator, **navigation systems,** intraoperative sonography and possibility of realization of electrophysiological monitoring. **Electrophysiological monitoring** requires appropriate instrumentation and personnel equipment that enhances the safety of the operation to the full possible extent in the eloquent areas of the CNS. Use of 5-aminolevulic acid is very helpful in operations of HGG. Patient ingests this acid prior to surgery, and then during surgery, with use of fluorescence on the microscope, high-grade glial cells begin to gleam, which also contributes to performance of accurate resection and representative tumor sampling for histological examination. **Awake operations** with the possibility of intraoperative stimulation, in which the patient is conscious either during the entire procedure or in a certain part of it, are used in adult patients, especially in tumors in motor, sensory and speech areas. In children, it is significantly limited by age and ability to cooperate. They are mainly performed in older age groups of children [15].

According to extent of resection, we divide surgical treatment into: **total resection, near-total resection**, **partial resection** and **biopsy.** In most tumors (except well-defined benign tumors or well-defined metastases), total resection is only a radiological rather than a biological term. The surgical approach can serve (though not as a standard treatment method) for the targeted administration of radiotherapy in the form of **intraoperative radiotherapy** with a single irradiation of the tumor bed directly after resection of the tumor [16] **or chemotherapy**—for example, intraoperative administration of biodegradable carmustine [17]. In addition to **craniotomy**, other techniques—for example, **endonasal trans-sphenoidal approach**—can also be used, including endoscopy for pituitary tumor tumors. Another option for biopsy or tumor removal (often when located in brain ventricles) is **endoscopic surgery**. From other surgical methods, shunts in hydrocephalus can be used, most commonly **ventriculoperitoneal shunt**. Another option is implantation of Ommaya reservoir, which is useful for repeated sampling of CSF for laboratory examinations, for therapeutic evacuation puncture of CSF, as well as for the local administration of chemotherapy.

Chemotherapy is part of adjuvant oncological treatment after surgical resection alone or along with radiotherapy. It can be administered **systemically** (intravenously or orally), **locally** during surgery, or postoperatively into an implanted reservoir. Most serious side effects of chemotherapy are: bone marrow depression, nausea, vomiting, diarrhea and temporary hair loss. Generally, children better tolerate high doses of chemotherapy compared to adults, which may increase the aggressiveness of treatment if necessary.

Targeted biological therapy is directed against the specific protein and gene targets of the tumor, or against the environment that affects its growth and survival. But even all tumors of the same histological type do not have the same alterations and the treatment goals. Therefore, it is essential to examine each tumor sample for the presence of altered genes and proteins in order to determine targeted individualized treatment. One of the best known drugs is bevacizumab with an antiangiogenic effect, which stops the nutrient intake into the tumor by blocking of angiogenesis. This treatment is used for HGG. However, the effect of this treatment is lower than expected. Therefore, it is reserved as supportive treatment in relapsing non-responding tumors. Also used is everolimus, the *mTOR* pathway blocker in the treatment of subependemal giant astrocytoma, or tyrosine kinase inhibitors, in particular *EGFR* (erlotinib and gefitinib) in the treatment of ependymomas [18]. Patients with HGG with a proven *BRAF V600E* mutation also receive *BRAF* inhibitors (vemurafenib and dabrafenib) with partial effects [19].

Radiotherapy is also often used in treatment of pediatric brain tumors, either alone or as part of concomitant therapy. It uses high energy RTG beams to damage tumor cell DNA. It can take various forms, using external radiotherapy as well as local forms. **External radiotherapy** is mostly accomplished with a linear accelerator by various techniques, such as conventional radiotherapy, 3D conformal radiotherapy, modulated beam intensities, stereotactic radiotherapy using stereotactic frames or radio-surgical methods (single irradiation) that use a linear accelerator, gamma knife or cyber knife as the source of radiation. **Local forms** of radiotherapy require an invasive approach. This group includes intraoperative radiotherapy, which is applied during surgery and interstitial brachytherapy requiring surgical delivery of emitters close to the tumor. Subsequently, radiotherapy is applied in the postoperative period. Local forms have, of course, a minor incidence of undesirable radiotherapy effects, of which the most common are: fatigue, hair loss, radiation dermatitis, brain edema and presence of post radiation necrosis and encephalopathy. Proton therapy is becoming increasingly popular.

The novelty in the treatment of HGG is the use of an **alternating electric field.** It appears to be the most effective in connection to concomitant chemoradiotherapy. It is recommended for treatment of recurrent tumors [20].

Very necessary is also **supportive medical treatment**, in particular corticosteroids which suppress perifocal and postoperative edema, anticonvulsants (in the presence of epileptic seizures), analgesics, antiemetic drugs, nutritional support and oncological rehabilitation [21].

7. Most common brain tumor types occurring in childhood

The most common CNS tumors in children are: gliomas, ependymomas, neuroglial tumors, embryonal tumors, choroid plexus tumors, craniopharyngiomas and germ cell tumors.

7.1. Gliomas

Glial tumors account for 55% of pediatric CNS tumors [3]. It is a heterogeneous group of tumors that varies from a well-defined, potentially curable low-grade pilocytic astrocytoma and diffusely growing astrocytomas (grade II) to high-grade, aggressive and incurable tumors, such as diffuse glioma of midline structures. They arise from CNS glial precursor cells: astrocytomas originate in astrocytes, oligodendrogliomas in oligodendrocytes, mixed gliomas are derived from astrocytes, oligodendrocytes and ependymal cells. The histologically most common glioma in children is astrocytoma.

7.1.1. Low-grade gliomas in children

The most common LGG in children are: pilocytic astrocytoma—PA (grade I), diffuse astrocytoma (grade II), oligodendroglioma (grade II), subependemal giant astrocytoma (SEGA) and pleomorphic xanthastrocytoma (PXA). The prognosis of LGG in children is relatively good, especially in well-defined grade I lesions with the possibility of total resection. Dissemination within the CNS is rare, but may be multifocal, especially in patients with neurofibromatosis type 1 syndrome [22]. Unfavorable prognostic factors include: low age, impossibility of total resection, diffuse growth (especially *IDH* mutated), diencephalic syndrome, presence of symptoms of intracranial hypertension and metastasis [23].

7.1.1.1. Pilocytic astrocytoma WHO grade I

This tumor is the most frequent LGG in children (up to 85%). Typical localizations are: cerebellum, diencephalon, optic tract, basal ganglia or brain stem [3]. Various localizations of this tumor also have their typical genetic characteristics. Its autosomal dominant forms are part of NF type 1 syndrome and tuberous sclerosis with typical localization over the course of the optical pathway, less often in hypothalamus. However, sporadic forms are more frequent. It may contain a *BRAF-KIAA* fusion that is connected to better prognosis. Conversely, the higher MIB-1 proliferation index is associated with shortened survival [24]. Therapy consists of surgical treatment. Despite the limited growth and the benign nature, the possibility of its removal is sometimes limited by its localization.

Its subtype is a **pilomyxoid astrocytoma** with a typical angiocentric array of myxoid matrix. It is most common in infants and children of pre-school age with a typical hypothalamus and chiasm localization. Due to its localization, total resection is less probable and thus has a slightly worse prognosis compared to pilocytic astrocytoma [25].

7.1.1.2. Diffuse gliomas WHO grade II

Diffuse low-grade gliomas account for 10% of all LGG in children [3]. Histologically, most common types are: **astrocytoma**, **oligodendroglioma** and **mixed oligoastrocytoma**. The most frequent group is the diffuse astrocytoma (DA), which is mainly located in hemispheres (especially in the frontal and temporal lobe), brain stem, optic pathway, hypothalamus and thalamus. Although they may appear to be similar to diffuse gliomas of adulthood, they have different genetic characteristics and typical biological behavior. Unlike DA of adulthood, for which the presence of *IDH1* and *IDH2* mutations is typical, these are very rare in children. *MAPK* pathway and *BRAF* gene alterations are more common [26]. Unlike diffuse adult LGG, DA of pediatric type usually do not undergo malignant transformation into higher grade glioma, so their prognosis is more favorable. Especially in older children it is important to provide genetic diagnostics of the tumor type and differentiation between the more favorable type of LGG (DA without *IDH* mutation or diffuse oligodendroglioma without *IDH* mutation and 1p/19q co-deletion) and adult LGG type that may occur in older children and adolescents [27]. Up to 75% of adult LGG types in childhood are subject of malignant transformation. Treatment consists of surgical removal of the tumor and subsequent observation, but their infiltrative growth pattern generally does not allow their total resection. In case of relapse and progress in tumor growth, chemotherapy with carboplatin (with or without vincristine) may be used. Alternatively, the TPCV regimen (thioguanine, procarbazine, lomustine and vincristine) may be used, rarely in the second line with vinblastine and temozolomide. In relapsing non-responding tumors, bevacizumab is given in combination with irinotecan [28] and in some cases accompanied with radiotherapy. For early and late side effects of radiation, chemotherapy is preferred in children (in opposite to adult treatment). In pediatric patients, tumor localization and age at diagnosis are stronger factors for choosing therapy modality than the histological characteristics of the tumor itself [29, 30].

7.1.1.3. Subependymal giant cell astrocytoma WHO grade I

This tumor type is most frequently diagnosed in patients with tuberous sclerosis and mutations in *TSC1* and *TSC2* genes. Its typical location is a lateral ventricle, mostly growing subependymal near the foramen Monroi [6]. Growth pattern is slow without infiltration of surrounding tissues. Surgical resection, if possible, is a modality of choice in treatment of this tumor. SEGA is one of few tumors with proven efficacy of targeted treatment with mTOR inhibitors, everolimus or sirolimus, which may also eliminate the necessity of surgical treatment [31].

7.1.1.4. Pleomorphic xanthoastrocytoma WHO grade II

PXA is relatively rare tumor, which accounts for 0.5–1% of all CNS tumors in childhood [3], typically occurring supratentorially, especially in the temporal lobe. It grows in the cortex, sometimes infiltrating meninges [6]. The most common symptoms are epileptic seizures. Frequently, *V600E* mutation of the *BRAF* gene occurs, especially in temporal lobe localization [32]. This tumor may undergo malignant transformation into an anaplastic form, which is classified as a separate type of tumor in the new WHO classification, has grade III and belongs to the HGG. Like grade II pleomorphic xanthastrocytoma, it often shows a *V600E* mutation of the *BRAF* gene [33].

7.1.2. High-grade gliomas in children

High-grade gliomas account for 15–20% of all pediatric CNS tumors [3]. HGG in children include **anaplastic astrocytoma (grade III), glioblastoma** and its variants **(grade IV)** and **diffuse gliomas of midline structures** (including diffuse pontine glioma). They are characterized by very high mitotic activity and in grade IV also with presence of microvascular proliferation and necrosis as it is in adult HGG. Despite these common histological features, children's HGG differ from adult tumors by their typical localization, genetic alterations and clinical behaviors. Pediatric HGG almost always grow as primary malignancies and their malignant transformation from LGG is extremely rare [34]. Besides localization in cerebral hemispheres, which is also typical for adult forms of HGG, pediatric HGG occur more often in midline structures, such as thalamus, cerebellum or pons. Pontine HGG are typical for pediatric age group (account for 50% of all HGG in children) and have even worse prognosis than hemispheric tumors [35]. Children's HGGs (especially tumors in children under 3 years of age) have significantly less genetic alterations than adult forms [36]. On the basis of a recurring combination of genetic and epigenetic features and characteristic biological and clinical behavior, 6 subtypes of HGG were determined (**Table 1**).

The *K27* subtype is characteristically found in pons, thalamus and cerebellum in younger children. Its typical alterations are: mutation of *K27*, *TP53* and *ATRX* genes, *PDGFRA* amplification, *ACVR1* mutation (typical for localization in pons) and mutation of *FGFR1* which is typical for thalamic site of tumor. Among all subtypes it has the shortest survival—from 6 to 9 months [37, 38].

The *G34* subtype is more frequent in adolescents and young adults and typically grows in cerebral hemispheres. It most commonly contains mutations of the *G34*, *TP53* and *ATRX* genes. The survival time is about 1 year after the diagnosis is determined [37].

The *IDH* subtype with typical *IDH1*, *IDH2*, *TP53* and *ATRX* mutations, grows usually in the hemisphere. Tumors with *IDH* mutations account for less than 10% of children's HGG, they occur more commonly in adults. This type can also arise from malignant transformation of

Type	K27	G34	IDH	RTK-I	Mesenchymal	Epitheloid
Age	Young child	Adolescent	Adolescent	All	Adolescent	Young child
Typical location	Cerebellum, pons, spinal cord, thalamus	Brain hemispheres	Brain hemispheres	Brain hemispheres	Brain hemispheres	Brain hemispheres
Typical alteration	*H3.3* or *H3.1* mut. *K27, TP53, ATRX, ACVR1* (pons), *FGFR1* (thalamus), ampl. *PDGFRA*	*H3.3*, mut. *G34, TP53, ATRX*	mut. *IDH1, IDH2, ATRX, TP53*	ampl. *PDGFRA, EGFR*, mut. *TP53*, del. *CDKN2A/CDKN2B*	mut. *NF1, TP53*, ampl. *PDGFRA, EGFR*, del. *CDKN2A/CDKN2B*	mut. *BRAF V600E*, del. *CDKN2A*
Gene expression	Proneural	Mixed	Proneural	Proneural	Mesenchymal	Unknown
Median survival	6 months	1 year	>2 years	1 year	1 year	>4 years

Mut., mutation; ampl., amplification, del., deletion [38].

Table 1. Characterization of pediatric HGG subtypes.

LGG, what is generally rare in children. According to prognosis, this type belongs to more favorable subtypes with a survival period of more than 2 years [34, 38].

The *RTK-I* (receptor tyrosine kinase inhibitor) subtype grows in cerebral hemispheres and occurs throughout the pediatric age spectrum. Typically, it includes: amplification of *PDGFRA* and *EGFR*, *TP53* mutation and *CDKN2A*/*CDKN2B* deletion. Patients with this tumor subtype have a worse prognosis of survival, generally within 1 year [36, 38].

Mesenchymal subtype is most common among adolescents and young adults. It also occurs in cerebral hemispheres and contains mutations of *NF1* and *TP53*, amplification of *PDGFRA* and *EGFR* and deletion of *CDKN2A*/*CDKN2B*. It also belongs to worse types according to prognosis, with a survival of up to 1 year [36, 38, 39].

The last subtype is **epithelioid glioblastoma** which is similar to pleomorphic xanthoastrocytoma. It grows in cerebral hemispheres, in younger children and typically displays *BRAF V600E* mutation and *CDKN2A* deletion. It belongs to most favorable subtypes with a survival of more than 4 years [6, 12].

The presence of oncogene amplification, such as *MYCN*, *PDGFR* and *EGFR*, is associated with a worse prognosis in all types [40]. The most important prognostic factor is histological tumor grading and the extent of surgical resection. Radiotherapy is used in subsequent oncological treatment. Its combination with chemotherapy with temozolomide is therapeutically less successful than in adults [35]. Lomustine, vincristine and prednisone may also be used in chemotherapy. In case of recurrent HGG, repeated resection is considered individually, depending on the histological nature of the original tumor, the recurrence localization or the length of the progression free period. Reoperation could be also necessary for obtaining of fresh tissue samples for targeted treatment or for local administration of chemotherapy. In patients whose initial treatment failed, high-dose chemotherapy with total bone marrow suppression and subsequent hematopoietic stem cell transplantation [41] or clinical trial of new treatment modalities may be attempted. Molecular targets are very limited. Patients with *BRAF V600E* mutation are tested for BRAF inhibitors (vemurafenib and dabrafenib) with partial effect [19].

7.1.2.1. Diffuse midline glioma, H3 K27 M-mutant

The previous WHO classification is also called diffuse intrinsic pontine glioma (DIPG). The new edition classifies this tumor as diffuse midline glioma because it also appears in thalamus, cerebellum and spinal cord. It is predominantly considered childhood tumor, although it may also occur in adults. It contains a typical *K27 M* mutation of the histone H3 gene *H3F3A* (less frequently the *HIST1H3B* gene) and grows typically diffusely and infiltrates surrounding tissues [37]. It is classified as WHO grade IV, regardless of the presence or absence of anaplastic features [12]. A tumor growing in the ventral pontine region is a highly aggressive, destructive neoplasm that accounts for up to 80% of all glioma in the brain stem of children. The mean age at diagnosis is 6–7 years and median survival is 9 months [42]. Cranial nerve lesions, long-tract lesion symptoms, ataxia and behavioral disorders appear as leading clinical symptoms. The first symptom is often the abducens nerve palsy, which is also a negative prognostic factor. Also facial nerve palsy may occur. Obstruction of CSF pathways could lead to hydrocephalus [43]. Typically, on MR image tumor occupies more than half of the axial diameter of the pons. It has no exact boarders and does not enhance after gadolinium administration. Due to the typical MRI image and its localization, biopsy is rarely indicated, but in some cases stereotactic biopsy could be beneficial [44]. This tumor is known to spread to the distal parts of the brain stem and along the white matter tract to both the cerebellum and the thalamus in over half of the patients. Supratentorial spreading and leptomeningeal dissemination are uncommon [39]. Total resection due to its localization and growth pattern is not possible, so the most common treatment is radiotherapy, which helps to control symptoms and generally prolongs patient's survival. Because of the known CNS spread, irradiation of the entire head or the entire neural axis is sometimes chosen [39]. Systemic administration of chemotherapeutic agents has been shown to be ineffective for insufficient passage through the hematoencephalic barrier to pons [45]. The administration of chemotherapy (especially topotecan) is also attempted locally, directly to the tumor, using a stereotactic catheter. However, the results are not yet clear [46]. Children under age of 3 have a slightly better prognosis, probably due to different molecular genetic characteristics [47].

7.1.3. Ependymomas

Ependymomas are tumors originating from ependymal cells, which form a lining of CSF pathways and produce cerebrospinal fluid. They form the second most common group of children's CNS malignancies. They occur supratentorially, in the posterior fossa and in the spinal cord, mostly in children under 10 years of age [48]. Clinical signs depend on localization. In the most frequent, infratentorial localization, they present with the development of obstructive hydrocephalus, ataxia, cervical spinal pain and symptoms of cranial nerve lesion can also be present. Supratentorial localization often causes headaches, epileptic seizures and depending on localization, the development of focal neurological deficit. In case of suspicion on ependymoma, it is necessary to realize the MRI of whole craniospinal axis even before surgery. If possible, lumbar puncture with CSF sampling is recommended.

Ependymomas could be histologically: **subependymoma (grade I), myxopapillary ependymoma (grade I), ependymoma (grade II), ependymoma, *RELA* fusion-positive (grade II—III)** and **anaplastic ependymoma (grade III)**. Subependymoma and myxopapillary ependymoma appear almost exclusively in adults. The existence of several molecular subtypes of ependymomas, which differ in their localization, molecular genetic characteristics, typical age group of patients and prognosis, are known.

Two genetically distinct subgroups are distinguished in **ependymomas of posterior fossa** localization [49]. **Group A** occurs more frequently (up to half the ependymomas of all localizations) affecting predominantly younger children (3 years of age) and has a worse prognosis. In these tumors, fewer gene alterations occur and the *VEGF, PDGFR,* integrin and *MAPK* signaling pathways are most commonly affected [50]. Epigenetic suppression of differentiation genes is often present in this group of tumors [51]. Duplication of 1q occurs in 25% of group A ependymomas and it is a common negative prognostic feature [52]. Less frequently occurring **group B** affects predominantly adolescents and young adults. It contains frequent chromosome changes and its prognosis is more favorable than in group A. In both groups, the mutation rate is relatively low and gene mutations occur sporadically [50].

Up to 70% of **supratentorially localized ependymomas** harbor fusion of *C11orf95-RELA* on chromosome 11q [50]. This change never occurs when locating in the posterior fossa. The discovery of the presence of this fusion was so significant that in the new WHO classification of brain tumors from 2016 the **ependymoma with the *RELA* fusion** was classified as a separate entity [12]. Homozygous deletion of *CDKN2A* with or without the presence of duplication of 1q is a negative prognostic factor [53]. The most frequent occurrence is in children with an average age of 8 years. **The fusion of *YAP1*** (with *MAMLD1* or *FAM118B*) occurs in supratentorially localized ependymomas without *RELA* fusion. These tumors are more common in younger children with an average age of 1.4 years. From all ependymomas, the worst prognosis has supratentorial *RELA* positive tumors and group A ependymomas in the posterior fossa. At the same time, they are the most common forms (together make up two-thirds of all ependymomas) that occur predominantly in children [53].

Therapeutic modality is extensive surgical removal followed by radiotherapy, which can only be used in the treatment of children aged more than 1 year. Currently, the use of chemotherapy (especially vincristine, cyclophosphamide, cisplatin and etoposide) is in clinical trials [38]. The choice of the treatment scheme determines the age of the child, the histological type of tumor, the extent of the resection performed and the presence of dissemination in the CSF pathways.

7.2. Neuronal and mixed neuronal-glial tumors

It is a heterogeneous group of tumors with neuronal or mixed neuroglial morphology. They are mostly grade I, but their anaplastic forms can also occur. Following tumors are most frequently present in children.

7.2.1. Desmoplastic infantile astrocytoma (DIA) and ganglioglioma (DIGG)

These grade I tumors account for 0.5% of CNS childhood tumors [3]. They occur almost exclusively in children under 2 years of age. MRI verifies a large cystic tumor, especially in the frontal or parietal lobe. They are histologically and genetically almost identical, the only difference between them is the neoplastic neuronal component. Approximately 40% of these tumors display *MET* amplification and about 10% also *BRAF V600E* mutation [54].

7.2.2. Ganglioglioma (GG)

These tumors are characterized by a combination of neoplastic ganglion cells with a glial component similar to PA or diffuse glioma (especially astrocytoma). They occur mainly supratentorially. Seizures are usually leading symptom [33]. GG often harbor *BRAF V600E* mutation. The glial component of GG can undergo malignant transformation to anaplastic form that has higher mitotic activity, endothelial proliferation and necrosis in 3–5%. Up to half of the anaplastic GG is characterized by the presence of the *BRAF V600E* mutation, a minor part of the *TP53* mutation [6].

7.2.3. Dysembryoplastic neuroepithelial tumor (DNET)

It is a low-grade tumor (grade I), which occurs mainly supratentorially in the temporal lobe. It often manifests as drug-resistant epilepsy. There are several histological subtypes, which do not differ in typical age of origin, the nature of epileptic seizures or prognosis. Most of these tumors show alterations of *FGFR1* and *BRAF V600E* mutation [27].

7.3. Embryonal tumors

This group of tumors originates from embryonal cells that remain present in the CNS after birth. They are the most common childhood malignant CNS tumors (15–20%) in children under the age of 14 [12]. In adults, they are extremely rare. Most frequently occurring embryonal tumors are: meduloblastoma, atypical teratoid/rhabdoid tumor and CNS embryonal tumors (better known under the older name CNS primitive neuroectodermal tumors—PNETs). All tumors of this group tend to spread along the CFS pathways. Therefore, it is recommended to perform MR of whole craniospinal axis prior to surgery. CSF sampling is also indicated, as the finding of circulating tumor cells can appear earlier than dissemination in MRI. The prognosis of embryonic tumors depends on the age of the patient, dissemination of the tumor within CNS at the time of diagnosis, the size of the postoperative residue and on the histopathological and molecular biological properties of the tumor.

7.3.1. Medulloblastoma (MB)

It is the most common malignant brain tumor type in children. MB is a group of lesions that differ significantly by their genetic alterations, histological features and prognosis. In all cases, however, they are grade IV and fast-growing. Characteristic localization is infratentorial and leptomeningeal spread is typical. MB often manifests by symptoms of intracranial hypertension and blockage of CSF pathways as well as other symptoms, such as ataxia and nystagmus. Medulloblastoma may also occur as part of hereditary syndromes: Turcot, Rubinstein-Taybi, Gorlin, Li-Fraumeni syndrome and Fanconi anemia. There are four **histological variants** (classic type, desmoplastic nodular type, medulloblastoma with extensive nodularity and large cell and anaplastic type) and four subtypes depending on the signal pathway involved or genes altered: *WNT* (10%), *SHH* (30%), group 3 (15%) and group 4 (45%). WHO classification of brain tumors from 2016 classifies genetically defined MB into: *WNT*-activated, *SHH*-activated and *TP53*-mutant, *SHH*-activated and *TP53*-wildtype and non-*WNT*/non-*SHH* medulloblastoma, which is divided into MB group3 and MB group 4 [12].

The *WNT* medulloblastoma is the less frequent group (10%), which is typically found in the brain stem area in children aged 10. Often displays classic histology. The incidence of CNS metastases is very low. Activation of the *WNT* signaling pathway is characteristic [55]. About 90% of these tumors present with *CTNNB1* mutation. Mutations of *DDX3X*, chromatin remodeling genes and *TP53* are also common. *TP53* mutation in this type of tumor is not associated with a worse prognosis as it is in *TP53* mutated *SHH* MB. In general, *WNT*-activated MB has a very good prognosis.

The *SHH* group of medulloblastomas accounts for 30% of all MB and is the most heterogeneous. All histological types could occur. Dominant localization is in cerebral hemispheres. The most commonly affected age group is up to 4 years of age and then adolescents over 17 years of age. In children up to 4 years of age, it is most commonly present MB with extensive nodularity and in group 4–17 years of age, it is classic and large cell anaplastic type.

Desmoplastic nodular type is typical for patients over 17 years of age [56]. Genetic alterations also vary by age category. Mutation of *SUFU* gene is commonly present in age group up to 4 years, whereas *SMO* mutation occurs mainly in patients over 17 years of age. Between 4 and 17 years of age, amplification of *MYCN* and *GLI2* occurs. *PTCH1* alterations and *TERT* promoter mutation occur in all age categories [57]. While MBs of children under 4 years with extensive nodularity generally have a better prognosis, MBs with large cell anaplastic characteristics, presence of *MYCN* amplification or *TP53* mutation are very aggressive. They tend to metastasize within the CNS, and therefore are associated with a very poor prognosis [55, 56]. *SHH*-activated MBs with *TP53* mutation are classified separately. In children with *TP53* mutation, it is often a germline mutation that is part of the Li-Fraumeni syndrome [58].

Non-*WNT*/non-*SHH* MB is divided into **group 3** and **group 4**. While group 3 forms 15%, group 4 45% of all MBs. Although genetically different, some characteristics and genetic alterations are common. There is a higher occurrence in boys in both groups, structural anomalies are common—especially the formation of isochromosome 17q. A structural alteration that aberrantly induces the activity of *GFI1* or *GF1B* proto-oncogenes is common in both groups, particularly in group 3 [59]. The worst prognosis of all types has group 3 (particularly in boys), with large cell anaplastic morphology and with proven *MYC* over-expression and amplification. Group 4 is the most common molecular type with a pronounced predominance in boys. Nearly all tumors in this group have classic morphology. The prognosis of patient survival is moderate—except those with proven *MYC* amplification, which have worse prognosis [55]. Patients with metastasis present at diagnosis have a high risk of relapse, with the exception of patients with isochromosome 17, who make up a subgroup with more favorable prognosis [60].

The diagnosis is based on preoperative MRI examination of the craniospinal axis. Over the past 30 years, the most fundamental shift has been made in treatment of MB among all CNS childhood tumors and has changed from a fatal disease to a tumor with a 70% curability. The basis is surgical treatment with the maximal possible extent of resection. In the postoperative period, MRI is again indicated to evaluate the postoperative residue and the examination of cerebrospinal fluid is also beneficial. Medulloblastoma has as one of the few CNS tumors **staging system** that has 5 degrees (M0 = not disseminated, M1 = positive cytology of CSF without MR image of dissemination, M2 = nodular proliferation in cerebellar and cerebral subarachnoid spaces and in ventricles, M3 = nodular proliferation in spinal subarachnoid spaces, M4 = extra-neural propagation). Surgery is followed by chemotherapy and radiotherapy with whole CNS irradiation for frequent dissemination of medulloblastoma within the CNS. The chemotherapy regimens use either a combination of cisplatin, lomustine and vincristine or a combination of cisplatin, cyclophosphamide and vincristine [61]. Radiotherapy is administered at a dose of 54 Gy targeted to the tumor bed, followed by irradiation of the craniospinal axis at a dose of 24–36 Gy. The introduction of chemotherapy into the treatment scheme reduced the dose necessary to irradiate the craniospinal axis, thereby reducing the incidence of side effects of radiation [62]. However, radiotherapy in children under 3 years of age is not used for serious adverse effects on brain development. To potentiate the effects of standard chemotherapy, methotrexate is concomitantly administered to children under 3 years, either systemically or locally [63].

7.3.2. Atypical teratoid/rhabdoid tumor (AT/RT)

This high-grade neoplasm (grade IV) accounts for 1–2% of pediatric CNS tumors. Typically, it occurs in the age category up to 5 years, and in children under 1 year of age, it is the most common malignant CNS tumor. As it grows very quickly, clinical manifestations occur early. AT/RT is often localized supratentorialy and also in the posterior fossa [3, 64]. About 20% of patients have already dissemination of the tumor at the time of diagnosis, usually along leptomeninges. Rare coincidence with renal tumors may occur [65]. Genetically, it is characterized by deletion on the 22nd chromosome and loss of *INI1/SMARCB1/BAF47* expression due to germline or somatic mutations. Evaluation of *SMARCB1* expression is necessary to distinguish AT/RT from other embryonic tumors [66]. This tumor was the first primary CNS tumor in which the major tumor suppressor gene was identified, namely *SMARCB1*. The presence of *SMARCB1* germline mutation is the basis for identifying the **syndrome predisposing to the rhabdoid tumor,** which is common in patients with coincidence of AT/RT with rhabdoid tumor of the kidney. The greatest risk of developing tumors in this syndrome is during the first year of age, which requires monitoring and active screening in children from these families. Immunohistochemical evidence of cytokeratin, epithelial membrane antigen, glial fibrillary acidic protein, synaptophysin, desmin and vimentin is also necessary. The MIB-1 proliferation index is high, 50–100% [67]. MRI of the entire craniospinal axis as well as examination of CSF for the presence of tumor cells is useful in diagnosis. There is no standard treatment regime for AT/RT. Treatment is based on surgical resection. The localization of the tumor and the extent of its spread is crucial for the choice of treatment modalities. Prolongation of survival requires a combination of postoperative systemic and intrathecal chemotherapy (methotrexate, cytarabine and hydrocortisone) with radiotherapy. Negative prognostic factors include: the presence of *SMARCB1* germline mutations, postoperative residues, dissemination at the time of diagnosis and the age under 2 years [64].

7.3.3. Embryonal tumor with multilayered rosettes, C19MC-altered (ETMR)

This tumor typically occurs in children under 3 years of age. It has a poor prognosis, most patients die within 1–2 years after diagnosis [68]. Characteristic is the 19q13.42 locus amplification, which contains a cluster of microRNA (C19MC) and a fusion between *TTYH1* and *C19MC* [69]. Treatment begins with a surgical resection, followed by adjuvant oncology treatment with chemotherapy and radiotherapy. In children under 3 years, radiotherapy is not indicated.

7.3.4. Neuroblastoma and ganglioneuroblastoma CNS

These two neoplasms belong to embryonal tumors but show neuronal differentiation, in the case of ganglioneuroblastoma also the presence of ganglionic cells. They most often occur in early childhood. In general, neuroblastomas are a frequent diagnosis, but especially in the chest and abdominal cavity (in the brain they are rare). Some of these include gene alterations leading to increased expression of the transcription factor *FOXR2* [70]. The treatment scheme is the same as for other embryonal tumors – surgery followed by chemotherapy in children less than 3 years of age and addition of radiotherapy in older children.

7.4. Pineoblastoma

In the past, this tumor was classified as embryonal, but in the new WHO classification it was reclassified to a group of pineal tumors. Its histological and molecular biological properties are similar to embryonal tumors. Because of its location, obstructive hydrocephalus is predominantly caused by blockage of CSF passages at the level of the third ventricle, and symptoms of the pressure on tectum—especially oculomotor disorder, poor reaction of pupils to light with present reaction to accommodation, later hemiparesis and ataxia. Often occur germline mutations of the *RB1* and *DICER1* genes [71]. Pineoblastoma is often found in children with congenital retinoblastoma. It can rarely disseminate along CSF pathways. A **staging system** similar to embryonal tumors is used. The primary therapeutic step is surgical resection. However, due to localization, total resection is unlikely, with only partial resection or biopsy performed in the majority of patients. This is followed by oncological treatment that combines chemotherapy and radiotherapy with a dose of 54 Gy on tumor bed and 24–36 Gy for craniospinal axis. A different therapy management is used in children under 3 years of age who undergo biopsy, followed by chemotherapy or high-dose chemotherapy with bone marrow ablation followed by hematopoietic stem cell transplantation.

7.5. Germ cell tumors

Intracranial germ cell tumors are a heterogeneous group that accounts for 3–4% of brain tumors with the exception of Japan where the incidence is higher, up to 15% [72]. Based on histopathological characteristics, they are divided into **germinomas** and **nongerminomas** (embryonal carcinoma, choriocarcinoma, mature or immature teratoma, teratoma with malignant transformation, yolk sac tumor and mixed germ cell tumor). In some countries, dividing into **secretory** and **non-secretory** tumors is also used—depending on the presence and absence, respectively, of elevation of serum and CSF tumor markers [12].

The most common localization is the pineal and suprasellar area, where they form either solitary or multiple lesions. The pineal region is much more frequent, but up to 10% of patients have both sites at the time of diagnosis, which is typical for pure germinomas [73]. Rare localities include basal ganglia, brain ventricles, cerebral hemispheres and thalamus. Tumor in the suprasellar region is often presented by hormonal expression. Often occur diabetes insipidus, enuresis, anorexia and also psychological changes [74]. Pineal localization has usually earlier manifestation, with hydrocephalus and diplopia developing from pressure to the tectal and aqueductal region. The most common germ cell tumor is germinoma. Mutations of the *KIT*, *KRAS* and *NRAS* genes are common [75]. Half of germinoma cases harbor deregulation of the *KIT/RAS* and *AKT/mTOR* pathways. The germline variations of *JMJD1C* occur more frequently in Japanese, which is probably related to the higher incidence of germinomas in this country. This gene is important for maintaining male germ cells [76].

In the diagnosis, apart from MRI, cytological examination of CSF and evaluation of **alpha-fetoprotein (AFP)** and **beta human chorionic gonadotropin (bHCG)** concentrations in both serum and in CSF is used [77]. In addition, hormonal examination of hypothalamic and pituitary function and examination of the visual field in suprasellar and hypothalamic tumors are necessary. The essentials of the treatment are chemotherapy and radiotherapy, but biopsy is required for reliable diagnosis. Only in tumors with unambiguous MRI image and positive tumor markers in CSF can be treated without biopsy.

7.6. Choroid plexus tumors

These rare intraventricular tumors account for 1% of all brain tumors and 2–4% of pediatric tumors. They arise from neuroectoderm and consist of differentiated epithelial plexus cells that produce CSF. They most often occur in the age group under 2 years of age. The most common site are lateral ventricles (less often the 3rd and 4th ventricle), but could also occur in the cerebellopontine angle and in the cerebral parenchyma. They mostly manifest by symptoms of intracranial hypertension from hydrocephalus, both from overproduction of the CSF as well as from obstruction of the CSF pathways. Sometimes, however, they can also manifest suddenly, in case of bleeding into the tumor [78]. This group of tumors consists of: **choroid plexus papilloma (grade I), atypical choroid plexus papilloma (grade II)** and **choroid plexus carcinoma (grade III).** There are no genetic differences between papilloma and atypical papilloma. In both, immunoreactivity to cytokeratin, vimentin, S100 protein and synaptophysin is present. On the other hand, carcinoma is genetically different. The germline mutations of *TP53* as part of the Li-Fraumeni syndrome predispose to the formation of plexus carcinoma. Somatic *TP53* mutations are present in up to 60% of the plexus carcinomas and the more copy of the mutated *TP53* is present, the worse is the prognosis [79]. Chromosome alterations are rarely detected.

MRI showing relatively well-defined extra-axial mass that does not invade the brain tissue with gadolinium enhancement and containing calcification and microhemorrhages is essential. Surgical treatment is the method of choice. Due to the rich vascular supply, preoperative tumor embolization is preferred in some cases. Hydrocephalus treatment is also necessary—sometimes requires external ventricular drainage. In some patients hydrocephalus is permanent, and therefore ventriculoperitoneal shunt or the endoscopic ventriculostomy of the 3rd ventricle are required [80]. There is no need for further treatment in the papilloma, radiotherapy, radiosurgery or chemotherapy with bevacizumab may be used in atypical or recurrent forms. Chemotherapy has been proven in choroid plexus carcinoma, which can spread along CSF pathways [81].

7.7. Craniopharyngioma

Craniopharyngiomas are rare tumors, accounting for 3–5% of pediatric brain tumors. They occur in two subtypes: adamantinomatous and papillary [12]. The **adamantinomatous variant** for which the *CTNNB1* mutation is typical, is often found in children [6]. Their congenital origin is assumed to be from the ectodermal residues of the Rathke capsule or from another embryonal epithelium. They most commonly occur in the suprasellar area with intrasellar propagation. Symptoms include: endocrine disorders, visual disturbances, hydrocephalus symptoms and very rarely when growing in the posterior fossa—headache, diplopia, ataxia and hearing loss [82]. The diagnosis is made by MRI that displays a tumor with a solid and cystic component and with intratumoral calcifications. Evaluation of hormonal function and visual field is also necessary. The therapy of newly diagnosed craniopharyngiomas is a combination of surgical treatment, radiotherapy and a drainage of the cyst. The prognosis is good, 90% of patients survive more than 10 years [83]. Total resection may have serious complications, including: need for hormone replacement therapy, severe obesity, behavioral disorders, blindness, epileptic seizures, postoperative CSF leak, pseudoaneurysms, oculomotor disorders, severe postoperative bleeding and hypothalamic injury [84]. While recurrent craniopharyngiomas are treated by resection, radiotherapy or radiosurgery, tumors with unresponsive cystic component can be treated by administration of P32, bleomycin or interferon alpha directly into the tumor bed. It can be supplemented by systemic administration of interferon [85].

7.8. Other pediatric CNS tumors

Schwannomas are in children rare, mostly benign neoplasms originating from Schwann cells of cranial or other nerves. Some of these tumors are present as a part of the NF2 type genetic syndrome, especially at bilateral occurrence. From cranial nerves, this tumor mostly affects VIII cranial nerve and is called vestibular schwannoma or acoustic neurinoma [86]. Vestibular schwannomas can cause loss of hearing and tinnitus. Diagnosis is mainly based on MRI. The method of choice is resection of the tumor, further treatment is usually not necessary. In rare cases, radiotherapy can be used in the presence of postoperative residues [87].

Meningiomas that grow from meninges are much rarer in children than in adults—they account for about 2.6–2.9% of CNS childhood tumors [2]. It occurs most often between 6 and 12 years of age. Children have a higher incidence of tumors growing from the skull base and a higher incidence of atypical (grade II) and anaplastic (grade III) meningiomas compared to adults. Chromosome 22 abnormalities are often present, also as a part of the NF2 type syndrome. Tumors connected with NF2 occur at younger age (about 2 years) and may also be the first symptom of this disease. In benign tumors, surgical treatment is largely sufficient, but in the case of incomplete resection and in tumors of higher grade, is usually combined with radiotherapy. Favorable prognostic factors include: age up to 10 years, superficial localization, total extirpation and absence of NF2 syndrome, where localization and resection extent are stronger predictive factors than histological grade [88].

Primary CNS lymphomas (PCNSL) are rare in children. Patients with immunodeficiency have an increased risk of developing CNS lymphomas [89]. They occur mainly in children around 14 years of age with moderate predominance in boys [90]. They are mostly localized in brain hemispheres. Clinical symptoms include symptoms of increased intracranial pressure, ataxia, hemiparesis, epileptic seizures and cranial nerve palsy. MRI and CSF sampling is used in diagnostics. MRI verifies solid lesion (even with a possible cystic component). Histologically, **mature aggressive B cell lymphoma (B-NHL),** as well as **anaplastic large cell lymphoma (ALCL)** or **peripheral T cell lymphoma (PTCL)** are most often present. Pediatric B-NHL has a low to moderate proliferation index, a lower Bc12 protein expression and a higher frequency of the Bc16 + GC fetal center phenotype, indicating a better prognosis [91]. While the prognosis of PCNSL in adults is very poor, in children is better. Interestingly, localization of PCNSL in deep brain structures does not affect the prognosis [90]. In chemotherapy, methotrexate or cytarabine at high doses are mostly used, usually providing satisfactory remission without need for use of radiotherapy (often used in ALCL form). It has been found that the exclusive use of chemotherapy is more effective than combined chemoradiotherapy. Explanation could be the use of lower doses of chemotherapy in combined therapy. High-dose therapy of methotrexate, which appears to be the most effective, is better tolerated by children compared to adults. Radiotherapy is therefore reserved for recurrent forms [89].

8. Conclusion

Pediatric CNS tumors are diagnostic and therapeutic challenge. A lot of specialists are involved in their management: pediatricians, neurologists, neurosurgeons, radiologists, radiation and clinical oncologists, endocrinologists and others. Due to the development of MRI and its techniques, use of invasive examinations is minimalized. Over the past decades, there has been a significant refinement of operational technologies, enabling the most extensive and yet safe resection of the tumor. Children CNS tumors are frequent, often with unfavorable prognosis. While in most malignant tumors the prognosis has not improved as hoped, in case of medulloblastoma there has been a significant survival prolongation during last decades. Undoubtedly, this is due to extensive research of the molecular genetic characteristics of tumors, which identified genetically defined subgroups of medulloblastoma with different treatment strategies. This change was also reflected in the new WHO classification, which also classifies medulloblastomas based on genetic alterations. Intense research also takes place in other tumor entities, where the discovery is yet about to come. Identifying molecular and genetic targets is the only possible way to target individualized therapy that appears both in treatment and in further prognosis improving in this age group as a key point.

Author details

Romana Richterová* and Branislav Kolarovszki

*Address all correspondence to: romana.richterova@gmail.com

Clinic of Neurosurgery, Jessenius Faculty of Medicine of Commenius University in Bratislava, University Hospital in Martin, Martin, Slovak Republic

References

[1] Siegel R, Naishadham D, Jemal A. Cancer statistics, 2013. CA: a Cancer Journal for Clinicians. 2013;**63**(1):11-30. DOI: 10.3322/caac.21166

[2] Ostrom QT, de Blank PM, Kruchko C et al. Alex's lemonade stand foundation infant and childhood primary brain and central nervous system tumors diagnosed in the United States in 2007-2011. Neuro-Oncology 2015;**16**(10):1-36. DOI: 10.1093/neuonc/nou327

[3] Ostrom QT, Gittleman H, Liao P, et al. CBTRUS statistical report: Primary brain and central nervous system tumors diagnosed in the United States in 2007-2011. Neuro-Oncology. 2014;**16**(4):1-63. DOI: 10.1093/neuonc/nou223

[4] Pui CH, Gajjar AJ, Kane JR, et al. Challenging issues in pediatric oncology. Nature Reviews. Clinical Oncology. 2011;**8**:540-549. DOI: 10.1038/nrclinonc.2011.95

[5] Ostrom QT, Gittleman H, de Blank PM et al. American Brain Tumor Association adolescent and young adult primary brain and central nervous system Tumors diagnosed in the United States in 2008-2012. Neuro-Oncology 2016;**18**(1):1-50. DOI: 10.1093/neuonc/nov297

[6] Chiang JC, Ellison DW. Molecular pathology of paediatric central nervous system tumours. The Journal of Pathology. 2017;**241**(2):159-172. DOI: 10.1002/path.4813

[7] Andersen TV, Schmidt LS, Poulsen AH, et al. Patterns of exposure to infectious diseases and social contacts in early life and risk of brain tumours in children and adolescents: An international case-control study (CEFALO). British Journal of Cancer. 2013;**108**:2346-2353. DOI: 10.1038/bjc.2013.201

[8] Partap S, MacLean J, Von Behren J, et al. Birth anomalies and obstetric history as risks for childhood tumors of the central nervous system. Pediatrics. 2011;**128**:652-657. DOI: 10.1542/peds.2010-3637

[9] Bjorge T, Sorensen HT, Grotmol T, et al. Fetal growth and childhood cancer: A population-based study. Pediatrics. 2013;**132**:1265-1275. DOI: 10.1542/peds.2013-1317

[10] Roncarolo F, Infante-Rivard C. Asthma and risk of brain cancer in children. Cancer Causes & Control. 2012;**23**:617-623. DOI: 10.1007/s10552-012-9928-7

[11] Shu X, Prochazka M, Lannering B, et al. Atopic conditions and brain tumor risk in children and adolescents--an international case-control study (CEFALO). Annals of Oncology. 2014;**25**(4):902-908. DOI: 10.1093/annonc/mdu048

[12] Louis DN, Perry A, Reifenberger G, et al. The 2016 World Health Organization classification of tumours of the central nervous system. Acta Neuropathologica. 2016;**131**(6):803-820. DOI: 10.1007/s00401-016-1545-1

[13] Pollack IF. Multidisciplinary management of childhood brain tumors: A review of outcomes, recent advances, and challenges. Journal of Neurosurgery. Pediatrics. 2011;**8**(2):135-148. DOI: 10.3171/2011.5.PEDS1178

[14] Wells EM, Packer RJ. Pediatric brain tumors. Continuum (Minneap Minn). 2015;**21**(2):373-396. DOI: 10.1212/01.CON.0000464176.96311.d1

[15] Balogun JA, Khan OH, Taylor M, et al. Pediatric awake craniotomy and intra-operative stimulation mapping. Journal of Clinical Neuroscience. 2014;**21**(11):1891-1844. DOI: 10.1016/j.jocn.2014.07.013

[16] Seddighi A, Esmaeil Akbari M, Seddighi AS, et al. First experience of intraoperative radiation therapy in cerebral high grade Glioma in Iran: A report of three cases and literature review. Iranian Journal of Cancer Prevention. 2015;**8**(5):e3795. DOI: 10.17795/ijcp-3795

[17] Xing W, Shao C, Qi Z, et al. The role of Gliadel wafers in the treatment of newly diagnosed GBM: A meta-analysis. Drug Design, Development and Therapy. 2015;**9**:3341-3348. DOI: 10.2147/DDDT.S85943

[18] Karajannis M, Allen JC, Newcomb EW. Treatment of Pediatric brain Tumors. Journal of Cellular Physiology. 2008;**217**(3):584-589. DOI: 10.1002/jcp.21544

[19] Kieran MW, Hargrave DR, Cohen KJ, et al. Phase 1 study of dabrafenib in pediatric patients (pts) with relapsed or refractory BRAF V600E high- and low-grade gliomas (HGG, LGG), Langerhans cell histiocytosis (LCH), and other solid tumors (OST). Journal of Clincal Oncology. 2015;**33**(15):A-10004. DOI: 10.1200/jco.2015.33.15_suppl.10004

[20] Green A, Foreman N, Levy JM, et al. HG-120case series of three pediatric brain tumor patients treated with tumor-treating fields. Neuro-Oncology. 2016;**18**:75-76. DOI: 10.1093/neuonc/now073.116

[21] Grob ST, Levy JMM. Improving diagnostic and therapeutic outcomes in Pediatric brain Tumors. Molecular Diagnosis & Therapy. 2017. DOI: 10.1007/s40291-017-0299-3

[22] Bandopadhayay P, Bergthold G, London WB, et al. Long-term outcome of 4,040 children diagnosed with pediatric low-grade gliomas: An analysis of the surveillance epidemiology and end results (SEER) database. Pediatric Blood & Cancer. 2014;**61**(7):1173-1179. DOI: 10.1002/pbc.24958

[23] Stokland T, Liu JF, Ironside JW, et al. A multivariate analysis of factors determining tumor progression in childhood low-grade glioma: A population-based cohort study (CCLG CNS9702). Neuro-Oncology. 2010;**12**(12):1257-1268. DOI: 10.1093/neuonc/noq092

[24] Hawkins C, Walker E, Mohamed N, et al. BRAF-KIAA1549 fusion predicts better clinical outcome in pediatric low-grade astrocytoma. Clinical Cancer Research. 2011;**17**(14):4790-4798. DOI: 10.1158/1078-0432.CCR-11-0034

[25] Colin C, Padovani L, Chappe C, et al. Outcome analysis of childhood pilocytic astrocytomas: A retrospective study of 148 cases at a single institution. Neuropathology and Applied Neurobiology. 2013;**39**:693-705. DOI: 10.1111/nan.12013

[26] Forshew T, Tatevossian RG, Lawson AR, et al. Activation of the ERK/MAPK pathway: A signature genetic defect in posterior fossa pilocytic astrocytomas. The Journal of Pathology. 2009;**218**(2):172-181. DOI: 10.1002/path.2558

[27] Qaddoumi I, Orisme W, Wen J, et al. Genetic alterations in uncommon low-grade neuroepithelial tumors: BRAF, FGFR1, and MYB mutations occur at high frequency and align with morphology. Acta Neuropathologica. 2016;**131**:833-845. DOI: 10.1007/s00401-016-1539-z

[28] Avery RA, Hwang EI, Jakacki RI, et al. Marked recovery of vision in children with optic pathway gliomas treated with bevacizumab. JAMA Ophthalmology. 2014;**132**(1):111-114. DOI: 10.1001/jamaophthalmol.2013.5819

[29] Wisoff JH, Sanford RA, Heier LA, et al. Primary neurosurgery for pediatric low-grade gliomas: A prospective multi-institutional study from the Children's oncology group. Neurosurgery. 2011;**68**:1548-1554. DOI: 10.1227/NEU.0b013e318214a66e

[30] Müller K, Gnekow A, Falkenstein F, et al. Radiotherapy in pediatric pilocytic astrocytomas: A subgroup analysis within the prospective multicenter study HIT-LGG 1996 by the German Society of Pediatric Oncology and Hematology (GPOH). Strahlentherapie und Onkologie. 2013;**189**:647-655. DOI: 10.1007/s00066-013-0357-7

[31] Weidman DR, Pole JD, Bouffet E, et al. Dose-level response rates of mTor inhibition in tuberous sclerosis complex (TSC) related subependymal giant cell astrocytoma (SEGA). Pediatric Blood & Cancer. 2015;**62**(10):1754-1760. DOI: 10.1002/pbc.25573

[32] Ida CM, Rodriguez FJ, Burger PC, et al. Pleomorphic xanthoastrocytoma: Natural history and long-term follow-up. Brain Pathology. 2015;**25**:575-586. DOI: 10.1111/bpa.12217

[33] Schindler G, Capper D, Meyer J, et al. Analysis of BRAF V600E mutation in 1,320 nervous system tumors reveals high mutation frequencies in pleomorphic xanthoastrocytoma, ganglioglioma and extra-cerebellar pilocytic astrocytoma. Acta Neuropathologica. 2011;**121**:397-405. DOI: 10.1007/s00401-011-0802-6

[34] Sturm D, Witt H, Hovestadt V, et al. Hotspot mutations in H3F3A and IDH1 define distinct epigenetic and biological subgroups of glioblastoma. Cancer Cell. 2012;**22**:425-437. DOI: 10.1016/j.ccr.2012.08.024

[35] Cohen KJ, Heideman RL, Zhou T, et al. Temozolomide in the treatment of children with newly diagnosed diffuse intrinsic pontine gliomas: A report from the Children'sOncology group. Neuro-Oncology. 2011;**13**:410-416. DOI: 10.1093/neuonc/noq191

[36] Wu G, Diaz AK, Paugh BS, et al. The genomic landscape of diffuse intrinsic pontine glioma and pediatric non-brainstem high-grade glioma. Nature Genetics. 2014;**46**:444-450. DOI: 10.1038/ng.2938

[37] Wu G, Broniscer A, McEachron TA, et al. Somatic histone H3 alterations in pediatric diffuse intrinsic pontine gliomas and non-brainstem glioblastomas. Nature Genetics. 2012;**44**:251-253. DOI: 10.1038/ng.1102

[38] Gajjar A, Bowers DC, Karajannis MA, et al. Pediatric brain Tumors: Innovative genomic information is transforming the diagnostic and clinical landscape. Journal of Clinical Oncology. 2015;**33**(27):2986-2998. DOI: 10.1200/JCO.2014.59.9217

[39] Buczkowicz P, Bartels U, Bouffet E, et al. Histopathological spectrum of paediatric diffuse intrinsic pontine glioma: Diagnostic and therapeutic implications. Acta Neuropathologica. 2014;**128**(4):573-581. DOI: 10.1007/s00401-014-1319-6

[40] Korshunov A, Ryzhova M, Hovestadt V, et al. Integrated analysis of pediatric glioblastoma reveals a subset of biologically favorable tumors with associated molecular prognostic markers. Acta Neuropathologica. 2015;**129**:669-678. DOI: 10.1007/s00401-015-1405-4

[41] Finlay JL, Dhall G, Boyett JM, et al. Myeloablative chemotherapy with autologous bone marrow rescue in children and adolescents with recurrent malignant astrocytoma: Outcome compared with conventional chemotherapy: A report from the Children's oncology group. Pediatric Blood & Cancer. 2008;**51**(6):806-811. DOI: 10.1002/pbc.21732

[42] Johung TB, Monje M. Diffuse intrinsic Pontine Glioma: New pathophysiological insights and emerging therapeutic targets. Current Neuropharmacology. 2017;**15**(1):88-97. DOI: 10.2174/1570159X14666160509123229

[43] Schroeder KM, Hoeman CM, Becher OJ. Children are not just little adults: Recent advances in understanding of diffuse intrinsic pontine glioma biology. Pediatric Research. 2014;**75**(1-2):205-209. DOI: 10.1038/pr.2013.194

[44] Roujeau T, Machado G, Garnett MR, et al. Stereotactic biopsy of diffuse pontine lesions in children. Journal of Neurosurgery. 2007;**107**(1):1-4. DOI: 10.3171/PED-07/07/001

[45] Jansen MH, van Vuurden DG, Vandertop WP, et al. Diffuse intrinsic pontine gliomas: A systematic update on clinical trials and biology. Cancer Treatment Reviews. 2012;**38**:27-35. DOI: 10.1016/j.ctrv.2011.06.007

[46] Anderson RC, Kennedy B, Yanes CL, et al. Convection-enhanced delivery of topotecan into diffuse intrinsic brainstem tumors in children. Journal of Neurosurgery. Pediatrics. 2013;**11**(3):289-295. DOI: 10.3171/2012.10.PEDS12142

[47] Broniscer A, Laningham FH, Sanders RP, et al. Young age may predict a better outcome for children with diffuse pontine glioma. Cancer. 2008;**113**(3):566-572. DOI: 10.1002/cncr.23584

[48] McGuire CS, Sainani KL, Fisher PG. Incidence patterns for ependymoma: A surveillance, epidemiology, and end results study. Journal of Neurosurgery. 2009;**110**:725-729. DOI: 10.3171/2008.9.JNS08117

[49] Hoffman LM, Donson AM, Nakachi I, et al. Molecular sub-group-specific immunophenotypic changes are associated with outcome in recurrent posterior fossa ependymoma. Acta Neuropathologica. 2014;**127**:731-745. DOI: 10.1007/s00401-013-1212-8

[50] Archer TC, Pomeroy SL. Defining the molecular landscape of ependymomas. Cancer Cell. 2015;**27**:613-615. DOI: 10.1016/j.ccell.2015.04.015

[51] Mack SC, Witt H, Piro RM, et al. Epigenomic alterations define lethal CIMP-positive ependymomas of infancy. Nature. 2014;**506**:445-450. DOI: 10.1038/nature13108

[52] Korshunov A, Witt H, Hielscher T, et al. Molecular staging of intracranial ependymoma in children and adults. Journal of Clinical Oncology. 2010;**28**(19):3182-3190. DOI: 10.1200/JCO.2009.27.3359

[53] Pajtler KW, Witt H, Sill M, et al. Molecular classification of ependymal tumors across all CNS compartments, histopathological grades, and age groups. Cancer Cell. 2015;**27**:728-743. DOI: 10.1016/j.ccell.2015.04.002

[54] Gessi M, Zur Muhlen A, Hammes J, et al. Genome-wide DNA copy number analysis of desmoplastic infantile astrocytomas and desmoplastic infantile gangliogliomas. Journal of Neuropathology and Experimental Neurology. 2013;**72**:807-815. DOI: 10.1097/NEN.0b013e3182a033a0

[55] Kool M, Korshunov A, Remke M, et al. Molecular subgroups of medulloblastoma: An international meta-analysis of transcriptome, genetic aberrations, and clinical data of WNT, SHH, group 3, and group 4 medulloblastomas. Acta Neuropathologica. 2012;**123**:473-484. DOI: 10.1007/s00401-012-0958-8

[56] Ellison DW, Dalton J, Kocak M, et al. Medulloblastoma: Clinicopathological correlates of SHH, WNT, and non-SHH/WNT molecular subgroups. Acta Neuropathologica. 2011;**121**:381-396. DOI: 10.1007/s00401-011-0800-8

[57] Remke M, Ramaswamy V, Peacock J, et al. TERTpromoter mutations are highly recurrent in SHH subgroup medulloblastoma. Acta Neuropathologica. 2013;**126**:917-929. DOI: 10.1007/s00401-013-1198-2

[58] Kool M, Jones DT, Jäger N, et al. Genome sequencing of SHH medulloblastoma predicts genotype-related response to smoothened inhibition. Cancer Cell. 2014;**25**:393-405. DOI: 10.1016/j.ccr.2014.02.004

[59] Northcott PA, Lee C, Zichner T, et al. Enhancer hijacking activates GFI1 family oncogenes in medulloblastoma. Nature. 2014;**511**:428-434. DOI: 10.1038/nature13379

[60] Shih DJ, Northcott PA, Remke M, et al. Cytogenetic prognostication within medulloblastoma subgroups. Journal of Clinical Oncology. 2014;**32**:886-896. DOI: 10.1200/JCO.2013.50.9539

[61] Nageswara Rao AA, Wallace DJ, Billups C, et al. Cumulative cisplatin dose is not associated with event-free or overall survival in children with newly diagnosed average-risk medulloblastoma treated with cisplatin based adjuvant chemotherapy: Report from the Children's oncology group. Pediatric Blood & Cancer. 2014;**61**(1):102-106. DOI: 10.1002/pbc.24670

[62] Mizumoto M, Murayama S, Akimoto T, et al. Proton beam therapy for pediatric malignancies: A retrospective observational multicenter study in Japan. Cancer Medicine. 2016;**5**(7):1519-1525. DOI: 10.1002/cam4.743

[63] Lafay-Cousin L, Smith A, Chi SN, et al. Clinical, pathological, and molecular characterization of infant Medulloblastomas treated with sequential high-dose chemotherapy. Pediatric Blood & Cancer. 2016;**63**(9):1527-1534. DOI: 10.1002/pbc.26042

[64] Lafay-Cousin L, Hawkins C, Carret AS, et al. Central nervous system atypical teratoid rhabdoid tumours: The Canadian paediatric brain tumour consortium experience. European Journal of Cancer. 2012;**48**:353-359. DOI: 10.1016/j.ejca.2011.09.005

[65] Biegel JA, Fogelgren B, Wainwright LM, et al. Germline INI1 mutation in a patient with a central nervous system atypical teratoid tumor and renal rhabdoid tumor. Genes, Chromosomes & Cancer. 2000;**28**(1):31-37. DOI: 10.1002/(SICI)1098-2264(200005)28

[66] Slavc I, Chocholous M, Leiss U, et al. Atypical teratoid rhabdoid tumor: Improved long-term survival with an intensive multimodal therapy and delayed radiotherapy—The Medical University of Vienna experience, 1992 to 2012. Cancer Medicine. 2014;**3**:91-100. DOI: 10.1002/cam4.161

[67] McLendon RE, Adekunle A, Rajaram V, et al. Embryonal central nervous system neoplasms arising in infants and young children: A pediatric brain tumor consortium study. Archives of Pathology & Laboratory Medicine. 2011;**135**(8):984-993. DOI: 10.5858/2010-0515-OAR1

[68] Spence T, Sin-Chan P, Picard D, et al. CNS-PNETs with C19MC amplification and/or LIN28 expression comprise a distinct histogenetic diagnostic and therapeutic entity. Acta Neuropathologica. 2014;**128**:91-103. DOI: 10.1007/s00401-014-1291-1

[69] Kleinman CL, Gerges N, Papillon-Cavanagh S, et al. Fusion of TTYH1with the C19MC microRNA cluster drives expression of a brain-specific DNMT3Bisoform in the embryonal brain tumor ETMR. Nature Genetics. 2014;**46**:39-44. DOI: 10.1038/ng.2849

[70] Sturm D, Orr BA, Toprak UH, et al. New brain tumor entities emerge from molecular classification of CNS-PNETs. Cell. 2016;**164**:1060-1072. DOI: 10.1016/j.cell.2016.01.015

[71] De Kock L, Sabbaghian N, Druker H, et al. Germ-line and somatic DICER1 mutations in pineoblastoma. Acta Neuropathologica. 2014;**128**(4):583-595. DOI: 10.1007/s00401-014-1318-7

[72] Millard NE, Dunkel IJ. Advances in the management of central nervous system germ cell tumors. Current Oncology Reports. 2014;**16**:393. DOI: 10.1007/s11912-014-0393-1

[73] Weksberg DC, Shibamoto Y, Paulino AC. Bifocal intracranial germinoma: A retrospective analysis of treatment outcomes in 20 patients and review of the literature. International Journal of Radiation Oncology, Biology, Physics. 2012;**82**(4):1341-1351. DOI: 10.1016/j.ijrobp.2011.04.033

[74] Afzal S, Wherrett D, Bartels U, et al. Challenges in management of patients with intracranial germ cell tumor and diabetes insipidus treated with cisplatin and/or ifosfamide based chemotherapy. Journal of Neuro-Oncology. 2010;**97**(3):393-399. DOI: 10.1007/s11060-009-0033-z

[75] Wang L, Yamaguchi S, Burstein MD, et al. Novel somatic and germline mutations in intracranial germ cell tumours. Nature. 2014;**511**:241-245. DOI: 10.1038/nature13296

[76] Kuroki S, Akiyoshi M, Tokura M, et al. JMJD1C, a JmjC domain-containing protein, is required for long-term maintenance of male germ cells in mice. Biology of Reproduction. 2013;**89**:93. DOI: 10.1095/biolreprod.113.108597

[77] Allen J, Chacko J, Donahue B, et al. Diagnostic sensitivity of serum and lumbar CSF bHCG in newly diagnosed CNS germinoma. Pediatric Blood & Cancer. 2012;**59**(7):1180-1182. DOI: 10.1002/pbc.24097

[78] Pandey S, Sharma V, Singh K, et al. Uncommon presentation of choroid plexus papilloma in an infant. Journal of Pediatric Neurosciences. 2016;**11**(1):61-63. DOI: 10.4103/1817-1745.181254

[79] Merino DM, Shlien A, Villani A, et al. Molecular characterization of choroid plexus tumors reveals novel clinically relevant subgroups. Clinical Cancer Research. 2015;**21**:184-192. DOI: 10.1158/1078-0432.CCR-14-1324

[80] Ogiwara H, Dipatri AJ Jr, Alden TD, et al. Choroid plexus tumors in pediatric patients. British Journal of Neurosurgery. 2012;**26**(1):32-37. DOI: 10.3109/02688697.2011.601820

[81] Gopal P, Parker JR, Debski R, et al. Choroid Plexus Carcinoma. Archives of Pathology & Laboratory Medicine. 2008;**132**:1350-1354. DOI: 10.1043/1543-2165(2008)132[1350:CPC]2.0.CO;2

[82] Zhou L, Luo L, Xu J, et al. Craniopharyngiomas in the posterior fossa: A rare subgroup, diagnosis, management and outcomes. Journal of Neurology, Neurosurgery, and Psychiatry. 2009;**80**(10):1150-1154. DOI: 10.1136/jnnp.2008.149088

[83] Zacharia BE, Bruce SS, Goldstein H, et al. Incidence, treatment and survival of patients with craniopharyngioma in the surveillance, epidemiology and end results program. Neuro-Oncology. 2012;**14**(8):1070-1078. DOI: 10.1093/neuonc/nos142

[84] Clark AJ, Cage TA, Aranda D, et al. Treatment-related morbidity and the management of pediatric craniopharyngioma: A systematic review. Journal of Neurosurgery. Pediatrics. 2012;**10**(4):293-301. DOI: 10.3171/2012.7.PEDS11436

[85] Maarouf M, El Majdoub F, Fuetsch M, et al. Stereotactic intracavitary brachytherapy with P-32 for cystic craniopharyngiomas in children. Strahlentherapie und Onkologie. 2016;**192**(3):157-165. DOI: 10.1007/s00066-015-0910-7

[86] Gaikwad N, Sathe NU, Wadkar G, et al. Schwannoma of the cervical Vagus nerve in a child: A case report. Indian Journal of Otolaryngology and Head & Neck Surgery. 2013;**65**:188-191. DOI: 10.1007/s12070-011-0475-4

[87] Vadivelu S, Prasad P, Adesina AM, et al. Giant invasive spinal schwannoma in children: A case report and review of the literature. Journal of Medical Case Reports. 2013;**7**:289. DOI: 10.1186/1752-1947-7-289

[88] Menon G, Nair S, Sudhir J, et al. Childhood and adolescent meningiomas: A report of 38 cases and review of literature. Acta Neurochirurgica. 2009;**151**(3):239-244. DOI: 10.1007/s00701-009-0206-8

[89] Thorer H, Zimmermann M, Makarova O, et al. Primary central nervous system lymphoma in children and adolescents: Low relapse rate after treatment according to non-Hodgkin-lymphoma berlin-Frankfurt-Münster protocols for systemic lymphoma. Haematologica. 2014;**99**(11):238-241. DOI: 10.3324/haematol.2014.109553

[90] Abla O, Weitzman S, Blay JY, et al. Primary CNS lymphoma in children and adolescents: A descriptive analysis from the international primary CNS lymphoma collaborative group (IPCG). Clinical Cancer Research. 2011;**17**(2):346-352. DOI: 10.1158/1078-0432.CCR-10-1161

[91] Miles R, Raphael M, McCarthy K, et al. Pediatric diffuse large B-cell lymphoma demonstrates a high proliferation index, frequent c-Myc protein expression, and a high incidence of germinal Center subtype: Report of the French-American-British (FAB) international study group. Pediatric Blood & Cancer. 2008;**51**:369-374. DOI: 10.1002/pbc.21619

6

Neuropsychiatry: Aspects of Childhood Cranial Tumours

Alexander Hegarty and Yulia Furlong

Abstract

More than 90 years have passed since Baily and Cushing first introduced a histogenetic classification for tumours of the cranial nervous system (CNS). More recently, our knowledge of the genetic and molecular basis of tumorigenesis has caused a major paradigm shift towards defining tumours genetically, thus allowing greater diagnostic accuracy and prognostication to better guide tumour management. Correspondingly, successes in integrated management and improved survival rates have shifted attention towards overall quality of life studies, where psychosocial sequelae and adjustment implications are of particular interest to mental health professionals. To date, research relevant to this field has focused on the identification of neuropsychiatric symptoms at manifestation of illness. Such studies indicate that mood, cognition and psychosocial functioning are important factors in early diagnosis, mediating health outcomes, especially following radical and risk-adapted antineoplastic treatment. In addition to psychological burden, the neuropsychiatric aspects of childhood CNS tumours, including posterior fossa syndrome and cerebellar cognitive affective syndrome, are increasingly recognised as crucial causes of poor outcomes. The chapter ahead will initially address the shifting landscape of neuro-oncology, and then provide an overview of the neuropsychiatric aspects of CNS tumours in childhood, highlighting the underlying neurobiological and pathogenic mechanisms, whenever possible.

Keywords: childhood CNS tumours, cerebellar cognitive affective syndrome, posterior fossa syndrome, cerebellar mutism, neuropsychiatric presentation, neuropsychiatric outcomes

1. Introduction

Central nervous system (CNS) tumours are one of the most common cancers among children and adolescents, with an incidence rate of 5.57 per 100,000 population [1]. Among children (aged 1–14 years) they account for 26% of all childhood cancers, and are thus second only to leukaemia (29%); in adolescents (aged 15–19 years) they remain the second most common cancer (17%), following lymphoma (21%). Overall, CNS tumours represent the leading cause of cancer mortality in all individuals aged <20 [2]. However, a multitude of advancements in early diagnosis and risk-adapted treatment has resulted in increased survival; the importance of psychological and neurocognitive outcomes is thus more apparent than ever. Of course, childhood neuropsychiatry remains a nascent discipline and therefore it is prudent to begin with an overview of the current landscape of neuro-oncology.

The most utilised classification system for brain tumours—the 4th edition of the 'World Health Organisation (WHO) Classification of Tumours of the CNS' (2007)—was recently updated in 2016 [3]. It marks a conceptual milestone, finally enhancing the century-old principle of histogenesis-based nosology; this is largely due to the addition of molecular markers into CNS tumour classification. Evidently, we are entering a new era of neuro-oncology, with promise of superior clinical, experimental and epidemiological methods that may bring 'personalised' or 'precision medicine', within reach [3, 4].

Previously, tumours of the CNS were exclusively recognised by their morphological resemblance to constituent cells, including astrocytes, oligodendrocytes and ependymal cells. However, this system had three major deficiencies: first, differentiation can co-exist within the tissue of a single tumour; second, the accuracy of the prognosis was suboptimal; and most crucially, inter-observer differences were very apparent among neuropathologists [5].

With regards to diagnostic concordance, the discovery of a codeletion of chromosome 1p and 19q in oligodendroglioma signalled marked progress; it likely contributed to the inspiration behind the molecular underpinning of 'WHO 2016' [6]. Indeed, oligodendroglia-like cells in various neuroepithelial tumours have always been a diagnostic challenge due to diverse differentiation and biological behaviour; alternatively, the 1p/19q codeletion correlated with the classic oligodendroglioma morphology as well as the clinical, radiological and biological characteristics, i.e., gliomas harbouring 1p/19q are a coherent single entity, and thus provide superior inter-observer reliability [5].

Moreover, these molecular stratifiers provide prognostic and predictive information: for example, Isocitrate dehydrogenase 1 and 2 (IDH1 and IDH2, respectively) mutations are found almost exclusively in infiltrating astrocytomas and oligodendrogliomas [7, 8]; conversely, a medulloblastoma with genetic alterations in the wingless (WNT) pathways suggests excellent long-term survival rates [9]. As these tumour sub-classifications are informed by transcriptomes with similar biological behaviour, they will likely respond to corresponding targeted treatments, an approach that will drive many other successful anti-neoplastic therapies in the future [10, 11].

1.1. CNS tumour classification

The new nomenclature in CNS tumour classification empowers a clinician to pragmatically and scientifically construct a diagnosis by combining the histopathological name with the genetic determinant (if unavailable, 'NOS' suffix is used, i.e., not otherwise specified): conventional histology determines the initial stratification (e.g., 'diffuse glioma'); and secondly, a molecular defined genotype is added to denominate the subset, e.g., IDH-mutant (note: the genotype follows a comma and includes an adjective). Therefore, examples read as follows: 'Diffuse astrocytoma, IDH-mutant'; 'Medulloblastoma, WNT-activated' and so forth. Of note, the WHO grading system remains informed by histology only; thus each tumour is graded between I and IV (note: Roman numerals), in accordance with the degree of anaplasia, mitotic activity with microvascular proliferation and/or necrosis [8].

1.2. Medulloblastoma

Medulloblastoma (MB), a small blue cell malignancy of the cerebellum, is an embryonal tumour and represents the most common malignant brain tumour of childhood. Asides from its importance in paediatric neuro-oncology, MB will be discussed frequently in this chapter due to its relevance in childhood and adolescent neuropsychiatry. The 'medulloblastoma'—originally named in 1925 for its anatomical and histopathological traits [12]—is nowadays defined by a genetic biomarker: namely, either 'WNT-activated', 'SHH-activated', 'group 3' or 'group 4'. Nevertheless, diagnosis is gleaned from genome-wide transcriptomic and DNA methylation patterns, in addition to these distinct clinicopathological and molecular features. The wingless (WNT) and Sonic Hedgehog (SHH) subgroups are named for the signalling pathways thought to play prominent roles in their individual – and eponymously titled - pathogenesis, i.e., these MB subgroups are underpinned by WNT or SHH-activating mutations [5]. In contrast, MB group 3 and MB group 4 have few mutations but exhibit multiple DNA copy number alterations [13]. MB typically develops in children aged between 4 and 9 years, with a higher rate in boys. This predilection for onset in childhood is illustrated by the US incidence rate of 6 per million in children (1–9 years), a rate 10 times higher than that seen in the adult population [14], a statistic underpinned by histological and genetic differences, with more mutations observed in medulloblastoma of childhood when compared to that of adult-onset [15].

The subgrouping of MB has been useful in facilitating direct treatment strategies and reducing long-term intellectual and neuro-endocrine impairments associated with existing multimodal therapies [16]. The subgroups also add prognostic and predictive value; for example, in contrast to adult WNT-activated MB, children in this subgroup have an excellent overall prognosis (>90%) [17, 18]. Therefore, individualised and reduced intensity risk-adapted therapies are in development [19]. Moreover, SHH pathway inhibitors have had success in treating SHH-activated disease in early-phase trials [20]. Of note, the prognosis of SHH-activated MB is dictated by the presence of TP53 mutations, half of which are underlined by germline mutations and thus associated with secondary tumours [21, 22]. Evidently, genetic counselling is paramount for all families of children with MB with SHH-activation [23].

There are other high risk clinical factors in MB, and include: metastatic disease; large-cell, anaplastic (LCA) pathology; incomplete surgical resection; and MYC amplification [16]. Of note, the histological subtypes of MB have not been dramatically changed in 'WHO 2016'. However, large cell and anaplastic variants have been married to reflect their typical co-occurrence; this single entity (LCA) has a very poor prognosis. Furthermore, molecular and histological subtypes co-exist in many cases, e.g., 'WNT-activated' MB almost always has classic histology (**Figure 1**).

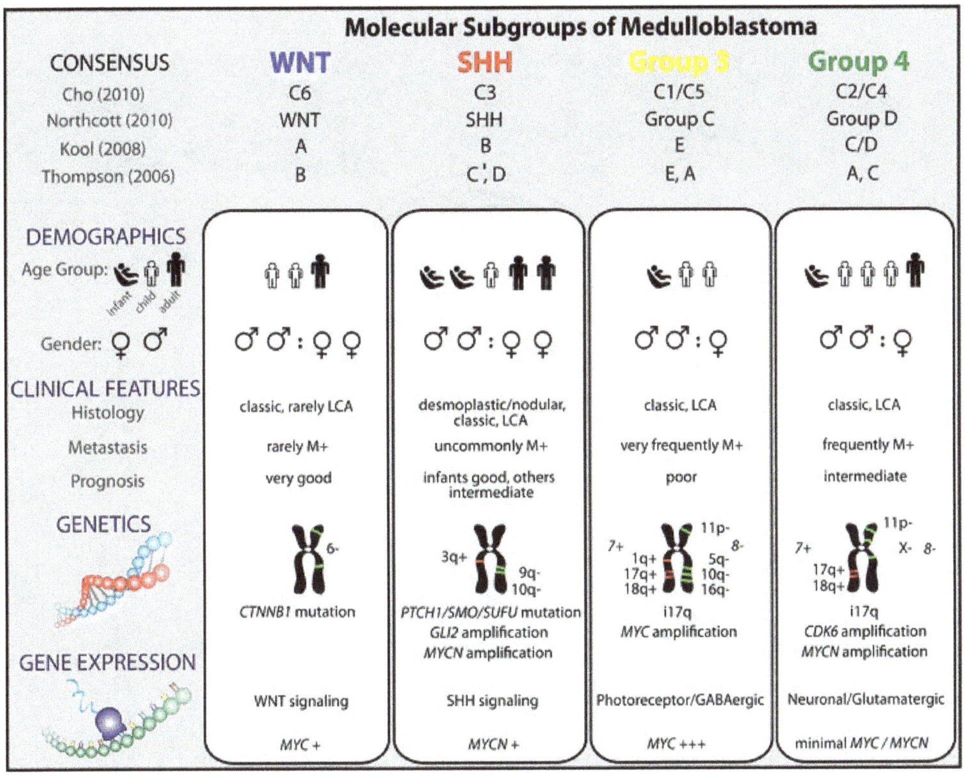

Figure 1. Molecular subgroups of medulloblastoma: A comparison of the various subgroups of medulloblastoma, adapted from Taylor et al. [10] with permission.

Evidently, the molecular era has sparked a rapidly propagating area of research which will further optimise CNS tumour diagnosis, treatment and outcomes. The latter is inextricably linked to psychological well-being; thus, it is crucial that psychiatric illness and neurocognitive deficits are investigated, recognised and addressed in order that a truly optimal and holistic clinical outcome is achieved. Therefore, the many guises of neuropsychiatry and its management will be the main focus of the remaining chapter.

1.3. Neuroanatomical correlates

The differential of a suspected CNS tumour can be narrowed by designating its location as 'supratentorial' or 'infratentorial', depending on whether it originates above or below the tentorium cerebella/cerebellar tentorium (Latin for 'tent of the cerebellum'); the tentorium is an extension of the dura matter that separates the cerebellum from the inferior portion of the occipital lobes [24]. A cancer's 'tentorial topography' varies across the lifespan: toddlers (aged 2–3 years) and adults are most likely to have supratentorial tumours; conversely, an infratentorial origin is more common in young children (aged 4–10); however, in older children and teenagers (i.e., aged 10–18 years) supratentorial and infratentorial tumours may occur with equal frequency [25] (**Figure 2**).

The supratentorial region—specifically the supra or (para)sellar area—hosts three main paediatric cancer types: craniopharyngioma, optic pathway/hypothalamic glioma and germ cell tumours. Several studies have shown that supratentorial tumours generally result in greater morbidity than infratentorial tumours in surviving children and adults [4].

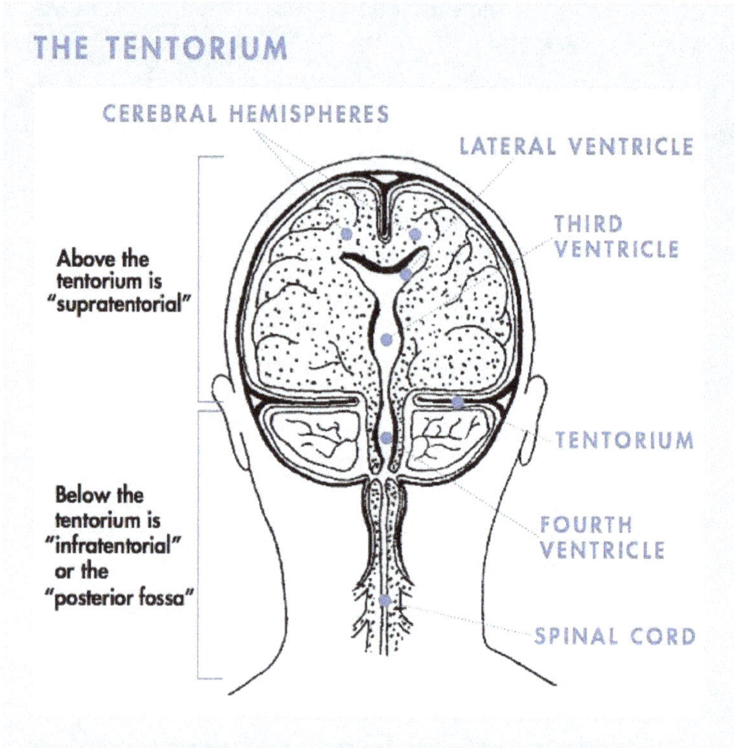

Figure 2. Illustration of the tentorium; including supratentorial and infratentorial view. Adapted from The American Brain Tumor Association with permission.

Supratentorial tumours are most commonly associated with the non-specific symptoms of raised intracranial pressure, seizures and papilledema. Any centrally localised neoplasm will also present vaguely (bar visual symptoms); headache, nausea and vomiting are commonly reported [26].

In the infratentorial region, the common tumours are MB, low-grade cerebellar astrocytoma, brain stem glioma and ependymoma; the commonest posterior fossa tumours of childhood are brainstem glioma, MB, ependymoma and cerebellar astrocytoma. When presenting as posterior fossa tumours, MB (and other cancers) cause vague symptoms such as nausea, vomiting, headache and papilledema. Additionally, they may present with gait disturbance and/or incoordination, i.e., signs that are also seen in brain stem and spinal cord tumours. Of note, back pain is a common manifestation of spinal cord tumours, whereas cranial nerve palsies and pyramidal signs would suggest brain stem tumours [26].

At times, clinical suspicion may be strengthened by comparatively specific signs and symptoms of infratentorial lesions: for example, brainstem involvement can cause extra-ocular muscle impairment, facial paresis, swallowing difficulties, hemiparesis, quadriparesis, ataxia or dysmetria; similarly, ataxia, dysmetria, headache, nausea, vomiting, neck pain or extra-ocular muscle impairment can correspond with posterior fossa involvement [27].

MB typically develops in the midline, within the vermis; however, paediatric MB is also characterised by growth into the fourth ventricle [28]. Radiologically, MB is hyperdense on CT but hypointense on T1-W MRI and T2-W MR [29] usually demonstrating homogeneous enhancement with gadolinium administration [30].

2. Neuropsychiatric presentation of brain tumour

Unsurprisingly, a child with a brain tumour rarely presents to a psychiatrist at the manifestation of illness. Nevertheless, neuropsychiatric presentations in children with brain tumours can, and do, come to the attention of psychiatrists, albeit infrequently. The psychiatric and behavioural presenting symptoms of CNS tumours and/or subsequent iatrogenic sequelae include internalising presentations (mood and anxiety disorders), mutism, pseudobulbar symptoms, somatic problems, externalising presentations (such as aggression), eating disorders, psychosis, and hyperkinetic disorders. The clinical course is multi-faceted: the symptoms may appear early as the presenting complaint; later, following a confirmed (tumour) diagnosis; as a complication of anti-neoplastic therapy; or as an 'adjustment disorder'. Nevertheless, there is a relative paucity of studies that describe the neuropsychiatric symptoms associated with this cohort of patients [26].A literature review was conducted by Zyrianova et al. [26] to address childhood CNS tumour presentations of a 'neuropsychiatric' nature; the many possible combinations of symptoms—from psychiatric to physical/neurological—largely depended on the location and extent of the tumour [26]. Interestingly, the location of the lesion strongly correlated to neuropsychiatric prognosis. Supratentorial, right-sided cerebellar and vermal lesions all demonstrated the poorest outcomes [31–34]. Specifically, lesions of the vermis were associated with dysregulation of affect [33].

In certain cases, neurobehavioural disorders are known to increase the risk of developing a childhood brain tumour. For example, children with Autism Spectrum Disorder are more likely than the general paediatric population to develop a CNS malignancy [34]. Furthermore, mere behavioural (and 'mental') symptoms existed pre-morbidly in a quarter of children with a subsequent diagnosis of thalamic tumours in a case series [35]. A retrospective case note review of 200 children with brain tumours demonstrated that neurological symptoms (present in 88% of patients) were only twice as common as 'educational or behavioural problems'; moreover, the latter represented the initial presentation in 10% of cases [36].

2.1. Case series

There are no large-scale studies that specifically assess the presenting symptoms of childhood brain tumours in a psychiatric context. Nevertheless, several case reports/small case series have highlighted specific psychiatric symptoms that heralded a brain cancer, as follows:

- An intracranial germinoma presented in an adolescent male as a first episode psychosis. This followed a 3-month history of negative symptoms, daytime somnolence, 'distorted thought processes' and memory loss; the only positive symptoms were 'sporadic visual sensations' at the edge of the visual field [37].

- A left temporal lobe tumour presented as psychosis in an 18-year-old girl. It was characterised by withdrawal, paranoia, ideas of reference and derealisation. Of note, her neurological examination had been normal [38].
- A case series of three paediatric patients illustrated cerebral malignancies which had imitated neuropsychiatric diagnoses, namely one case of Giles de la Tourette Syndrome(GTS) and two cases of obsessive-compulsive disorder (OCD) [39]. The first patient, initially diagnosed at 18 months with a malignant hypothalamic tumour (with local spread), developed vocal and facial tics in childhood. Surgery successfully resolved the tics; nevertheless, compulsions, such as 'rocking', 'skin picking' and hyperphagia emerged post-operatively. The second case, parietal malignancy in a male child, was heralded by a worsening of a pre-morbid obsessive-compulsive syndrome, although eye signs and seizures ultimately developed. The third case, a 4-year-old boy with pre-morbid diagnoses of OCD, GTS and attention deficit hyperactivity disorder (ADHD), developed a severe depressive illness and worsening ('incapacitating') motor and verbal tics prior to a diagnosis of midbrain glioma.
- Anorexia, including cognitive distortions—'feeling fat and ugly'—preceded the diagnosis of a 'lobular mass within the pituitary fossa' in a 14-year-old girl. Although she had demonstrated possible seizure activity (i.e., 'eyes would roll back into her head' and 'staring' were reported), the patient had initially presented to an eating disorder specialist unit [40]. Of note, a review article in 2005 described 54 previously published case reports about 'eating disorders in brain damage' (the majority of these cases were brain tumours) [41]. Many of these cases, among all age groups, described the typical presentation of an eating disorder, i.e., the classic behaviours and expected cognitions. However, almost all the subjects had co-existing positive neurological signs and/or complications, including headache, seizures, visual impairment, diabetes insipidus and hypopituitarism.

2.2. Posterior fossa syndromes

Of particular relevance to neuropsychiatrists are lesions within the posterior fossa (PF), a portion of the intracranial cavity that contains the cerebellum and brainstem. Over half of childhood tumours are located in the PF [42]. These lesions account for the largest number of cancer deaths in children and may initially present with neuropsychiatric signs and symptoms [43]. Within the PF, in addition to the co-ordination of balance and motor functions, the cerebellum has a role in functions such as cognition, emotion and language [44]. Indeed, the independent role of the cerebellum in higher order brain function is expansive: internal architecture and wide connectivity co-ordinate and integrate this crucial regulation of neuropsychiatric functions. Such orchestration is only possible due to the cerebellum's connections to prefrontal cortex, subcortical limbic structures, and catecholamine-containing brainstem nuclei [45]. Similarly, the brainstem—once almost exclusively known for its involvement in vital functions (breathing, heart rate, sleeping)—is increasingly recognised for affective and cognitive functioning. A recent critical review of the literature published (between 1950 and 2012) on the affective and cognitive symptoms that follow brainstem lesion has revealed neuropsychiatric symptoms in almost half the cases: apathy, emotional lability, irritability, mania, executive dysfunction, memory impairment, and inattention were among the symptoms listed; moreover, the authors hypothesised that the brainstem constitutes an inherent part of the cerebello-cerebral network that subserves cognition and affect. Therefore, isolated brainstem damage can cause symptoms that resemble the cerebellar cognitive affective syndrome (CCAS) [46]. Furthermore, children with midline tumours with brainstem invasion are at increased risk of posterior fossa syndrome (PFS) [47].

Of note, CCAS consists of neuropsychological and lingusitic deficits but does not include verbal mutism or neurological/motor symptoms. Conversely, posterior fossa syndrome (PFS) is a sprawling spectrum of neuropsychological, neurological and lingusitic symptoms [47]. Thus, lesions in the brainstem, but mostly those involving the fourth ventricle and cerebellum – or their surgical removal – can engender a variety of clinical outcomes. Confusingly, the literature has a formidable tapestry of definitions. Excluding both CCAS and 'Cerebellar Syndrome' (i.e. isolated cereballar signs), it is 'Cerellar Mutism' (a verbal mutism also known as 'Transient Cerebellar Mutism' or TCM) that is the defining hallmark of the relevant post-operative syndromes: (the aforementioned) Posterior Fossa Syndrome (PFS); the less expanisive 'Cerebellar Mutism Syndrome' (CMS) – which is limited to mutism, ataxia, hypophonia and irritability; and finally, the self-explanatory 'Mutism and Subsequent Dysarthri'a (MSD). Importantly all of the aforementioned syndromes (i.e. CM or TCM, CMS, CCAS, MSD and Cerebellar syndrome) are subsumed by the term Posterior Fossa Syndrome, i.e. they can be a presentation of PFS (**Figure 3**) [48].

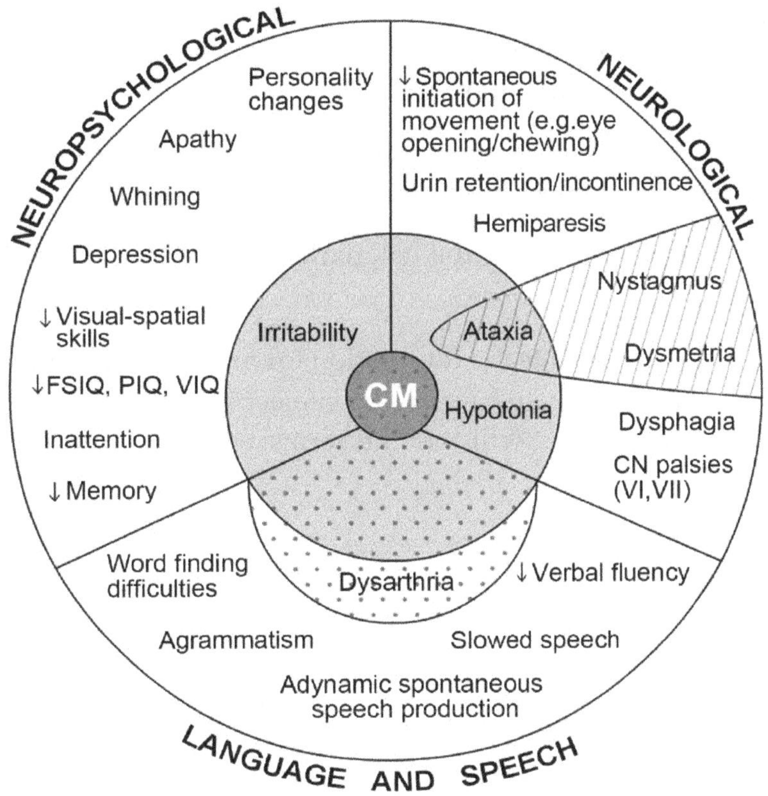

Figure 3. Symptomatic spectrum and relationship between the PFS, CCAS and related conditions. Adapted with permission from the Posterior Fossa Society [48]. Entire Figure = PFS, Left Half (Excluding CM) = CCAS, Inner Circle (Light Grey) = CMS, Dotted Area = MSD, Core (Dark Grey) = CM or TCM, Stripped Area = Cerebellar Signs or Cerebellar Syndrome.

The reader is also informed that in 2016 a new definition, 'Post-operative pediatric CMS' (POP-CMS), was devised by experts ('Iceland Delphi group') in the feld: "Post-operative pediatric cerebellar mutism syndrome is characterized by delayed onset mutism/*reduced speech* and emotional lability after cerebellar or 4th ventricle tumour surgery in children. Additional common features include hypotonia and oropharyngeal dysfunction/dysphagia. It may frequently be accompanied by the *cerebellar motor syndrome, cerebellar cognitive affective syndrome* and brain stem dysfunction including long tract signs and cranial neuropathies. The mutism is always transient, but recovery from CMS may be prolonged. Speech and language may not return to normal, and other deficits of cognitive, affective and motor function often persist"[49].

The Posterior Fossa Society has provided further guidance for clinicians when following this definition:

1. *Reduced speech*: "speech production that is severely reduced and limited to single words or short sentences that can only be elicited after vigorous stimulation".

2. *Cerebellar motor syndrome*: "impairment of gait (ataxia), extremity coordination (dysmetria), disordered eye movements, poor articulation (dysarthria), impaired swallowing (dysphagia) and tremor".

3. *Cerebellar cognitive affective syndrome*: "a pattern of behavioural abnormalities that includes impairments of executive function (planning, set-shifting, abstract reasoning, verbal fluency, working memory), often with perseveration, distractibility or inattention; visual-spatial disorganization and impaired visual-spatial memory; personality change with blunting of affect or disinhibited and inappropriate behaviour; and difficulties with language production including dysprosodia, agrammatism and mild anomia".

4. *Long tract signs*: "symptoms such as urinary retention/incontinence and hemiparesis, which are frequently observed in this patient population" [48].

Of note, like many of its predecessors, the hallmark of POP-CMS is CM (see discussion on CM below).

POP-CMS as a definition represents the foundation for more consistent research. However, its validity requires more testing and it may be subject to further revision. Therefore, for the remainder of the chapter, we will use the terms which are more established in the literature.

2.3. Cerebellar mutism

The term 'cerebellar mutism' refers to a muteness which results from lesions of the cerebellum as opposed to the cerebrum or lower cranial nerves. A severe dysregulation of volitional motor functions of speech creates a recognizable clinical signature: an absence of speech (verbal mutism) is seen, rather than an absence of non-verbal sounds (i.e. whining, laughter, crying) [49]. Although most commonly seen after resection of posterior fossa tumours, there are reports of non-surgical cases of paediatric CM, including trauma, vascular incidents, infections and inflammatory syndromes [48, 50, 51]. CM has been reported to resolve after as little as 6 days or as long as 52 months [52]. Indeed, a hallmark of CM is its idiosyncratic temporality: the onset is typically delayed, often emerging 24–48 hours post-operatively. The duration is variable, albeit self-limiting and usually resolving in weeks; the resolution often occurs rapidly, i.e. over days. However, many patients experience dysarthria throughout the recovery period and then suffer long-term speech and language dysfunction; this includes ataxic dysarthria, dysfluency and slowed speech rate [26]. Crucially, the duration of CM (i.e., whether 4 weeks or 4 months) will correlate with the functional prognosis. An absence of speech after PF tumour surgery was first described as "akinetic mutism" (AM) by Daly and Love in 1958 following the removal of a cerebellar tumour in a child [53]. However, a 1985 case series reporting on six children with cerebellar lesions is credited for the first reports of CM [54]. A complete absence of speech and up to 3 months of dysarthria was described following each posterior fossa craniectomy ('or a complication thereof'). The authors concluded that 'transient muteness may result from acute bilateral cerebellar injury' [55].

Since then, over 400 cases of CM have been reported in the literature. Law et al. [52] compared three groups of children—PF tumours with CM, PF tumours without CM, and healthy controls—to examine the clinical and neuroanatomical predictors of CM. The results of this study concluded that there was a statistically significant positive correlation between tumour size and the likelihood of developing CM. It also found that a greater proportion of children with CM were left-handed, compared to those without CM. However, medulloblastoma and/or brainstem invasion appear to pose the greatest risk of CM, while cerebellar hemisphere involvement is associated with highest risk of permanent motor and non-motor-speech related deficits [54]

In 2011, Di Rocco et al. [56] carried out a study on 34 children with PF tumours with the aim of determining whether there was a correlation between pre-operative language impairment (PLI) and post-operative development of CM. In their study, 11 out of 34 children had PLI; all 11 of these patients were among the subjects that ultimately developed CM (20.6%). Other pre-operative findings in this study included behavioural disorders (sleep, hyperkinetic and somatic complaints). As well as a number of neuropsychological deficits [56]. The children with pre-operative behavioural problems continued to experience these difficulties post-operatively. The primary status of CM as a neuro-surgical sequela is thought to be due to bilateral perturbation of the dentate nuclei and their efferent pathway. As we will discuss, the pathophysiological mechanisms of delayed onset and resolution of CM are hypothesised to be due to axonal damage, oedema, perfusional defects and metabolic disturbances [54].

In 1994, Crutchfield et al. [57] were the first to appreciate the role of the dentato-thalamo-cortical (DTC) pathway as an anatomical substrate in CM. They illustrated a phenomenon called bilateral crossed cerebello-cerebral diaschisis (BCCCD): a cerebellar lesion causes a lack of excitatory impulses from the cerebellum and hypoperfusion, decreased oxygen consumption, hypometabolism and functional inhibition subsequently occur in anatomically connected supratentorial structures [58].

Essentially, symmetrical dentate nuclei that are located in the paravermal regions of lobules VI and VII of the cerebellum give rise to a cerebello-cerebral connection (see **Figure 4**), a complex

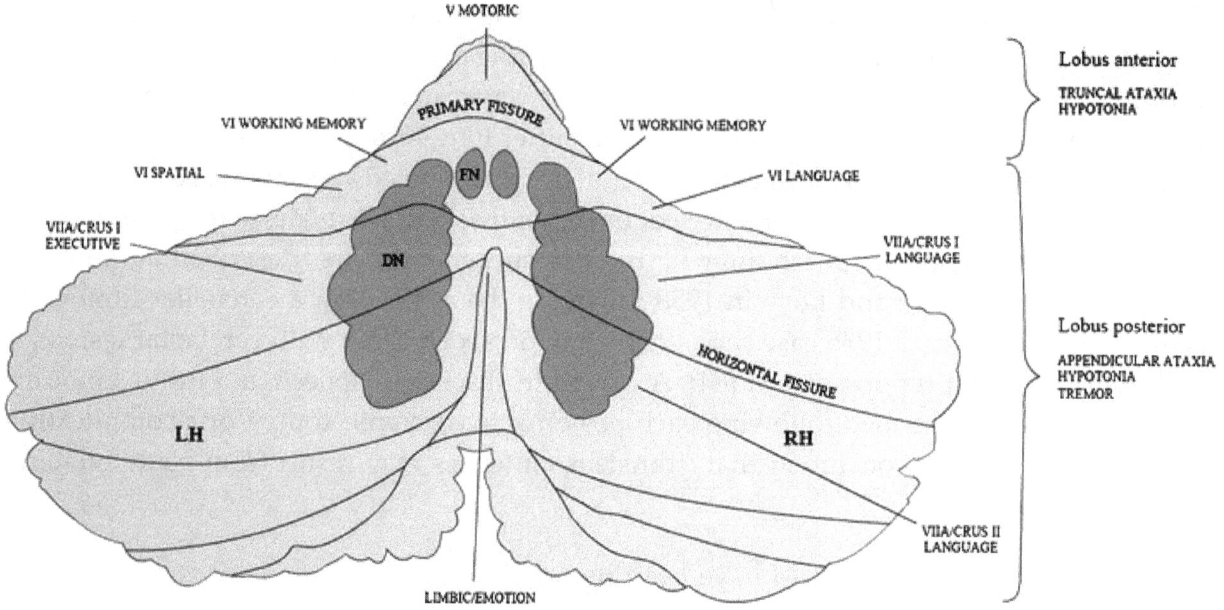

Figure 4. The topographic arrangement of functions in and around the vermis, dentate and fastigial nuclei. Language is lateralised to the right cerebellar hemisphere, executive functions and spatial processing to the left hemisphere and limbic/emotional functions to the vermis. Lesions of the anterior lobe result in truncal ataxia and hypotonia, while lesion of the posterior lobe result in appendicular ataxia, hypotonia and tremor. DN = dentate nucleus, FN = fastigial nucleus, LH = left hemisphere, RH = right hemisphere. Reprinted with permission from Gudrunardottir et al. [54].

system required for initiating voluntary movement and higher cognitive functions, including speech [54]. A literature review by Gudrunardottir et al. [54] highlights evidence that bilateral lesions of the dentate nuclei and their connections (i.e., a bilateral interruption of the DTC pathway) are the principal causes of CM [59–62].

Under normal circumstances, the cerebral cortex and cerebellum are in circuit via afferent and efferent signalling. Impulses originating within the cerebral cortex travel along axons via the cortico-ponto-cerebellar pathway to deliver input to the cerebellum, i.e., ultimately synapsing on the Purkinje cell layer of the cerebellum. Axons from these neurons form inhibitory synapses on the deep cerebellar nuclei, from which excitatory projections carry efferent signals travel throughout the CNS—to the spinal cord, brainstem and cerebral cortex—i.e., areas known for co-ordination of movement. The efferent pathway which finally communicates with the cerebral cortex is the DTC pathway. The tract is comprised of axons originating within the dentate nuclei (DN). The DN act as relay stations and send efferent signals back to the cerebral cortex via the DTC pathway; this tract travels through the ipsilateral superior cerebellar peduncle, and after decussation in the midbrain tegmentum, synapses within the contralateral ventrolateral nucleus of the thalamus. From the thalamus, second order axons terminate in the primary motor cortex as well as secondary and tertiary association areas within the frontal and parietal lobes. Thus, via the DTC pathway/tract, cognition and behaviour are likely modulated, a theory supported by the cognitive, linguistic and behavioural-affective impairments seen with an injury of the cerebellum and/or proximal DTC tract [63, 64].

Indeed, it is this vulnerable (i.e., peri-operatively) efferent white matter DTC tract that, if damaged, may be responsible for CM: therefore, any direct (i.e., trauma) or indirect (i.e., oedema) circulatory disturbance may cause hypoperfusion and metabolic related hypofunction in both cerebellar hemispheres, and a loss of function (diaschisis) in the areas mediated by the DTP [65]. CM thus results from a lesion anywhere along this path: bilateral thalamotomies; SMA lesions; bilateral oedema in the brachium pontis; and finally, superior cerebellar peduncles are also potential lesions. Nevertheless, bilateral injury to the dentate nuclei is the most frequently implicated cause [54].

Clinically, anatomical correlates of cerebellar lesions are relatively distinct: anterior lesions cause ataxia and hypotonia; while those in the posterior induce appendicular ataxia, hypotonia and tremor [66] (see **Figure 4**). The origin of the hemiparesis and lower cranial nerve dysfunction seen in the PFS is not known, although brainstem injury and/or damage to the dentate nuclei/DTC pathway are hypothesised [54]. In addition to its role in balance and co-ordination, the cerebellum is integral to higher cognitive processses (the cerebellar hemispheres) and regulation of affect (the vermis) [66]. The left cerebellar hemisphere is designated spatial and executive responsibility, and the right is tasked with language [64, 67]. The disruption between the right cerebellum and left frontal cortex likely contributes to the linguistic difficulties observed in CM. Interestingly, a study also found that all left-handed patients with MB had a 100% risk of developing CM post-operatively. It is possible that such correlates will pave the way for pre-op clinical profiles to inform post-operative rehabilitation, across the allied health spectrum [68]. As discussed, the dentate nuclei, the vermis, and the right cerebellar hemisphere are all important in cognitive performance; accordingly, damage to these structures, informed by MRI, can be used to predict the degree of post-operative neurological and neuropsychological impairment in children following PF tumour resection [69].

Of note, mutism that occurs immediately after surgery is indicative of bulbar dysfuction from damage to cranial nerve nuclei in the nuclie, rather than CM [70]. However, in typical CM, 'secondary processes' initiated by the tumour resection, are the likely underlying pathophysiological mechanism, and four have been described in literature: (1) dynamic perfusional disturbances, (2) oedema, (3) transient disturbances in neurotransmitter release, and (4) axonal injury.

First, dynamic perfusional disturbances in the cerebellum and the cerebrum are suspected causes of CM due to the delayed onset (i.e., possible vasospasms), type of disturbance (i.e., transient ischemia) and resolution (i.e., normalisation of blood flow). Surgical manipulation of the cerebellum [71], intra-operative coagulation of perforating vessels [72] and arterial embolic occlusion [73] are the suspected catalysts of such disturbances; cerebello-cerebral diaschisis is implicated when the proximal DTC pathway is damaged [54]. In fact, two small single proton emission computed tomography (SPECT) studies demonstrated a cerebellar hypoperfusion in mute patients which resolved as speech returned [72, 73]. Two other possible mechanisms of recovery are neuronal plasticity and reassignment of speech function within the cortical processing network.

Secondly, the latency of CM reflects post-operative swelling, with imaging studies (CT, MRI and DTI) demonstrating mutism occurring with bilateral oedema in the superior cerebellar peduncles and/or the pons or mesencephalon after PF tumour resection. Indeed, corticosteroids may prove useful in the context of this mechanism. Thirdly, dysregulation of neurotransmitter release has been postulated by Siffert et al. [74] in their concept that the cerebellum and its connections are tantamount to a 'modulatory system', controlling motor and non-motor functions. Finally, imaging studies imply that pathogenesis of CM could be from surgical manipulation, traction and release of tumour compression, resulting in axonal distortion and/or injury [63, 75].

CM risk is increased by several tumour-related factors: brainstem involvement [76]; (iatrogenic) brainstem compression; and midline (vermal and fourth ventricle) location [77]—i.e., MB is by far the most common cause of CM in the paediatric population. To illustrate this, two large studies found that the incidence of CM in children with medulloblastoma was 24% [78], and 44% if brainstem was involved [76]. Radical tumour removal [77] and young age at diagnosis [76] have inconsistent evidence [78], although some reports these as risk factors for CM [79]. Conversely, theories such as hydrocephalus, post-operative CNS infection (like meningitis), gender, length of vermal incision, type of neurosurgeon (paediatric vs. adult) and oedema/swelling have been refuted over recent years [80].

The prognosis and course of recovery in CM is variable, albeit largely unfavourable, even in spite of the resolution of mutism: two-thirds of patients will still suffer motor-speech deficits even after 12 months [81]; one-third will have persistent dysarthria; the remainder show a residual phonological impairment (including adynamic spontaneous speech production, impaired verbal fluency, word-finding difficulties and grammatical disturbances) [58]. Dysarthric features are more protracted and less amenable to recovery in children with associated combined procedural memory and defective neurocognitive functions present at diagnosis.

With regards preventing CM, surgical mitigation is a possibility: piecemeal removal (to protect the vermis) [82]; sparing of (cognitively significant) right cerebellar hemisphere [69], and finally, using a specific (telovelar) approach to access the fourth ventricle and avoid splitting the vermis [83]. In support of this approach, a series of telovelar cases showed no incidence of mutism; splitting the vermis reduced rates in one hospital and at another site similar surgical practices (e.g., less aggressive retraction) resulted in fewer cases of CM [84, 85].

2.4. Posterior fossa syndrome

Once regarded as an isolated deficit, CM is now well recognised as the predominant feature of the more expansive 'posterior fossa syndrome' (PFS; see below). Although CM and PFS appear to have separate anatomical substrates, topographical proximity ensures posterior fossa surgery can result in any combination of the shared phenomena.

In the relevant literature, across almost four decades, CM has been confused with other terms, including TCM, CMS [86] and MSD [87]. Furthermore, some authors use two or more of these terms interchangeably, including CM and PFS [48].

The essence of PFS is the constellation of four core symptoms: mutism, ataxia, behavioural disturbance and emotional lability; they occur in about 25% of children after the surgical resection of a posterior fossa tumour (**Figure 5**).

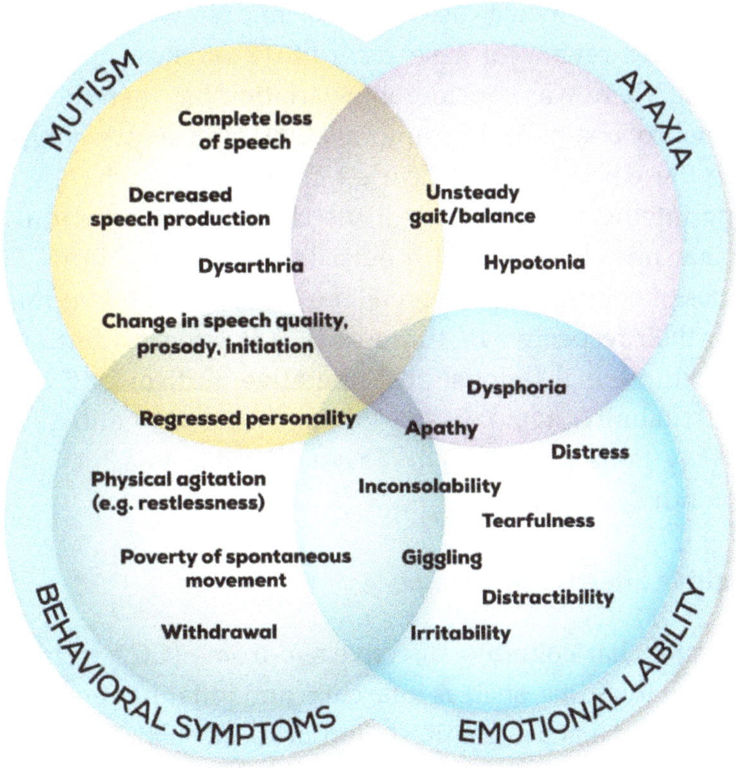

Figure 5. Posterior fossa syndrome. Reprinted with permission from Lanier et al. [84].

2.5. Posterior fossa syndrome cases

In a review of PFS, Lanier and Abrahams [88] summarised proposed theories/risk facors for PFS: 1. involvement of the vermis, 2. brainstem involvement, 3. bilateral edema within the cerebellar peduncles post surgery, 4.aggressive surgery of the cerebellum, 5. transient impairment of the DTC pathways, 6. midline location of the tumor, 7. focal vasospasms, 8. neurotransmitter dysfunction and 9. hydrocephalus. As expected, most overlap with those already discussed with regards to CM. These authors also presented a case series of PFS from their own institution, the Massachussetts General Hospital for Children. Three cases of resected medulloblastoma are described with regards boys aged 7–13 years. Post-operatively, two of the four cases suffered from mutism and another two cases had paucity of speech (e.g. monosyllabic) and dysarthria, respectively. All four cases had evidence of ataxia, emotional lability and behavioural symptoms. Of the mutism cases, both fully resolved with complete return of speech and good emotional stability; however, both had ongoing ataxia and one later died of a tumour recurrence. The third case (post-op paucity of speech) had screaming episodes with "screeching" and subsequently developed depression. At follow-up 5 years later, although in school he continued to have social and emotional difficulties. The final case (post-op dysarthria) initially had serious emotional dyscontrol with self-harming behaviour; this resolved with low dose risperidone. At her 5 year follow-up, she had no speech or behavioural issues, although balance remained problematic. Of note, three of these cases required psychotropic medication (low dose risperidone or lorazepam) to manage the emotional lability and behavioural issues.

In 1995, Pollack et al. [89] described a case series of children with open resection of infratentorial tumours. Following review of case records, 12 of these patients manifested with post-operative mutism. There was considerable variation between the clinical presentation, (i.e., pseudobulbar, neurobehavioural symptoms); however, a "stereotypical response" was observed in 11 cases; these patients were "curled up in bed and whining inconsolably, without actually uttering intelligible speech". All the children achieved full recovery within 4 months of surgery, bar one exception with persistent mild dysarthria. This finding is supported by a case series of children with cerebellar astrocytoma and vermal lesions who were surgically treated for their respective PF tumours [90]. Positive findings were seen in a number of the children with vermal lesions: post-operative mutism in six; behavioural disturbances in five, e.g., irritability, avoidance of others; and severe autistic behaviours in one. Similar to the study by Pollack et al. [89], almost all subjects achieved full or almost full recovery within a month.

2.6. Cerebellar cognitive affective syndrome

Another syndrome, cerebellar cognitive affective syndrome (CCAS), has been reported following acquired cerebellar lesions, such as infarction and inflammation [91, 92]. Some authors consider PFS to represent the acute manifestation of CCAS [92]. CCAS is primarily characterised by a deficit in emotional regulation that causes personality change; thus, a flattening or blunting of affect, and disinhibited/inappropriate behaviour are commonly seen. The syndrome also manifests as impairment of executive function (planning, set-shifting, verbal fluency, abstract reasoning and working memory difficulties) and visuospatial cognition. Finally, language deficits, including agrammatism and dysprosody are recognised features. This syndrome, described originally by Schmahmann et al. [93], is neurobiologically underpinned by the cerebellar organisation of higher order function, and more specifically, the associated modulatory role in mental and social function, operative early in childhood [26]. Hopyan et al. [91] compared cognitive control of emotions in cerebellar tumours against healthy matched controls. In their study, they tested the ability to identify happy and sad emotions in music. Contrary to their hypothesis, this study demonstrated largely normal emotional identification in both groups, but the control group performed better at emotional regulation tasks. The fact that in the study, childhood acquired cerebellar tumours disrupted cognitive control of emotion, rather than identification of emotion, provides support for a hypothesis of CCAS as a disorder not so much of emotion, but more so the regulation of emotion by cognition. A case series of 19 patients with cerebellar lesions also succeeded in illustrating cases of emotional dyscontrol in cerebellar tumours: an acute syndrome of inattention, dysphoria and emotional distress followed surgery of midline PF [92].

A case series by Hargrave et al. [94] described a slightly different manifestation of emotional dyscontrol in paediatric patients (aged 3–11) with pontine glioma. In 36% of the cases, outbursts of inappropriate laughter (i.e., "pathological laughter") were observed in wakefulness and sleep. Of note, symptoms improved in all cases following treatment but often returned in cases of tumour recurrence. Beckwitt-Turkel et al. [95] compared PFS symptoms before and after paediatric PF surgery in a naturalistic study. PFS was associated with midline and vermis involvement (and not lateral involvement) and was characterised by mutism, apathy and dysphoria. These symptoms presented early post-operatively, although affective and behavioural disturbances appeared at a later stage, with all symptoms, bar depression, resolving over time. In 2010, Larysz et al. [96] looked at a group of 34 children (mean age 12.3 years) with PF tumours (14 cerebellar, 20 extracerebellar) to establish whether neuropsychological deficits related to tumour location: neoplasms in the brainstem and vermis had a better outcome than those in the cerebellum. This finding was consistent with Riva et al. [97] whose sample showed an association between non-vermal tumours with language dysfunction; in the same sample, vermal tumours were more likely to present with neurobehavioural changes (emotional lability, irritability, weepiness, impulsiveness and shyness).

2.7. Psychological and adjustment disorder

In 2013, an article published by Pastore et al. [98] compared the neuropsychological profiles and behavioural symptoms in pre-school children with brain lesions: 18 of the 55 patients were brain tumour survivors and the remainder had traumatic, vascular or infectious lesions. The brain tumour group had high levels of internalising problems (77.8%); specifically, a combination of anxiety and/or depression and/or somatic symptoms and withdrawal were present in about half of the sample. However, the group with traumatic brain injury and non-cancerous brain lesions presented with externalising behaviours and aggression. These findings are consistent with those from a study of paediatric brain tumour survivors, in which the child behaviour checklist indicated that internalising behaviours (depression/anxiety) were the most common (48.4%) psychological disorder, while externalising behaviours were present in just 11.8%. Furthermore, those aged 7–13 were most predisposed to psychological problems, whereas social maladjustment was more frequent in those older than 13. These findings were relevant as they indicated the long-term psychosocial outcome of these individuals [99].

Campen et al. [100] found a high rate of depression and adjustment disorders (30.4%) in 56 children treated for MB, particularly if they were older and male. Importantly, the multimodal therapy in MB—which is generally a protracted process—influences the neurodevelopmental maturation that is implicated in the pathogenesis of depression. Therefore, their low mood is not just explainable as an expected psychological burden; rather, it is also engendered by neurobiological mechanisms such as a disruption of hippocampal cell formation and the saturation of the limbic system. Therefore, Campen et al. found a significant difference in age at diagnosis between those who developed depression, anxiety and adjustment disorder (median 9.5 years) and those who did not (median 5.9 years), with a median time to first psychiatric symptom of 7 months. Similarly, a study of children treated for craniopharyngioma highlighted a high rate of psychiatric morbidity in the study population; 100% of subjects experienced depression; 75% suffered poor frustration tolerance and 40% had anger dyscontrol [22]. Likewise, a case series of 20 subjects described poor neurobehavioural outcomes in post-operative paediatric craniopharyngioma: 85% of subjects had some degree of internalising (apathy, poor motivation) and externalising (irritability, hyperactivity, aggression) behaviour, as well as neuropsychological deficits, social maladjustment and poor school performance [23]. Finally, a study of paediatric and adult survivors of childhood brain tumours in 2013 revealed that more than 1 in 10 had reported suicidal ideation on at least one occasion, as documented in their medical records. The older patients, with greater co-morbidities (i.e., seizure disorder) were at highest risk [24].

2.8. Clinical guidelines

Around 9000 new primary brain and CNS tumours (CNST) are diagnosed every year in the UK, suggesting that a GP will diagnose a case every 3–5 years. Presenting complaints range from well recognised symptoms (i.e., headaches, new-onset seizures) to the more insidious, such as personality change. A combined retrospective and prospective study of 104 consecutive paediatric patients with brain tumours found that the median time from symptom onset to diagnosis was 3 months. However, diagnosis of CNST (whether primary or secondary) can be performed with the GP retaining clinical responsibility, i.e., ordering necessary diagnostic neuro-imaging tests [101].

'NICE alert symptoms' (e.g., neurological, headache, fatigue, back pain, bruising, lymphadenopathy, lump/mass/swelling, urinary symptoms, hepatosplenomegaly) and any new pattern of recurrent attendances to the GP are ominous warning signs for childhood CNST [102]. Ansell et al. [103] advised that 'the key to identifying the one child among many who merits prompt investigation is recognition of unusual symptoms, or specific symptom patterns'; these included head tilt, odd head movements, odd posture, back or neck stiffness and unsteadiness without obvious cause [103]. In concert with clinical acumen and intuition, the GP must respect the value of a parent's instinct that their child 'is not right', regardless of a specific problem *per se* [104].

The 2015 NICE guidelines, entitled 'Suspected Cancer: Recognition and Referral', features a section on 'Brain and CNS cancer' that informs clinicians about which specific symptoms in children and adolescents require investigation and/or neuro-oncological referral. Based on these symptoms, the positive predictive values (PPV) of having CNST varied in range: from <0.013% (for vomiting or headache, with loss of appetite) to 0.15 (for vomiting, in combination with unsteadiness) for patients aged 0–14 years old; and, from 0% (for primary headache) to 0.03% (for undifferentiated headache) for patients aged 5–17 years; and from 0.0029% (for pain) to 0.0238% (for seizure) for patients aged 15–24 years [101].

Adult referral was recommended for those symptoms with a PPV of 3% or above, i.e., the advantages of a suspected CNST pathway referral outweighed any disadvantages. However, in childhood cancer, such a threshold was deemed too stringent for the following reasons: (1) the high levels of treatability of these cancers, (2) early diagnosis can reduce mortality and morbidity, and (3) the number of life-years gained.

Referral at lower levels of risk than 3% is therefore permitted in children and adolescents. Accordingly, GPs/physicians/psychiatrists 'should consider a very urgent referral (for an appointment within 48 h) for a suspected brain or central nervous system cancer in children and young people with newly abnormal cerebellar or other central neurological function'. Furthermore, referral should be for urgent specialist assessment (and not a cancer pathway) in order to circumnavigate any issues with weekend cover, differences in local service configuration, etc.

The guidelines point out that trade-off between net health benefits and resource utilisation are not supported by published economic analysis. It is likely that the above recommendations will result in an increase in MRI scanning with a subsequent reduction in GP attendance, because of fast-tracking medical clearance or diagnosis. In fact, the guidelines predict that such action will actually constitute a small decrease in overall costs [101].

An evidence-based clinical guideline, 'Diagnosis of Brain Tumours in Children', was developed in 2010 by Wilne et al. [105]; it was informed by a systematic literature review, meta-analysis and cohort study [36]. As a result, six main categories of symptoms were identified: headache, nausea and vomiting, visual abnormalities, motor abnormalities, growth, development and behavioural abnormalities. Within the category of behavioural symptoms, lethargy and withdrawal were important neuropsychiatric signs of childhood CNS tumours. The importance of lethargy in diagnosing paediatric CNST has been highlighted by other studies [106, 107]. In fact, the prominence of lethargy in a series of 'sudden death from obstructive hydrocephalus due to intracranial lesions' prompted the authors to conclude that persistent lethargy should be considered a neurological symptom instead of a non-specific clinical sign [108].

The relevance of such symptoms in childhood CNST was also highlighted by an earlier study by Wilne et al. [36], in which 'behavioural and educational' symptoms were the presenting feature of brain tumours in children in 10% of cases, and were apparent in 44% of the patients. The behavioural symptoms included: lethargy (majority), irritability, personality change, aggression and emotional lability; and the educational symptoms included deterioration in reading and writing (majority), memory difficulty, poor concentration, global deterioration and decrease in school attendance.

Nevertheless, lethargy remains an unspecific symptom with many faces: it is prominent among physical syndromes relating to malignancy, infection, and inflammation; it is also a core psychiatric symptom in both affective (i.e., depression) and psychotic disorders (i.e., negative syndrome of schizophrenia). Despite such diagnostic opaqueness, the guidelines produced by Wilne et al. [105]—which recommend CNS imaging if lethargy or withdrawal persists for 4 weeks or more—have demonstrated promising results in initial UK studies. These successes include a reduction in median symptom interval, time between symptom onset, and ultimately, the diagnosis of brain tumours in children [105].

In addition to knowledge about when to suspect a brain tumour, it is important for those practicing in primary and secondary care to be familiar with the most comprehensive and current guidelines for childhood neuropsychiatric presentation of brain tumours, as outlined below [26].

3. Summary

3.1. Red flags

Recommendations for detecting malignancy in a childhood neuropsychiatric case:

- Childhood cancer is rare and may present initially with symptoms and signs associated with common conditions, e.g., headache, nausea and vomiting. Repeated presentation with the same problem and with no clear diagnosis should raise the suspicion and facilitate further assessment and referral.
- Psychiatric symptoms are best to be considered dynamically and in combination with other signs and symptoms that are listed here. It is very rare for a childhood cranial malignancy to present with only psychiatric symptoms.
- Common psychiatric symptoms:
  - internalising behaviour,
  - withdrawal,
  - social problems,
  - somatic complaints,
  - externalising problems,
  - depression and/or anxiety
  - hyperactivity.
- Rare psychiatric symptoms:
  - eating disorder and
  - first episode of psychosis.
- Also watch for:
  - atypical psychiatric symptoms,
  - unexplained behavioural and/or mood changes,
  - unexplained deteriorating school performance or developmental milestones,
  - personality change,
  - disinhibited or inappropriate behaviour,
  - pathological laughter,
  - emotional lability,

- especially emotional reactions disproportionate to significance or severity of trigger,
- flattening or blunting of affect,
- impairment of working memory,
- agrammatism and dysprosody of speech,
- impaired executive function and
- poor attention.

- Psychiatric symptoms (including behavioural) with a headache (i.e., advised to directly enquire about presence of a headache) constitute a red flag. Persistent headache that can occur at any time of the day or night requires a neurological examination. Younger children and those with communication difficulties may not be able to report headache, thus watch for behavioural representation, e.g., pointing at, holding or squeezing head.
- Headache and vomiting that cause early morning waking or occur on awakening are classical signs of raised intracranial pressure and an immediate referral should be made. In cases of persistent vomiting, exclude pregnancy where appropriate. Psychiatric symptoms (including behavioural) with neurological signs warrants a neurological examination. However, a normal neurological examination does not exclude a brain tumour.
- Neurological and motor symptoms:
  - new-onset seizures—including focal (with/without loss of awareness) and generalised onset
  - altered consciousness,
  - cranial nerve abnormalities,
  - regression in motor skills,
  - gait abnormalities and/or abnormal motor co-ordination,
  - focal motor weakness and
  - swallowing difficulties.
- Visual symptoms and signs including:
  - papilledema,
  - reduced visual acuity,
  - reduced visual fields,
  - new-onset nystagmus,
  - new-onset paralytic squint,
  - optic atrophy,

  - abnormal fundoscopy
  - proptosis.
- Visual assessment including fundoscopy:
  - acuity,
  - eye movements,
  - pupil responses,
  - visual fields in school age children and older and
  - optic disc appearance.
- Growth and developmental abnormalities:
  - growth failure and
  - delayed, arrested or precocious puberty.
- Diabetes insipidus presenting with polyuria and polydipsia.
- Persistent back pain can be a symptom of cancer.

In children aged younger than 2 years, any of the following symptoms may suggest a CNS tumour and require following:

- Immediate referral:
  - new-onset seizures,
  - bulging fontanelle,
  - extensor attacks and
  - persistent vomiting.
- Urgent referral:
  - abnormal increase in head size,
  - arrest or regression of motor development,
  - altered behaviour,
  - abnormal eye movements,
  - lack of visual following and
  - poor feeding/failure to thrive.
  - Urgency contingent on other factors: squint.

Following the diagnosis

- Screening for internalising problems in children and adolescents with brain tumours.
- Baseline and follow-up screening/assessment for ADHD symptoms prior to treatment
    - Externalising problems are less common than internalising problems but, if missed, will have significant implications for educational abilities.
- In those for whom the symptoms represent an adjustment reaction, there is an improved outcome if a truthful, complete and consistent approach to communication is taken.

When considering posterior fossa tumour resection

- The complication of cerebellar mutism is rarely mentioned to parents during the consent for surgery of a posterior fossa tumour. It is a common syndrome and, reassuringly, to the authors' knowledge there have been no reported cases of a child with cerebellar mutism not returning to some functional speech.

4. Conclusion

The era of molecular informed neuro-oncology has set a foundation for precise diagnosis and tailored anti-neoplastic therapy. Such changes may lead to great improvements in overall survival of paediatric patients and so inadvertently marks an auspicious time for neuropsychiatry, which has never been more relevant. In concert with an optimal medical model, neuropsychiatric informed care is required to ensure a truly holistic and integrated approach. In their ability to weave together so many disparate perspectives—psychiatric, neurological, cognitive, psychosocial and many more—these specialists will be invaluable in leading multidisciplinary rehabilitation programs. Contemporary studies indicate that mood, cognition and psychosocial functioning are important factors in early diagnosis, as well as mediating health outcomes following radical and risk-adapted anti-neoplastic treatment. In addition to psychological burden, the neuropsychiatric aspects of childhood CNS tumours, including posterior fossa syndrome and cerebellar cognitive affective syndrome, are increasingly recognised as crucial causes of poor outcomes. Current research highlights the necessity for routine psychological and psychiatric screenings of children with suspected brain tumours and at follow-up of childhood brain tumour survivors. Thus, we provided a review of the available neuropsychiatric guidelines for identification of brain tumours in primary, secondary and tertiary health services. However, further progress is still required in these areas and in the sphere of public awareness. In the future, neuropsychiatric intervention should aim to complement the anticipated challenges of neuro-oncological management, e.g., a left-handed child treated for medulloblastoma would have intensive neuropsychiatric screening and linguistic rehabilitation.

As our understanding of the neuroscience relevant to childhood neuro-oncology expands, neuropsychiatric input will be invaluable at crucial stages of care, including at time of diagnosis, pre- and post-operatively. Earlier intervention will consolidate a child's resilience through a multi-axial combination of psychometrics, psychoeducation, psychosocial support, psychotherapy and psychopharmacological intervention. Specifically, neuropsychological profiling will enrich the clinical pre-operative prognostication and determine treatment goals post-operatively.

Author details

Alexander Hegarty[1,2] and Yulia Furlong[1,2*]

*Address all correspondence to: alexander.hegarty@health.wa.gov.au

1 Perth Children's Hospital, Perth, WA, Australia

2 University of Western Australia, Crawley, WA, Australia

References

[1] Ostrom QT, Gittleman H, Fulop J, Liu M, Blanda R, Kromer C, et al. CBTRUS statistical report: Primary brain and central nervous system tumors diagnosed in the United States in 2008-2012. Neuro-Oncology. Oxford University Press. 2015;**17**(Suppl 4):iv1-iv62. DOI: 10.1093/neuonc/nov189

[2] Siegel RL, Miller KD, Jemal A. Cancer statistics, 2017. CA: a Cancer Journal for Clinicians. 2017;**67**(1):7-30. DOI: 10.3322/caac.21387

[3] Louis DN, Perry A, Reifenberger G, von Deimling A, Figarella-Branger D, Cavenee WK, et al. The 2016 World Health Organization classification of Tumors of the central nervous system: A summary. Acta Neuropathologica. Springer Berlin Heidelberg. 2016;**131**(6):803-820. DOI: 10.1007/s00401-016-1545-1

[4] Ramkissoon SH, Bandopadhayay P, Hwang J, Ramkissoon LA, Greenwald NF, Schumacher SE, et al. Clinical targeted exome-based sequencing in combination with genome-wide copy number profiling: Precision medicine analysis of 203 pediatric brain tumors. Neuro-Oncology. Oxford University Press. 2017;**19**(7):now294. DOI: 10.1093/neuonc/now294

[5] Komori T. The 2016 WHO classification of tumours of the central nervous system: The major points of revision. Neurologia Medico-Chirurgica (Tokyo). 2017;**57**(7):301-311. DOI: 10.2176/nmc.ra.2017-0010

[6] Reifenberger J, Reifenberger G, Liu L, James CD, Wechsler W, Collins VP. Molecular genetic analysis of oligodendroglial tumors shows preferential allelic deletions on 19q and 1p. The American Journal of Pathology. American Society for Investigative Pathology. 1994; **145**(5):1175-1190

[7] Hartmann C, Meyer J, Balss J, Capper D, Mueller W, Christians A, et al. Type and frequency of IDH1 and IDH2 mutations are related to astrocytic and oligodendroglial differentiation and age: A study of 1,010 diffuse gliomas. Acta Neuropathologica. 2009; **118**(4):469-474. DOI: 10.1007/s00401-009-0561-9

[8] Ichimura K. Molecular pathogenesis of IDH mutations in gliomas. Brain Tumor Pathology. 2012;**29**(3):131-139. DOI: 10.1007/s10014-012-0090-4

[9] Ellison DW, Kocak M, Dalton J, Megahed H, Lusher ME, Ryan SL, et al. Definition of disease-risk stratification groups in childhood medulloblastoma using combined clinical, pathologic, and molecular variables. Journal of Clinical Oncology. 2011;**29**(11):1400-1407. DOI: 10.1200/JCO.2010.30.2810

[10] Taylor MD, Northcott PA, Korshunov A, Remke M, Cho Y-J, Clifford SC, et al. Molecular subgroups of medulloblastoma: The current consensus. Acta Neuropathologica. 2012;**123**(4): 465-472. DOI: 10.1007/s00401-011-0922-z

[11] Wen PY, Kesari S. Malignant gliomas in adults. The New England Journal of Medicine. 2008;**359**(5):492-507. DOI: 10.1056/NEJMra0708126

[12] Bailey P. Medulloblastoma cerebelli. Archives of Neurology and Psychiatry. 1925;**14**(2): 192. DOI: 10.1001/archneurpsyc.1925.02200140055002

[13] Jones DTW, Jäger N, Kool M, Zichner T, Hutter B, Sultan M, et al. Dissecting the genomic complexity underlying medulloblastoma. Nature. 2012;**488**(7409):100-105. DOI: 10.1038/nature11284

[14] Smoll NR, Drummond KJ. The incidence of medulloblastomas and primitive neurectodermal tumours in adults and children. Journal of Clinical Neuroscience. 2012;**19**(11):1541-1544. DOI: 10.1016/j.jocn.2012.04.009

[15] Parsons DW, Li M, Zhang X, Jones S, Leary RJ, Cheng J, et al. The genetic landscape of the childhood cancer medulloblastoma. Science. 2011;**331**(6016):435-439. DOI: 10.1126/science.1198056

[16] Schwalbe EC, Lindsey JC, Nakjang S, Crosier S, Smith AJ, Hicks D, et al. Novel molecular subgroups for clinical classification and outcome prediction in childhood medulloblastoma: A cohort study. The Lancet Oncology. 2017;**18**(17):958-971. DOI: 10.1016/S1470-2045(17)30243-7

[17] Zhao F, Ohgaki H, Xu L, Giangaspero F, Li C, Li P, et al. Molecular subgroups of adult medulloblastoma: A long-term single-institution study. Neuro-Oncology. 2016;**18**(7):982-990. DOI: 10.1093/neuonc/now050

[18] Gajjar A, Pfister SM, Taylor MD, Gilbertson RJ. Molecular insights into pediatric brain tumors have the potential to transform therapy. Clinical Cancer Research. 2014;**20**(22): 5630-5640. DOI: 10.1158/1078-0432

[19] Pizer BL, Clifford SC. The potential impact of tumour biology on improved clinical practice for medulloblastoma: Progress towards biologically driven clinical trials. British Journal of Neurosurgery. 2009;**23**(4):364-375. DOI: 10.1080/02688690903121807

[20] Robinson GW, Orr BA, Wu G, Gururangan S, Lin T, Qaddoumi I, et al. Vismodegib exerts targeted efficacy against recurrent sonic hedgehog–subgroup medulloblastoma: Results from phase II Pediatric brain tumor consortium studies PBTC-025B and PBTC-032. Journal of Clinical Oncology. 2015;**33**(24):2646-2654. DOI: 10.1200/JCO.2014.60.1591

[21] Zhukova N, Ramaswamy V, Remke M, Pfaff E, Shih DJH, Martin DC, et al. Subgroup-specific prognostic implications of *TP53* mutation in medulloblastoma. Journal of Clinical Oncology. 2013;**31**(23):2927-2935. DOI: 10.1200/JCO.2012.48.5052

[22] Kool M, Jones DTW, Jäger N, Northcott PA, Pugh TJ, Hovestadt V, et al. Genome sequencing of SHH medulloblastoma predicts genotype-related response to smoothened inhibition. Cancer Cell. 2014;**25**(3):393-405. DOI: 10.1016/j.ccr.2014.02.004

[23] Pickles JC, Hawkins C, Pietsch T, Jacques TS. CNS embryonal tumours: WHO 2016 and beyond. Neuropathology and Applied Neurobiology. 2017. DOI: 10.1111/nan.12443

[24] Bican O, Pruitt AA. The spinal cord: A review of functional neuroanatomy. Neurologic Clinics. Elsevier. 2013;**31**(1):1-18. DOI: 10.1016/j.ncl.2012.09.009

[25] Raybaud CBA. Intracranial, orbital and neck masses of childhood. In: Barkovich AJRC, editor. Pediatric Neuroimaging. Philadelphia: Lippincott Williams & Wilkins; 2012. pp. 637-807

[26] Zyrianova Y, Alexander L, Faruqui R. Neuropsychiatric presentations and outcomes in children and adolescents with primary brain tumours: Systematic review. Brain Injury. 2016;**30**(1):1-9. DOI: 10.3109/02699052.2015.1075590

[27] Pollack IF, Jakacki RI. Childhood brain tumors: Epidemiology, current management and future directions. Nature Reviews. Neurology. Nature Publishing Group. 2011;**7**(9):495-506. DOI: 10.1038/nrneurol.2011.110

[28] Koci TM, Chiang F, Mehringer CM, Yuh WT, Mayr NA, Itabashi H, et al. Adult cerebellar medulloblastoma: Imaging features with emphasis on MR findings. American Journal of Neuroradiology (AJNR). 1993;**14**(4):929-939

[29] Meyers SP, Kemp SS, Tarr RW. MR imaging features of medulloblastomas. American Journal of Roentgenology. American Public Health Association. 1992;**158**(4):859-865. DOI: 10.2214/ajr.158.4.1546606

[30] Poussaint TY, Panigrahy A, Huisman TAGM. Pediatric brain tumors. Pediatric Radiology. Springer Berlin Heidelberg. 2015;**45**(S3):443-453. DOI: 10.1007/s00247-015-3326-8

[31] Larner AJ. Referral guidelines for suspected central nervous system or brain tumours. Journal of Neurology, Neurosurgery, and Psychiatry. BMJ Publishing Group. 2006;**77**(12): 1305-1306. DOI: 10.1136/jnnp.2005.077453

[32] Fuemmeler BF, Elkin TD, Mullins LL. Survivors of childhood brain tumors: Behavioral, emotional, and social adjustment. Clinical Psychology Review. 2002;**22**(4):547-585. DOI: 10.1016/S0272-7358(01)00120-9

[33] Levisohn L, Cronin-Golomb A, Schmahmann JD. Neuropsychological consequences of cerebellar tumour resection in children: Cerebellar cognitive affective syndrome in a paediatric population. Brain. 2000;**123**(Pt 5):1041-1050

[34] Lumsden DE, Woodthorpe C, Hargrave D, Hedderly TJ. Pre-existing neurodevelopmental and neuropsychiatric difficulties in children with brain tumours: Implications for future outcome studies. Developmental Medicine and Child Neurology. Blackwell Publishing Ltd. 2011;**53**(1):93-93. DOI: 10.1111/j.1469-8749.2010.03822.x

[35] Martínez-Lage JF, Pérez-Espejo MA, Esteban JA, Poza M. Thalamic tumors: Clinical presentation. Child's Nervous System. 2002;**18**:405-411. DOI: 10.1007/s00381-002-0605-0

[36] Wilne SH, Ferris RC, Nathwani A, Kennedy CR. The presenting features of brain tumours: A review of 200 cases. Archives of Disease in Childhood. 2006;**91**(6):502-506. DOI: 10.1136/adc.2005.090266

[37] Undurraga J, Baeza I, Valentí M, Lázaro ML. Brain germinoma presenting as a first psychotic episode in an adolescent male. European Child & Adolescent Psychiatry. 2010; **19**(9):741-742. DOI: 10.1007/s00787-010-0107-7

[38] Zugman A, Pan PM, Gadelha A, Mansur RB, Asevedo E, Cunha GR, et al. Brain tumor in a patient with attenuated psychosis syndrome. Schizophrenia Research. 2013;**144**(1-3):151-152. DOI: 10.1016/j.schres.2012.11.036

[39] Peterson BS, Bronen RA, Duncan CC. Three cases of symptom change in Tourette's syndrome and obsessive-compulsive disorder associated with paediatric cerebral malignancies. Journal of Neurology, Neurosurgery, and Psychiatry. BMJ Publishing Group. 1996;**61**(5):497-505. DOI: 10.1136/jnnp.61.5.497

[40] Sokol MS, Fujimoto CK, Jackson TK, Silberberg PJ. Anorexia nervosa and brain tumor in a 14-year-old girl. CNS Spectrums. Cambridge University Press. 2006;**11**(9):669-673. DOI: 10.1017/S1092852900014759

[41] Uher R, Treasure J. Brain lesions and eating disorders. Journal of Neurology, Neurosurgery, and Psychiatry. BMJ Publishing Group. 2005;**76**(6):852-857. DOI: 10.1136/jnnp.2004.048819

[42] Zakrzewski K, Fiks T, Polis L, Liberski PP. Posterior fossa tumours in children and adolescents. A clinicopathological study of 216 cases. Folia Neuropathologica. 2003;**41**(4): 251-252

[43] Varela M, Liakopoulou M, Alexiou GA, Pitsouni D, Alevizopoulos GA. Presurgical neuropsychological and behavioral evaluation of children with posterior fossa tumors. Journal of Neurosurgery. Pediatrics. American Association of Neurological Surgeons. 2011;**8**(6):548-553. DOI: 10.3171/2011.8.PEDS11223

[44] Riva D, Giorgi C. The cerebellum contributes to higher functions during development: Evidence from a series of children surgically treated for posterior fossa tumours. Brain. 2000;**123**(Pt 5):1051-1061. DOI: 10.1093/brain/123.5.1051

[45] Konarski JZ, McIntyre RS, Grupp LA, Kennedy SH. Is the cerebellum relevant in the circuitry of neuropsychiatric disorders? Journal of Psychiatry & Neuroscience. 2005; **30**(3):178-186

[46] Daes T, Mariën P. Cognitive and affective disturbances following focal brainstem lesions: A review and report of three cases. Cerebellum. 2015. DOI: 10.1007/s12311-014-0626-8

[47] Korah MP, Esiashvili N, Mazewski CM, Hudgins RJ, Tighiouart M, Janss AJ, et al. Incidence, risks, and Sequelae of posterior fossa syndrome in pediatric medulloblastoma. International Journal of Radiation Oncology. 2010;**77**(1):106-112. DOI: 10.1016/j.ijrobp.2009.04.058

[48] Posterior Fossa Society [Internet]. [cited 2018 May 6]. Available from: http://www.posteriorfossa.org/posterior-fossa-syndrome-cerebellar-mutism-definitions/

[49] Gudrunardottir T, Morgan AT, Lux AL, Walker DA, Walsh KS, Wells EM, et al. Consensus paper on post-operative pediatric cerebellar mutism syndrome: The Iceland Delphi results. Child's Nerv Syst. 2016. Jul 3;**32**(7):1195-203. DOI: 10.1007/s00381-016-3093-3. [Epub 2016 May 3]

[50] Papavasiliou AS, Kotsalis C, Trakadas S. Transient cerebellar mutism in the course of acute cerebellitis. Pediatric Neurology. 2004;**30**(1):71-74. DOI: 10.1016/S0887-8994(03)00420-X

[51] Drost G, Verrips A, Thijssen MHO, Gabreëls MFJ. Cerebellar involvement as a rare complication of pneumococcal meningitis. Neuropediatrics. 2000;**31**(2):97-99. DOI: 10.1055/s-2000-7474

[52] Law N, Greenberg M, Bouffet E, Taylor MD, Laughlin S, Strother D, et al. Clinical and neuroanatomical predictors of cerebellar mutism syndrome. Neuro-Oncology. 2012;**14**(10):1294-1303. DOI: 10.1093/neuonc/nos160

[53] Daly DD, Love JG. Akinetic mutism. Neurology. 1958;**8**:238-242. DOI: 10.1212/WNL.8.3.238

[54] Gudrunardottir T, Sehested A, Juhler M, Schmiegelow K. Cerebellar mutism. Child's Nervous System. 2011;**27**(3):355-363. DOI: 10.1007/s00381-010-1328-2

[55] Rekate HL, Grubb RL, Aram DM, Hahn JF, Ratcheson RA. Muteness of cerebellar origin. Archives of Neurology. 1985;**42**(7):697-698. DOI: 10.1001/archneur.1985.04060070091023

[56] Di Rocco C, Chieffo D, Frassanito P, Caldarelli M, Massimi L, Tamburrini G. Heralding cerebellar Mutism: Evidence for pre-surgical language impairment as primary risk factor in posterior fossa surgery. The Cerebellum. 2011;**10**(3):551-562. DOI: 10.1007/s12311-011-0273-2

[57] Crutchfield JS, Sawaya R, Meyers CA, Moore BD. Postoperative mutism in neurosurgery. Report of two cases. Journal of Neurosurgery. 1994;**81**(1):115-121. DOI: 10.3171/jns.1994.81.1.0115

[58] De Smet HJ, Baillieux H, Wackenier P, De Praeter M, Engelborghs S, Paquier PF, et al. Long-term cognitive deficits following posterior fossa tumor resection: A neuropsychological and functional neuroimaging follow-up study. Neuropsychology. 2009;**23**(6):694-704. DOI: 10.1037/a0016106

[59] Erşahin Y, Mutluer S, Çaǧli S, Duman Y. Cerebellar Mutism: Report of seven cases and review of the literature. Neurosurgery. 1996;**38**(1):60-66. DOI: 10.1097/00006123-199601000-00015

[60] van Dongen HR, Catsman-Berrevoets CE, van Mourik M. The syndrome of "cerebellar" mutism and subsequent dysarthria. Neurology. 1994;**44**(11):2040-2046. DOI: 10.1212/WNL.44.11.2040

[61] Kotil K, Eras M, Akçetin M, Bilge T. Cerebellar mutism following posterior fossa tumor resection in children. Turkish Neurosurgery. 2008;**18**(1):89-94

[62] Wells EM, Walsh KS, Khademian ZP, Keating RF, Packer RJ. The cerebellar mutism syndrome and its relation to cerebellar cognitive function and the cerebellar cognitive affective disorder. Developmental Disabilities Research Reviews. 2008;**14**(3):221-228. DOI: 10.1002/ddrr.25

[63] Morris EB, Phillips NS, Laningham FH, Patay Z, Gajjar A, Wallace D, et al. Proximal dentatothalamocortical tract involvement in posterior fossa syndrome. Brain. 2009;**132**(Pt 11):3087-3095. DOI: 10.1093/brain/awp241

[64] Baillieux H, De SHJ, Paquier PF, De Deyn PP, Mariën P. Cerebellar neurocognition: Insights into the bottom of the brain. Clinical Neurology and Neurosurgery. 2008;**110**(8):763-773. DOI: 10.1016/j.clineuro.2008.05.013

[65] Sagiuchi T, Ishii K, Aoki Y, Kan S, Utsuki S, Tanaka R, et al. Bilateral crossed cerebello-cerebral diaschisis and mutism after surgery for cerebellar medulloblastoma. Annals of Nuclear Medicine. 2001;**15**(2):157-160. DOI: 10.1007/BF02988609

[66] Stoodley CJ, Schmahmann JD. Evidence for topographic organization in the cerebellum of motor control versus cognitive and affective processing. Cortex. 2010;**46**(7):831-844. DOI: 10.1016/j.cortex.2009.11.008

[67] Stoodley CJ, Schmahmann JDJ. Functional topography in the human cerebellum: A meta-analysis of neuroimaging studies. NeuroImage. 2009;**44**(2):489-501. DOI: 10.1016/j.neuroimage.2008.08.039

[68] Law N, Greenberg M, Bouffet E, Taylor MD, Laughlin S, Strother D, et al. Clinical and neuroanatomical predictors of cerebellar mutism syndrome. Neuro-Oncology. 2012 Oct;**14**(10):1294-1303. DOI: 10.1093/neuonc/nos160

[69] Puget S, Boddaert N, Viguier D, Kieffer V, Bulteau C, Garnett M, et al. Injuries to inferior vermis and dentate nuclei predict poor neurological and neuropsychological outcome in children with malignant posterior fossa tumors. Cancer. 2009;**115**(6):1338-1347. DOI: 10.1002/cncr.24150

[70] Robertson PL, Muraszko KM, Holmes EJ, Sposto R, Packer RJ, Gajjar A, et al. Incidence and severity of postoperative cerebellar mutism syndrome in children with medulloblastoma: A prospective study by the Children's oncology group. Journal of Neurosurgery. Pediatrics. 2006;**105**(6):444-451. DOI: 10.3171/ped.2006.105.6.444

[71] Pollack IF. Posterior fossa syndrome. International Review of Neurobiology. 1997;**41**:411-432. DOI: 10.1016/S0074-7742(08)60362-1

[72] Asamoto M, Ito H, Suzuki N, Oiwa Y, Saito K, Haraoka J. Transient mutism after posterior fossa surgery. Child's Nervous System. 1994;**10**(4):275-278. DOI: 10.1007/BF00301168

[73] Nishikawa M, Komiyama M, Sakamoto H, Yasui T, Nakajima H. Cerebellar Mutism after basilar artery occlusion —Case report—. Neurologia Medico-Chirurgica. 1998;**38**(9):569-573. DOI: 10.2176/nmc.38.569

[74] Siffert J, Poussaint TY, Goumnerova LC, Scott RM, LaValley B, Tarbell NJ, et al. Neurological dysfunction associated with postoperative cerebellar mutism. Journal of Neuro-Oncology. 2000;**48**(1):75-81. DOI: 10.1023/A:1006483531811

[75] McMillan HJ, Keene DL, Matzinger MA, Vassilyadi M, Nzau M, Ventureyra ECG. Brainstem compression: A predictor of postoperative cerebellar mutism. Child's Nervous System. 2009;**25**(6):677-681. DOI: 10.1007/s00381-008-0777-3

[76] Doxey D, Bruce D, Sklar F, Swift D, Shapiro K. Posterior fossa syndrome: Identifiable risk factors and irreversible complications. Pediatric Neurosurgery. 1999;**31**(3):131-136. DOI: 10.1159/000028848

[77] Catsman-Berrevoets CE, Van Dongen HR, Mulder PG, Paz y Geuze D, Paquier PF, Lequin MH. Tumour type and size are high risk factors for the syndrome of cerebellar mutism and subsequent dysarthria. Journal of Neurology, Neurosurgery, and Psychiatry. 1999;**67**(6):755-757. DOI: 10.1136/jnnp.67.6.755

[78] Robertson PL, Muraszko KM, Holmes EJ, Sposto R, Packer RJ, Gajjar A, et al. Incidence and severity of postoperative cerebellar mutism syndrome in children with medulloblastoma: A prospective study by the Children's oncology group. Journal of Neurosurgery. Pediatrics. 2006;**105**(6):444-451. DOI: 10.3171/ped.2006.105.6.444

[79] Korah MP, Esiashvili N, Mazewski CM, Hudgins RJ, Tighiouart M, Janss AJ, et al. Incidence, risks, and Sequelae of posterior fossa syndrome in pediatric medulloblastoma. International Journal of Radiation Oncology. 2010;**77**(1):106-112. DOI: 10.1016/j.ijrobp.2009.04.058

[80] Gudrunardottir T, Sehested A, Juhler M, Schmiegelow K. Cerebellar mutism. Child's Nervous System. 2011;**27**(3):355-363. DOI: 10.1007/s00381-010-1328-2

[81] Gelabert-González M, Fernández-Villa J. Mutism after posterior fossa surgery. Review of the literature. Clinical Neurology and Neurosurgery. 2001;**103**(2):111-114. DOI: 10.1016/S0303-8467(01)00125-1

[82] Aguiar PH, Plese JP, Ciquini O, Marino R. Transient mutism following a posterior fossa approach to cerebellar tumors in children: A critical review of the literature. Child's Nervous System. 1995;**11**(5):306-310

[83] Mussi ACM, Rhoton AL. Telovelar approach to the fourth ventricle: Microsurgical anatomy. Journal of Neurosurgery. 2000;**92**(5):812-823. DOI: 10.3171/jns.2000.92.5.0812

[84] Grill J, Viguier D, Kieffer V, Bulteau C, Sainte-Rose C, Hartmann O, et al. Critical risk factors for intellectual impairment in children with posterior fossa tumors: The role of cerebellar damage. Journal of Neurosurgery. Pediatrics. 2004;**101**(2):152-158. DOI: 10.3171/ped.2004.101.2.0152

[85] El-Bahy K. Telovelar approach to the fourth ventricle: Operative findings and results in 16 cases. Acta Neurochirurgica. 2005;**147**(2):137-142. DOI: 10.1007/s00701-004-0407-0

[86] Van Calenbergh F, Van de Laar A, Plets C, Goffin J, Casaer P. Transient cerebellar mutism after posterior fossa surgery in children. Neurosurgery. 1995;**37**(5):894-898. DOI: 10.1227/00006123-199511000-00007

[87] Catsman-Berrevoets CE, Van Dongen HR, H Mulder PG, Paz Geuze D, Paquier PF, Lequin MH. Tumour type and size are high risk factors for the syndrome of "cerebellar" mutism and subsequent dysarthria. Journal of Neurology, Neurosurgery, and Psychiatry. 1999;**67**:755-757. DOI: 10.1136/jnnp.67.6.755

[88] Lanier JC, Abrams AN. Posterior fossa syndrome: Review of the behavioral and emotional aspects in pediatric cancer patients. Cancer. 2017;**123**(4):551-559. DOI: 10.1002/cncr.30238

[89] Pollack IF, Polinko P, Albright AL, Towbin R, Fitz C. Mutism and pseudobulbar symptoms after resection of posterior fossa tumors in children: Incidence and pathophysiology. Neurosurgery. 1995;**37**(5):885-893. DOI: 10.1227/00006123-199511000-00006

[90] Netson KL, Conklin HM, Ashford JM, Kahalley LS, Wu S, Xiong X. Parent and teacher ratings of attention during a year-long methylphenidate trial in children treated for cancer. Journal of Pediatric Psychology. 2011;**36**(4):438-450. DOI: 10.1093/jpepsy/jsq102

[91] Hopyan T, Laughlin S, Dennis M. Emotions and their cognitive control in children with cerebellar Tumors. Journal of the International Neuropsychological Society. 2010;**16**(6):1027-1038. DOI: 10.1017/S1355617710000974

[92] Turkel SB, Shu Chen L, Nelson MD, Hyder D, Gilles FH, Woodall L, et al. Case series: Acute mood symptoms associated with posterior fossa lesions in children. The Journal of Neuropsychiatry and Clinical Neurosciences. 2004;**16**(4):443-445. DOI: 10.1176/jnp.16.4.443

[93] Schmahmann JD, Sherman JC. The cerebellar cognitive affective syndrome. Brain. 1998;**121**(Pt 4):561-579. DOI: 10.1093/brain/121.4.561

[94] Hargrave DR, Mabbott DJ, Bouffet E. Pathological laughter and behavioural change in childhood pontine glioma. Journal of Neuro-Oncology. 2006;**77**(3):267-271. DOI: 10.1007/s11060-005-9034-8

[95] Beckwitt Turkel S, Krieger MD, O'Neil S, Jubran R, Tavaré CJ. Symptoms before and after posterior fossa surgery in pediatric patients. Pediatric Neurosurgery. 2012;**48**(1):21-25. DOI: 10.1159/000337730

[96] Larysz D, Blamek S, Larysz P, Pietras K, Mandera M. Posterior Fossa Brain Tissue Injury: Developmental, Neuropsychological, and Neurological Consequences of Brain Tumors in Children. Vienna: Springer; 2010. pp. 271-274

[97] Riva D, Giorgi C. The cerebellum contributes to higher functions during development: Evidence from a series of children surgically treated for posterior fossa tumours. Brain. 2000;**123**(5):1051-1061. DOI: 10.1093/brain/123.5.1051

[98] Pastore V, Colombo K, Villa F, Galbiati S, Adduci A, Poggi G, et al. Psychological and adjustment problems due to acquired brain lesions in pre-school-aged patients. Brain Injury. 2013;**27**(6):677-684. DOI: 10.3109/02699052.2013.775482

[99] Poggi G, Liscio M, Galbiati S, Adduci A, Massimino M, Gandola L, et al. Brain tumors in children and adolescents: Cognitive and psychological disorders at different ages. Psycho-Oncology. 2005;**14**(5):386-395. DOI: 10.1002/pon.855

[100] Campen C, Ashbey D, Fisher PG, MM. Psychiatric symptoms in children with medullolblastoma. Neuro-Oncology. 2012;**14**(Suppl 1):i25-i39

[101] National Institute for Health and Care Excellence. Suspected Cancer: Recognition and Referral. London: NICE; 2015 Available from: https://www.nice.org.uk/guidance/ng12

[102] Dommett RM, Redaniel MT, Stevens MC, Hamilton W, Martin RM. Features of childhood cancer in primary care: A population-based nested case-control study. British Journal of Cancer. 2012;**106**(5):982-987. DOI: 10.1038/bjc.2011.600

[103] Ansell P, Johnston T, Simpson J, Crouch S, Roman E, Picton S. Brain tumor signs and symptoms: Analysis of primary health care records from the UKCCS. Pediatrics. 2010; **125**(1):112-119. DOI: 10.1542/peds.2009-0254

[104] Dixon-Woods M, Findlay M, Young B, Cox H, Heney D. Parents' accounts of obtaining a diagnosis of childhood cancer. Lancet. 2001;**357**(9257):670-674. DOI: 10.1016/S0140-6736(00)04130-1

[105] Wilne S, Koller K, Collier J, Kennedy C, Grundy R, Walker D. The diagnosis of brain tumours in children: A guideline to assist healthcare professionals in the assessment of children who may have a brain tumour. Archives of Disease in Childhood. 2010;**95**(7): 534-539. DOI: 10.1136/adc.2009.162057

[106] Edgeworth J, Bullock P, Bailey A, Gallagher A, Crouchman M. Why are brain tumours still being missed? Archives of Disease in Childhood. 1996;**74**(74):148-151

[107] Mehta V, Chapman A, McNeely PD, Walling S, Howes WJ. Latency between symptom onset and diagnosis of pediatric brain tumors: An eastern Canadian geographic study. Neurosurgery. 2002;**51**(2):365-72-3. DOI: 10.1097/00006123-200208000-00012

[108] Shemie S, Jay V, Rutka J, Armstrong D. Acute obstructive hydrocephalus and sudden death in children. Annals of Emergency Medicine. 1997;**29**(4):524-528. DOI: 10.1016/S0196-0644(97)70227-0

7

Neurocognitive Effects of Primary Brain Tumors

Mohammad Abu-Hegazy and
Hend Ahmed El-Hadaad

Abstract

Cognitive impairment, a common finding with the brain tumors, may result from the tumor itself or the treatment used: surgery, chemotherapy, or radiotherapy. Surgery for brain tumors improves the cognitive function due to reduction of compression as in case of removal of noninvasive tumors. Stability of cognitive function also was observed after tumor resection, such as tumors of third ventricle. Postoperative cognitive worsening was observed. Postoperative worsening of executive functions may correlate to volume of the operated area. Cognitive deficits may follow radiotherapy by several months to many years. These deficits may be due to vascular injury, local radionecrosis, and cerebral atrophy. This usually involves multiple domains, including memory, attention, executive function, and intelligence. The irradiated volume of brain tissue has great impact on cognition. Intensity-modulated radiotherapy (IMRT) and proton beam therapy result in greater sparing of healthy brain tissue and allow for a more-targeted delivery of radiation and smaller penetration of tissue beyond the tumor consequently reduce the risk of cognitive deficit after radiotherapy. Chemotherapy treatment in brain tumor seems to have a role in cognitive dysfunction deficits. The toxicity of chemotherapy increased when was given during or after radiotherapy. Chemotherapeutic agents, such as BCNU, CDDP, cytosine arabinoside, and intrathecal or intravenous methotrexate, have toxic effect to the CNS. Glioblastoma patients undergoing radiotherapy with concomitant and adjuvant temozolomide treatment do not develop cognitive deterioration. Patients with brain tumors face the challenge of cognitive impairment due to the tumor itself or treatments. Cognitive deficits in processing speed, memory, attention, and executive functions interfere with patients' daily life activities. Cognitive rehabilitation program has proven to be effective in patients with primary brain tumors. Cognitive impairments have a large impact on self-care, social and professional functioning, and consequently on quality of life. Preventing these late effects is a challenge for the medical team, psychologists, and rehabilitation specialists. Prevention depends in part on being able to predict those at greatest risk. Advances in neurosurgery, chemotherapy, and radiotherapy techniques are helping to a great extent, but may not be totally successful at preventing these late effects.

Keywords: Cognition, cognitive deficits, brain tumor, cognitive rehabilitation, brain tumor treatment

1. Introduction

1.1. Background

The term intellect designates the totality of the mental or cognitive operations that comprise human thought, and the higher cortical functions that make up the human mind. Memory is a specific cognitive function: the storage and retrieval of information. Other "higher" functions, such as language, calculations, spatial topography and reasoning, music, and creativity, all represent the functions of specific brain systems [1].

Cognitive functioning of brain tumor patients is an increasingly important outcome measure, because cognitive impairments can have a large impact on self-care, social and professional functioning, and consequently on quality of life (QOL) [2]. Patients with brain tumors often experience cognitive dysfunction associated with the disease itself and its treatment, as well, including surgery, radiotherapy (RT), and chemotherapy. Cognitive dysfunction has been recognized as the most frequent complication among long-term survivors. Despite the many advances made in the treatment modalities and surgical techniques, primary malignant brain cancer is a devastating illness, characterized by poor survival rates and significant morbidity as the disease progresses [3]. For many patients, cognitive changes are part of the disease process, but the pattern of impairment can vary markedly in different patients.

Resection of brain tumors may result in improvement of cognitive functions. Teixidor et al. [4] reported long-term improvement of verbal memory, after a transient immediate postoperative worsening, following frontal premotor and anterior temporal area resection, usually after a transient immediate postoperative worsening. Cognitive improvement has also been observed after surgical resection of high-grade gliomas [5], and in some studies stable, cognitive performance was observed after brain tumor resection, for instance, patients with tumors of the third ventricle [6].

Specific cognitive domain deficits after brain tumor removal were observed in some studies. A study conducted by Goldstein et al. [7] reported minimal deterioration in attention after right parenchymal frontal or precentral tumors resection. Another study [8] concluded that right rather than left prefrontal cortex resection was associated with, stroop performance test, selective attentional decline.

Radiation-induced cognitive impairment in some series is reported to occur in up to 50–90% of adult patients with brain tumor who survive >6 months after fractionated partial or whole-brain irradiation [9]. Moreover, because patients with brain tumor are surviving longer because of improved radiation therapy techniques and systemic therapies [10], the patient population experiencing these significant late effects is growing rapidly. Radiation-induced cognitive impairment is marked by decreased verbal memory, spatial memory, attention, and novel problem-solving ability [11]. Modern radiation therapy techniques have resulted in decreased acute and early delayed brain injury as well as late demyelination and white matter necrosis with less cognitive functional deficits, including progressive memory impairments, attention, and executive function that finally led to less impact on QOL of most survivors [12].

Neurocognitive sequelae of chemotherapy are less well documented than radiation effects [13]. Chemotherapy-related neurotoxicity to the central nervous system may be increased by intra-arterial administration, especially in combination with osmotic blood–brain barrier disruption, meant to increase the local concentration of chemotherapy in the brain [14]. Neurotoxicity may also be increased by chemotherapy given after, or even during, RT [15]. Primary central nervous system lymphoma is chemoresponsive, such as anaplastic oligodendroglioma (AO) and oligoastrocytoma (OA) tumors, chemotherapeutic agents are often ineffective due to limited ability to cross the BBB. Use of radiation therapy is often associated with significant neurotoxicity [16].

Advances in neurosurgery, chemotherapy, and RT are helping to a great extent in preventing cognitive deficit. Prevention depends in part on being able to predict the risky factors [17].

1.2. Objectives

The chapter examines:

- Cognition and its evaluation
- Brain tumors and cognition
- Brain tumor surgery and cognition
- Effect of adjuvant therapies (radio/chemotherapy) on cognition
- Prevention or reduction of cognitive deficits during the treatment of brain tumors
- Follow-up care and cognitive rehabilitation

2. Cognition and its evaluation

2.1. Cognition

Higher brain function may be subclassified into: (a) distributed functions, which do not localize to a particular brain region but instead require the concerted action of multiple parts on both sides of the brain, for example, attention and concentration, memory, higher-order executive function, social conduct, and personality; (b) localized functions, which are dependent on the normal structure and function of a particular part of one cerebral hemisphere, for example, language and praxis in dominant hemisphere the nondominant hemisphere hemisphere is largely, though not exclusively, responsible for visuospatial skills [18]. Cognitive impairment without crossing the threshold for dementia has been termed "mild cognitive impairment" (MCI) [19]. The MCI syndrome, as an expression of an incipient neurodegenerative disorder that may lead to dementia, is extremely heterogeneous and may coexist with systemic, neurologic, or psychiatric disorders that can cause cognitive deficits [20]. The criteria for MCI encompassed all possible cognitive manifestations of the syndrome and four subgroups have been proposed: deficits only in memory functions; memory deficits plus deficits in another cognitive domain; deficits in a single nonmemory domain; and deficits in more than one nonmemory domain [21].

2.2. Evaluation of cognitive functions

2.2.1. The Montreal cognitive assessment (MoCA)

MOCA was used as test of cognition, measure cognitive function, its cognitive domains: visuospatial/ executive function; naming; memory; language; abstraction; and attention. MoCA is scored out of 30 points. A normal score is 26 or above [22].

2.2.2. Mini Mental State Examination (MMSE)

MMSE is used for global cognitive functioning measurement [23].

2.2.3. Other cognitive domain-specific areas neuropsychological tests: focus on domain-specific areas of cognition:

(1) Hayling Sentence Completion Test, Word Span and Corsi's Test to test working memory [24], verbal and visual memory—Recognition Memory Tests, Words, and Topography [25]. (2) Rey Auditory Verbal Learning Test—RAVLT and logical memory to assess episodic memory, immediate and delayed recall [26], abstract reasoning: nonverbal—Raven's advanced progressive matrices [27, 28], verbal—Proverb Interpretation Test [29]. (3) Attention—Digit Span sub-test from the Wechsler Adult Intelligence Scale-III [30], Elevator Counting with Distraction from the Test of Everyday Attention [31], Trail Making test, part A and part B to test simple speed processing and complex attention, respectively, [32]. (4) Visual perception—Incomplete Letters Test from the Visual Object and Space Perception Battery [33], Rey–Osterrieth Complex Figure recall, to test visuospatial long-term memory, Rey–Osterrieth Complex Figure, copy to test visuoconstructional abilities [34]. (5) Phonemic and semantic fluency [35], language—Graded Naming Test [36], Word Comprehension—Synonyms Test [37]. (6) Executive functions—phonemic word fluency [38]. (7) Frontal Assessment Battery—FAB to assess frontal functionality [39].

For neuropsychological measures, age-, gender-, and education-corrected scores and equivalent scores should be calculated from the raw scores according to normative standards.

3. Brain tumors and cognition

Cognitive impairment, a common finding with the brain tumors, may result from the tumor itself or the treatment used surgery, chemotherapy, or RT.

3.1. Cognitive impairment due to tumor

More than 90% of patients with brain tumors showed impairments in the cognition at least in one area. The reported impairments of executive function were observed in 78%, while impairments of memory and attention were presented in more than 60% of patients [40].

Zucchella et al. [41] reported cognitive impairment in 54.4% of brain tumor patients, (53.75%) presented with multidomain impairment, while (46.25%) of the patients revealed cognitive deficits 16.25% of them limited to language, 13.75% to memory, 8.75% to attention, 6.25% to logical-executive functions, and 1.25% to visuospatial abilities.

Talacchi et al. [5] reported cognitive impairment in glioma patients 79% of patients have cognitive deficit in at least one test, (24, 3, 31, and 21% in one, two, three, four, or more tests, respectively, and this was correlated with edema, tumor grade, and size. Verbal memory, visuospatial memory, and word fluency were the most frequently affected functions.

3.2. Pathophysiology

Cognitive impairment associated with brain tumors can be induced by direct or indirect compression of normal brain tissue by reactive edema [42].

Tumor tissue can also invade directly into functional brain regions or indirectly disconnect the structures which can further contribute to cognitive deficits [43].

The mechanisms via which brain tumors affect brain function varied, highly malignant tumors grow quickly so they tend to infiltrate and displace the normal brain tissue, while the lower grade tumors tend to grow and infiltrate slowly disrupting brain function causing cognition deficit.

Tumors of ventricular system causes increase in intracranial pressure and hence affect the cognitive function; also large ventricular tumors affect the cognition directly through its compression effect. Functioning brain tumors which secrete hormones may have role in cognitive deficit through endocrine disturbance [44].

The main pathophysiology causes of cognitive dysfunction are not well known, different hypotheses were placed; progression of brain tumors seems to be the predominant one [45], also late treatment effects, for example, surgery, RT, chemotherapy, uses of antiepileptic drugs or corticosteroids), the psychological distress also may contribute in cognitive dysfunction [46].

The cognitive function disturbance in brain tumors may be due to combination of these factors.

4. Brain tumor surgery and cognition

In brain tumors, the first treatment modality is surgery. The aim was to balance the neurological outcomes (minimize the neurological deficits) and oncological outcome [2].

- Does brain surgery improve cognitive deficit?

Surgery for brain tumors improves the cognitive function due to the reduction of compression as after removal of noninvasive tumors, such as meningiomas, improvement of attentional function occur [42]. Patients with high-grade glioma have worse cognitive dysfunction than patients with low-grade glioma (LGG) [47]. The worse cognitive deficits in patients with high-grade gliomas have been attributed to higher incidence of intracranial hypertension, the rapid growth, and the infiltrative nature.

Sweet et al. [48] reported that the localization is associated with cognitive effects. Tumors of the pineal region associated with memory impairment, visuospatial function, attention, visuomotor function, problem-solving, and affective disorders.

Medial temporal lobe epilepsy caused by tumor is associated with cognitive deficit (long-term memory dysfunction, difficulties in learning, attention, naming, visuospatial abilities, executive functions, and intelligence) [49].

Less extensive surgery of the mesiotemporal structures correlates with better memory outcome than in the extensive temporal lobe surgery [50].

Verbal memory decline was observed in dominant temporal lobe resection [51], while visuospatial memory decline associated with nondominant temporal lobe resection [52].

Cognitive improvement has been observed after tumor resection, and improvement of verbal memory has been observed after LGG resections in frontal premotor and anterior temporal areas [4], usually after a transient postoperative worsening. This improvement was related to tumor lateralization [53].

Some studies reported postoperative cognitive worsening in (38%) of patients versus 24% rate of improved patients. Worsening associated with executive functions while improvement was observed with memory function. This worsening may correlate to volume of the operated area (tumor size) rather than the location. The postoperative improvement of memory function, the most frequent preoperative cognitive deficit, occurs due to release of the mass effect [54].

Teixidor et al. [4] reported immediate postoperative worsening for working memory in 96% of cases, and Giovagnoli et al. [55] reported that postoperative scores for cognitive tests were not significantly lower than the preoperative.

Talacchi et al. [5] found unexpected low incidence of additional deficits (38%) immediate postoperative and a considerable rate of early improvement (24%), and this correlated with tumor size and histology. This study reported also that postoperative worsening seems to be due to a generic mechanical effect and to manipulation/removal of tumor periphery rather than to discrete focal injury.

Yoshii et al. [53] reported that the cognitive functions in patients with LGG and meningiomas (MGs) in the right brain were normal preoperative and postoperative whereas it decreased preoperative and did not return to the normal scores postoperative in left brain MGs. Temporal and spatial orientation, similarities, first recall, writing, mental reversal decreased after operation.

The explanation of mild cognitive effects in MGs preoperatively is the ability of normal brain tissue to compensate as the slow growth of tumor provides enough time for this compensation, but after surgical decompression decline in brain function occurs due to remodeling of normal brain tissue [56]. Another explanation is that extracerebral tumor causes compression on brain tissues but local anatomical and functional integrity maintained before surgery.

Stability of cognitive function also was observed after tumor resection, like tumors of third ventricle; the preoperative cognitive impairment in executive function, memory, and fine manual speed did not improve or worsen postoperatively [57].

Postoperative cognitive defects in specific domains were observed, for example, some patients with frontal or precentral tumors showed postoperative minor deterioration in attention [58].

Right prefrontal cortex resection in one study [8] was associated with selective attention impairment (Stroop test performance).

5. Effect of brain RT on cognition

Cognitive deficits following RT are irreversible and progressive complication that may follow RT by several months to many years. These deficits may be due to vascular injury, local radionecrosis, and cerebral atrophy, the severity ranges from mild or moderate to progressive mental slowing, occurring in at least 12% of patients who were treated with radiation therapy [59].

5.1. Hypothesis of radiation-induced cognitive impairment

There are many hypotheses that explain how the cognitive deficits following radiation therapy occur, direct damage and subsequent death of parenchymal cells (oligodendrocytes, neurons, astrocytes, and microglia) or indirect through reactive oxygen species (ROS) production.

Dynamic interactions between the multiple cell types (astrocytes, endothelial cells, microglia, neurons, and oligodendrocytes) within the brain may be the cause of radiation-induced cognitive impairment [60]. Another hypothesis is that the RT can inhibit hippocampal neurogenesis causing the cognitive impairment.

Irradiation of the hippocampus results in loss of neuronal stem cells (NSCs) which are responsible on self-renewal and generating neurons, astrocytes, and oligodendrocytes [61]. The radiation injury to NSCs is dose-dependent [62] and results in decrease in proliferation of NSCs and decrease in its differentiation into neurons [63]. Radiation therapy for brain tumors may lead to a significant reduction in the number of neurogenic cells [64].

Direct damage of parenchymal brain cells due to RT and subsequent death of these leads to cognitive impairment; damage to oligodendrocytes, responsible for myelination, has been thought to play a role [65]. Neuronal irradiation of rodent causes altered expression of the gene activity-regulated cytoskeleton-associated protein, N-methyl-D-aspartate (NMDA) receptors, glutaminergic transmission, and also hippocampal long-term potentiation [66].

Disruption of the blood–brain barrier (BBB) as a result of brain RT has been associated with impaired cognition. This disruption and alteration of the BBB is likely due to imbalance between matrix metalloproteinase-2 and the metalloproteinase-2 tissue inhibitor levels [67], activation of microglial cells plays an important role in phagocytosis of dead cells, sustained activation is thought to contribute to a chronic inflammatory state in the brain [68]. Subsequent inflammation following RT and cell death usually associated with up regulation of cytokines, which are thought to be expressed by microglia, and pro-inflammatory transcription factors in the brain which contribute to endothelial cell dysfunction [69]. Glial and endothelial cells appear to have independent and overlapping roles in the pathogenesis.

Ionizing radiation produces its effect by direct DNA damage or indirect through generating ROS, leading to DNA damage to and activation of early response transcription factors and signal transduction pathways [70]. Activation of these pathways leads to the following: changes in cytokine milieu; the activation/influx of inflammatory cells, particularly microglia; marked increase in expression of the pro-inflammatory genes tumor necrosis factor (TNF)-α, interleukin (IL)-1β, IL-6, and Cox-2, and the chemokines, Monocyte Chemoattractant Protein-1 (MCP-1), intercellular adhesion molecule (ICAM)-1 and the development of post-irradiation complications [71].

Radiation injury to astrocytes makes them to undergo proliferation, exhibit hypertrophic nuclei/cell bodies, and show increased expression of glial fibrillary acidic protein .These reactive astrocytes secrete a host of pro-inflammatory mediators such as cyclooxygenase (Cox)-2 and the ICAM-1, which may lead to infiltration of leukocytes into the brain via BBB breakdown [72].

RT affects large- and medium-sized blood vessels of the brain. Vascular hypothesis predicts that blood-vessel dilatation, wall thickening with hyalinization, endothelial cell loss and a decrease in vessel density, all these finally lead to white-matter necrosis [73].

The severity of cognitive deficit following radiation therapy appears to be proportional to the dose of radiation therapy received by the hippocampus region [74].

5.2. Predisposing factors

Older ages more than 60 years and in some studies more than 40 years old have increased risk to develop leukoencephalopathy specifically in patients with genetic predisposition to leukoencephalopathy [75] with subsequent cognitive deficit. Also patient with white matter disease such as multiple sclerosis have increased risk, also vascular diseases such as hypertention carry risk [76].

Beside the previous patient-related factors, also there are factors related to treatment include the dose of RT received, dose per fraction and volume of irradiated brain, 5% of patients treated with more than 5000 cGy develop radiation necrosis [77], high radiation dose increases the risk of leukoencephalopathy, daily doses >200 cGy have a significantly increased risk of cognitive damage [75]. The large irradiated volume of brain tissues carries increased risk of cognitive impairment, and whole brain radiation has threefold to fourfold increased risk of encephalopathy [76].

Additional treatments to RT such as chemotherapy have increased risk on cognition than RT alone, systemic and intrathecal treatments have been implicated. Methotrexate chemotherapy when received intravenously or intrathecally after cranial irradiation has an effect on cognition in children and also on adults [78].

5.3. Neuropsychological assessments

Folstein MMSE is brief test that assess delirium or significant dementia. It does not adequately measure all the cognitive areas affected by radiation, and it is not a sensitive tool for detecting cognitive impairment in patients receiving RT [79].

Among the patients who have impaired cognitive function by neuropsychological testing, only 50% were considered abnormal on the MMSE [80].

The National Cancer Institute (NCI) Radiation Oncology Branch adapted the Meyers et al. [45] test battery by adding few measures to assess processing speed, working memory, and attention, which are functions that can be affected by RT [81].

Measurement of quality of life and daily activities of living is an important issue beside the neuropsychological testes, such as the Barthel index to assess the daily living skills and the Functional Assessment of Cancer Therapy-Brain (FACT-Br), to address the quality of life issues concerning brain tumor patients undergoing treatment The Barthel Index assesses daily living skills [82], and the FACT-Br was developed specifically to address the quality of life issues concerning brain tumor patients undergoing treatment [83].

5.4. Cognitive impairment following RT

RT is the leading cause of cognitive deficits involving multiple domains, including memory, attention, executive function, and intelligence.

Patients who received RT performed worse in measures of executive function and information processing speed. Worse cognitive functioning also observed with white-matter hyperintensities and global cortical atrophy [84].

Several studies assed cognitive defects to specific tumor-type and tumor location. Aarsen et al. [85] reported cognitive deficit, with sustained speech and speed of speech in children treated with RT for pilocytic astrocytoma, 60% of patients had difficulty with academics 3 years after treatment.

Cognitive impairment observed in children with medulloblastoma who had treated with RT. These deficits were prominent attention deficits correlated with impaired math and reading performance [86].

Hoppe-Hirsch et al. [87] conducted a study comparing intellectual outcomes of children diagnosed with ependymomas or medulloblastomas, treated with whole-brain radiotherapy (WBRT), and found that only 10% of medulloblastoma patients had an IQ above 90 after 10 years compared to 60% of ependymoma patients, and this result attributed to cerebral hemisphere radiation.

Posteroir fossa irradiation with 35 Gy was associated with lower cognitive scores than that irradiated with a dose 25 Gy, and IQ and verbal comprehension seems to be dose-dependent in posterior fossa tumors [88].

Large-sample controlled clinical trial conducted by Klein et al. [75] assed mid-term and long-term neuropsychological function following the RT in LGG. In the study, 195 patients with LGG compared with 195 healthy controls and 100 patients with hematological malignancies with mean follow-up period of 6 years. The results revealed that patients with LGG had lower scores in all cognitive domains than the controls and hematological patients, and the main cause of cognitive deficits was the tumor, but cognitive deficits of memory domain was observed only in patients who received RT with dose per fraction more than 2 Gy.

Another study was conducted on those patients after 12-year follow-up and found that the attentional deficits deteriorated in patients who received RT. The progressive decline was found even in patients received <2 Gy dose per fraction [89].

Decline in nonverbal memory was observed in patients with LGGs years post-RT, despite the long-term improvements which observed in verbal memory, attention, and executive function [84]. Postoperative RT in LGG was found to have a significant risk of long-term leukoencephalopathy and cognitive impairment [90].

The irradiated volume of brain tissue has great impact on cognition. A study conducted by Jalali et al. [91] reported that patients who treated with stereotactic conformal RT presented with unchanged overall mean full-scale IQ, while one third of patients showed a >10% decline in full-scale IQ as compared to baseline.

Chang et al. [92] found that cognitive deficits after the treatment with sterotactic radiosurgery (SRS) had lower incidence than that in patients treated with whole-brain radiotherapy (WBRT). The cognitive deficit in learning and memory function was (24%) in patients treated with SRS and (52%) in patients treated with WBRT and SRS.

Intensity-modulated radiotherapy (IMRT) is a type RT technique in which more sparing of normal brain tissue can be achieved and precise contouring to the tumor tissue.

Hippocampal sparing with IMRT reduced doses delivered to hippocampus by 87% (0.49 Gy) and 81% (0.73 Gy) [93].

Proton beam therapy results in greater sparing of healthy brain tissue and allows for a more-targeted delivery of radiation and smaller penetration of tissue beyond the tumor [94]. The mean dose of radiation to the hippocampus could be reduced much more, and it could be half that of IMRT and consequently reduce the risk of cognitive deficit after RT [95].

6. Effect of chemotherapy on cognition

Chemotherapy treatment in brain tumor seems to have a role in cognitive deficits. There is association between chemotherapy used in the treatment of brain tumor and an increased risk for cognitive dysfunction especially, if it is administered with RT.

6.1. Pathogenesis of cognitive impairment

The mechanisms by which chemotherapy-induced cognitive impairment are unclear [96].

Chemotherapy may reduce the number of neural stem/progenitor cells, which have role in memory and learning ability [97], and neural precursor cells are chemo-sensitivity, neural stem, and line age-restricted progenitor cells that form, among other cell types, the myelinating oligodendrocytes in the frontal white matter [98].

Primary pathological lesions including demyelination, inflammation, and microvascular injury [99]. Also mature oligodendrocytes are chemo-sensitive at lower dosage than those required to kill tumor cells [100].

Multiple chemotherapeutic agents affect hippocampal neurogenesis causing decrease in cell proliferation within the germinal region of the hippocampus and development of cognitive deficit [101].

Genetic role in chemotherapy-induced cognitive decline may be impilicated, and there is increased risk of cognitive impairment after RT with the apolipoprotein E4 alleles [102].

6.2. Cognitive impairment of chemotherapeutic agents

Chemotherapy added to slow the tumor progression especially in children to postpone radiation therapy or to reduce the dose of radiation therapy to decrease the neurocognitive sequelae of increasing doses of RT. Neurotoxic side-effects of chemotherapy alone can be difficult, because most patients of brain tumor have been treated with RT and chemotherapy [103].

The evidence that chemotherapy alone causes neurocognitive effects is not consistent. Studies have concluded that chemotherapy effects are negligible and not clinically significant compared to craniospinal irradiation (CSI) [104].

Neurotoxicity of chemotherapy arises during, or shortly after, chemoterapy. RT causes disturbance in BBB, so the toxicity of chemotherapy increased when was given during or after RT. In these cases, the chemotherapeutic drugs reach higher concentrations in brain tissue because of leakage of the blood–brain barrier due to RT. Intrathecal chemotherapy has higher CNS toxicity compared to systemic chemotherapy [105].

Chemotherapeutic agents, such as BCNU, CDDP, cytosine arabinoside, and intrathecal or intravenous methotrexate, have toxic effect to the CNS. Chemotherapy-related cognitive impairment in primary CNS lymphoma was observed in one or more domains: (attention, executive function, memory, psychomotor speed, and language). Other studies have shown that cognitive stability or cognitive improvement during chemotherapy provided that the tumor was responsive to chemotherapy treatment [106, 107]. Uses of high-dose IV methotrexate or interathecal methotrexate with radiation therapy result in dementia particularly when the radiation is given prior to the methotrexate. Leukoencephalopathy more commonly occurs. MRI shows bilateral periventricular white matter changes. The radiation therapy disrupts the BBB and results in increased permeability of the white matter to the methotrexate [108].

Copeland et al. [109] concluded that chemotherapy had only a slight effect on neurocognitive status and was confined to perceptual motor skills with observed age effect on performance IQ.

Chemotherapeutic agents, such as BCNU, cisplatin, and cytarabine, have proved to be more toxic to neural precursor cells than cancer cells [110]. Carmustine, methotrexate, and cytarabine have been found to induce central neurotoxicity to neural stem cell populations located in the subventricular zone and dentate gyrus [99].

Prabhu et al. [111] conducted a study on LGG patients and concluded that the addition of chemotherapy procarbazine, lomustine, and vincristine (PCV) to RT for LGGs did not result in significant MMSE score decline when compared to RT alone.

Regarding the HRQOL, there is a short-lasting negative impact of PCV chemotherapy on HRQOL during and shortly after treatment, but no long-term effects on HRQOL have been established [112].

Patients with previously untreated anaplastic astrocytoma, OA, or oligodendroglioma were evaluated for the long-term efficacy and safety of accelerated fractionated RT combined with intravenous carboplatin. In a phase II study conducted by Levin et al. [113], they found that after RT, patients received procarbazine, lomustine (CCNU), and vincristine (PCV) for 1 year or until tumor progression, 10% of those patients developed serious clinical neurologic deterioration and/or dementia requiring full-time caregiver attention.

Hilverda et al. [114] reported that glioblastoma patients undergoing RT with concomitant and adjuvant temozolomide treatment did not develop cognitive deterioration.

In LGG patients, temozolomide is not only successful in terms of extending the survival duration but also has been proven to maintain or even improve HRQOL while patients are on treatment [115].

Patients with recurrent high-grade glioma (HGG), successfully treated with temozolomide, achieved significant improvement in the HRQOL domains, whereas patients with disease progression had significant deterioration in most HRQOL domains [116].

7. Prevention or reduction of cognitive deficits during treatment of brain tumors

Reduction in treatment-related brain tissue toxicity has occurred with advances in neurosurgical techniques, advances in radiation therapy techniques, and use of neuroprotective agents.

7.1. Pharmacological prevention of neurocognitive impairment

Neuroprotective agents may be used to protect healthy tissue against neuronal cell death or degeneration caused by the treatment of brain tumor.

Lithium can be used to protect progenitor cells in the hippocampus through inhibition of radiation-induced apoptosis and induction of the DNA repair, and the tumor cells not included in this protection process. A study conducted by Yang et al. [117] found that neurocognitive performance in mice was improved after receiving lithium concomitant with RT, anthor neuroprotective drug; fenofibrate which prevents activation of microglia. Administration of fenofibrate during whole-brain RT prevents effects on hippocampal neurogenesis in mice, as it enhances survival of newborn neurons in the dentate gyrus [118].

7.2. New treatment techniques

The use of image-guided surgery such as the intraoperative magnetic resonance imaging resulted in improvement in tumor resection and reduction of residual [119]. The use of endoscopic biopsy is a minimally invasive method can be performed safely in conjunction with diversion of cerebrospinal fluid in cases of obstructive hydrocephalus and decrease neurocognitive decline [120].

New radiation techniques such as IMRT are able to minimize the radiation to healthy brain structures. With using IMRT, hippocampus can be localized and hence the dentate gyrus can be spared, resulting in prevention or decrease neurocognitive decline to some extent [121]. Lin et al. [122] reported significantly lower rates of memory loss posttreatment and with no treatment-related decline in quality of life with IMRT RT.

Insignificant neurocognitive decline was found in a study conducted by Wahba et al. [123] after use of reduced CSI followed by adjuvant chemotherapy in patients with average-risk medulloblastoma.

With proton beam RT, there is less radiation to surrounding normal brain tissues and decrease the area at risk for radiation injury, therefore, sparing of neurocognitive functioning [124].

7.3. Stem cell implantation

Mesenchymal stem cell implantation may reduce the cognitive impairment by two mechanisms: First, reversal of inflammatory process, as implanted mesenchymal stem cells can migrate to the site of damaged brain tissue and then release growth factors, [125]. Second, human mesenchymal stem cells can differentiate into neurons in the hippemocampal area and prevent radiation-induced late cognitive impairment [126].

8. Rehabilitation

Patients with brain tumors face the challenge of cognitive impairment due to the tumor itself or treatments. Cognitive deficits in processing speed, memory, attention, and executive functions interfere with patients' relationships, occupational activities and daily life activities.

8.1. Pharmacologic treatment of neurocognitive impairment

Methylphenidate (MPH) is a CNS stimulant that increases synaptic concentration of dopamine and noradrenaline in the brain [127]. De-Long et al. [128] conducted a pilot study on children with ALL or brain tumor, they found that approximately 75% of those patients had response to treatment with MPH regarding neuropsychological dysfunction.

Meyers et al. [129] reported significant improvements in processing speed, memory, mental flexibility, and even mood, in adult patients with brain tumors and receiving MPH. Conklin et al. showed encouraging results in the use of psychostimulant medication. On 122 survivors of childhood brain tumors or ALL who were enrolled in a double-blinded, cross-over trial comparing the acute efficacy and adverse effects of MPH and placebo.

Donepezil is acetylcholinesterase inhibitor and has efficacy in the treatment of cognitive functions impairment; uses of donepezil in adult patients with brain tumors treated with RT demonstrate improvements in cognition impairment such as attention, concentration, and verbal memory [130].

However, stimulant medication is short-acting and is not expected to result in long-term improvement in academic achievement and neurocognitive functioning once it is discontinued; on the other hand, newer pscyhostimulant medications have been widely used in children with attention-deficit hyperactivity disorder (ADHD) and have proven to have fewer side effects and a longer half-life than MPH, for these reasons further studies are needed [131].

8.2. Cognition rehabilitation program

Cognitive rehabilitation program has proven to be effective in in-patients with primary brain tumors. The program consists of psychoeducation, teaching of strategies to compensate for problems in attention, memory, and executive functioning in daily life.

Cognitive remediation program (CRP) highly structured and individualized regimen, included traditional massed practice rehabilitation, instruction in metacognitive strategies, and cognitive-behavioral psychotherapy focused primarily on improving resistance to distraction. Butler and Copeland tested the effectiveness of CRP. Thirty-one subjects who had been treated from CNS tumors included in the study, and they were suffering from cognitive impairment such as attention deficits documented by continuous performance test (CPT). Cognitive behavioral psychotherapy was used. Significant improvement in focused attention and attention/concentration was observed in those who underwent the CRP, but no significant benefit was measured with regard to arithmetic computation. The authors concluded that the intervention produced improved neurocognitive functioning on measures of attention, but that it was too early to expect a downstream effect on the desired end result of improved academic achievement [132].

A study conducted by Butler et al. all patients was offered the CRP treatment, improvement neurocognitive variables were observed but this was not statistically significant. The study results demonstrated highly significant improvement in academic achievement for those who completed the CRP, and significant gains in their child's or adolescent's attention/concentration in activities of daily living [133].

The majority of the participants of cognitive rehabilitation program found the program to be useful. However, older participants found the program more burdensome than younger participants [134].

Richard et al. [135] conduct a study to compare two cognitive rehabilitation program, goal management training (GMT) which is a neuroscience-based integration of mindfulness and strategy training and the Brain Health Workshop (BHW) which offers supportive psychoeducation about living with a brain tumor. They found that significant improvement in executive functions and greater attainment of pre-training functional goals in the GMT group while The BHW group showed in significant improvement in mood and behavioral regulation.

Author details

Mohammad Abu-Hegazy[1,3*] and Hend Ahmed El-Hadaad[2]

*Address all correspondence to: mhegazy@mans.edu.eg

1 Neurology Department, Mansoura University, Mansoura, Egypt

2 Clinical Oncology and Nuclear Medicine Department, Mansoura University, Mansoura, Egypt

3 Faculty of Medicine, Mansoura University, Mansoura, Egypt

References

[1] Kirshner HS. Approaches to Intellectual and Memory Impairments. In: Bradley WG, Daroff RB, Fenichel GM, Jankovic J, editors. Neurology in Clinical Practice: Principles of Diagnosis and Management. 4th Ed. Chichester: Elsevier Inc; 2004. pp. 65–74

[2] Klein M, Duffau H, Hamer PD. Cognition and resective surgery for diffuse infiltrative glioma: an overview. J Neurooncol. 2012;108:309–318

[3] Wrensch M, Minn Y, Chew T, Bondy M, et al. Epidemiology of primary brain tumors: current concepts and review of the literature. Neuro-oncology. 2002;4:278–299

[4] Teixidor P, Gatignol P, Leroy M, et al. Assessment of verbal working memory before and after surgery for low-grade glioma. J Neurooncol. 2007;81:305–313

[5] Talacchi A, Santini B, Savazzi S, et al. Cognitive effects of tumour and surgical treatment in glioma patients. J Neurooncol. 2011;103:541–549

[6] Friedman MA, Meyers CA, Sawaya R. Neuropsychological effects of third ventricle tumor surgery. Neurosurgery. 2003;52:791–798

[7] Goldstein B, Armstrong CL, John C, et al. Attention in adult intracranial tumors patients. J Clin Exp Neuropsychol. 2003;25:66–78

[8] Vendrell P, Junque C, Pujol J, et al. The role of prefrontal regions in the Stroop task. Neuropsychologia. 1995;33:341–352

[9] Meyers CA, Brown PD. Role and relevance of neurocognitive assessment in clinical trials of patients with CNS tumors. J Clin Oncol. 2006;24:1305–1309

[10] Cochran DC, Chan MD, Aklilu M, et al. The effect of targeted agents on outcomes in patients with brain metastases from renal cell carcinoma treated with Gamma Knife surgery. J Neurosurg. 2012;116:978–983

[11] Roman DD, Sperduto PW. Neuropsychological effects of cranial radiation: current knowledge and future directions. Int J Radiat Oncol Biol Phys. 1995;31:983–998

[12] Greene-Schloesser D, Robbins ME. Radiation-induced cognitive impairment from bench to bedside. Neuro-oncology. 2012;14:iv37–iv44. doi:10.1093/neuonc/nos196

[13] Anderson FS, Kunin-Batson AS, Perkins JL, et al. White versus gray matter function as seen on neuropsychological testing following bone marrow transplant for acute leukemia in childhood. Neuropsychiatr Dis Treat. 2008;4:283–288

[14] Shapiro WR, Green SB, Burger PC, et al. A randomized comparison of intra-arterial versus intravenous BCNU, with or without intravenous 5-fluorouracil, for newly diagnosed patients with malignant glioma. J Neurosurg. 1992;76:772–781

[15] DeAngelis LM, Yahalom J, Thaler HT, et al. Combined modality therapy for primary CNS lymphoma. J Clin Oncol. 1992;10:635–643

[16] Angelov L, Doolittle ND, Kraemer DF, et al. Blood–brain barrier disruption and intra-arterial methotrexate-based therapy for newly diagnosed primary CNS lymphoma: a multi-institutional experience with 149 patients. J Clin Oncol. 2009;27:3503–3509

[17] Askins MA, Moore BD 3rd. Preventing neurocognitive late effects in childhood cancer survivors. J Child Neurol. 2008;23:1160–1171

[18] Ginsberg L. Lecture Notes: Neurology, Lionel Ginsberg, 9th Ed. Chichester: John Wiley & Sons, Ltd., India, New delhi; Printed in Singapor; 2010. pp. 11–16.

[19] Lopez OL, Jagust WJ, DeKosky ST, et al. Prevalence and classification of mild cognitive impairment in the Cardiovascular Health Study Cognitive Study: part 1. Arch Neurol. 2003;60(10):1385–1389

[20] Ganguli M, Dodge HH, Shen C, DeKosky ST. Mild cognitive impairment, amnestic type: an epidemiologic study. Neurology. 2004;63(1):115–121

[21] Winblad B, Palmer K, Kivipelto M, et al. Mild cognitive impairment beyond controversies, towards a consensus: report of the International Working Group on Mild Cognitive Impairment. J Intern Med. 2004;256(3):240–246

[22] Nasreddine ZS, Phillips NA, Bédirian V, Charbonneau S, Whitehead V, Collin I, et al. The Montreal cognitive assessment, MoCA: a brief screening tool for mild cognitive impairment. J Am Geriatr Soc. 2005;53:695–9

[23] Folstein MF, Folstein SE, Mc Hugh PR. "Mini-mental state". A practical method for grading the cognitive state of patients for the clinician. J Psychiatry Res. 1975;12:189–198

[24] Orsini A, Grossi D, Capitani E, Laiacona M, Papagno C, Vallar G. Verbal and spatial immediate memory span: normative data from 1355 adults and 1112 children. Ital J Neurol Sci. 1987;8(6):539–548

[25] Warrington EK. The Camden Memory Tests. Hove: Psychology Press; 1996

[26] Carlesimo GA, Buccione I, Fadda L, Graceffa A, Mauri M, Lo Russo S, Bevilacqua G, Caltagirone C. Standardization of two memory tests for clinical use: short story and figure rey. Nuova Rivista Neurol. 2002;12:1–13

[27] Raven J. Advanced Progressive Matrices Set 1. Oxford: Oxford Psychologists Press; 23, 1976

[28] Caffarra P, Vezzadini G, Zonato F, Copelli S, Venneri A. A normative study of a shorter version of Raven's progressive matrices. Neurol Sci. 2003;24(5):336–339

[29] Murphy P, Shallice T, Robinson G, Mac Pherson SE, Turner M, Woollett K, etal. Impairments in proverb interpretation following focal frontal lobe lesions. Neuropsychologia. 2013;51(11):2075–86. doi:10.1016/j.neuropsychologia.2013. 06.029

[30] Wechsler D. Adult Intelligence Scale—Third Edition. San Antonio, TX: The Psychological Corporation; 1997

[31] Robertson IH, Ward T, Ridgeway V, Nimmo-Smith I. The structure of normal human attention: the test of every day attention. J Int Neuropsychol Soc. 1996;2(6):525–534

[32] Giovagnoli AR, Del Pesce M, Mascheroni S, Simoncelli M, Laiacona M, Capitani E. Trail making test: normative values from 287 normal adults controls. Ital J Neurol Sci. 1996;17:305–309

[33] Warrington EK, James M. The Visual Object and Space Perception Battery. Bury St Edmunds: Thames Valley Test Company; 1991

[34] Caffarra P, Vezzadini G, Dieci F, Zonato F, Venneri A. Rey–Osterrieth complex figure: normative values in an Italian population sample. Neurol Sci. 2002;22:443–447

[35] Novelli G, Papagno C, Capitani E, Laiacona M, Cappa SF, Vallar G. Tre test clinici di ricerca e produzione lessicale. Taratura su soggetti normali. Arch Psicol Neurol Psichiatr. 1986;47:477–506

[36] McKenna P, Warrington EK. Testing for nominal dysphasia. J Neurol Neurosurg Psychiatry. 1980;43:781–788. doi:10.1136/jnnp.43.9.781

[37] Warrington EK, McKenna P, Orpwood L. Single word comprehension: a concrete and abstract words synonym test. Neuropsychol Rehabil. 1998;8(2):143–154. doi: 10.1080/713755564

[38] Benton AL. Differential behavioral effects in frontal lobe disease. Neuropsychologia. 1968;6(1):53–60. doi:10.1016/0028-3932(68)90038-9

[39] Apollonio I, Leone M, Isella V, Piamarta F, Consoli T, Villa ML, Forapani E, Russo A, Nichelli P. The Frontal Assessment Battery (FAB): normative values in an Italian population sample. Neurol Sci. 2005;26:108–116

[40] Tucha O, Smely C, Preier M, Lange KW. Cognitive deficits before treatment among patients with brain tumors. Neurosurgery. 2000;47:324–334

[41] Zucchella C, Bartolo M, Di Lorenzo C, Villani V, Pace A. Cognitive impairment in primary brain tumors outpatients: a prospective cross-sectional survey. J Neurooncol. 2013;112(3):455–460. doi:10.1007/s11060-013-1076-8. Epub 2013 Feb 16

[42] Tucha O, Smely C, Preier M, Becker G, Paul GM, Lange KW. Preoperative and postoperative cognitive functioning in patients with frontal meningiomas. J Neurosurg. 2003;98(1):21–31

[43] Bosma I, Vos MJ, Heimans JJ, Taphoorn MJB, Aaronson NK, Postma TJ, van der Ploeg HM, Muller M, Vandertop WP, Slotman BJ, Klein M. The course of neurocognitive functioning in high-grade glioma patients. Neuro-oncology. 2007;9(1):53–62

[44] Kayl AE, Meyers CA. Does brain tumor histology influence cognitive function? Neuro-oncology. 2003;5(4):255–60

[45] Meyers CA, Smith JA, Bezjak A, Mehta MP, Liebmann J, Illidge T, Kunkler I, Caudrelier JM, Eisenberg PD, Meerwaldt J, Siemers R, Carrie C, Gaspar LE, Curran W, Phan SC, Miller RA, Renschler MF. Neurocognitive function and progression in patients with brain metastases treated with whole-brain radiation and motexafin gadolinium: results of a randomized phase III trial. J Clin Oncol. 2004;22:157–165

[46] Taphoorn MJ, Klein M. Cognitive deficits in adult patients with brain tumours. Lancet Neurol. 2004;3(3):159–168

[47] Busch E. Psychical symptoms in neurosurgical disease. Acta Psychiatr Neurol. 1940;15:257–290

[48] Sweet JJ, Nies KJ, Lorber R, Vick NA. Relative absence of neuropsychological deficit in patients with low-grade astrocytomas. J Clin Psychol Med Settings. 1994;1:83–104

[49] Allegri RF, Drake M, Thomson A. Neuropsychological findings in patients with middle temporal lobe epilepsy. Rev Neurol. 1999;29:1160–1163

[50] Helmstaedter C, Richter S, Roske S, Oltmanns F, Schramm J, Lehmann TN. Differential effects of temporal pole resection with amygdalohippocampectomy versus selective amygdalohippocampectomy on material-specific memory in patients with mesial temporal lobe epilepsy. Epilepsia. 2008;49(1):88–97

[51] Joo EY, Han HJ, Lee EK, Choi S, Jin JH, Kim JH, Tae WS, Seo DW, Hong SC, Lee M, Hong SB. Resection extent versus postoperative outcomes of seizure and memory in mesial temporal lobe epilepsy. Seizure. 2005;14(8):541–551

[52] Dulay MF, Levin HS, York MK, Mizrahi EM, Verma A, Gold smith I, Grossman RG, Yoshor D. Predictors of individual visual memory decline after unilateral anterior temporal lobe resection. Neurology. 2009;72(21):1837–1842

[53] Yoshii Y, Tominaga D, Sugimoto K, Tsuchida Y, Hyodo A, Yonaha H, et al. Cognitive function of patients with brain tumor in pre- and postoperative stage. Surg Neurol. 2008;69:51–61

[54] Broglio PS, Puetz TW. The effect of sport concussion on neurocognitive function, self-report symptoms and postural control. Sports Med. 2008;38(1):53–67

[55] Giovagnoli AR, Boiardi A. Cognitive impairment and quality of life in long-term survivors of malignant brain tumors. Ital J Neurol Sci. 1994;15:481–488

[56] Shen C, Bao WM, Yang BJ, Xie R, Cao XY, Luan SH, Mao Y. Cognitive deficits in patients with brain tumor. Chin Med J (Engl). 2012;125(14):2610–2617

[57] Petrucci RJ, Buchheit WA, Woodruff GC, et al. Transcallosal parafornicial approach for third ventricle tumors: neuropsychological consequences. Neurosurgery. 1987;20:457–464

[58] Braun V, Albrecht A, Kretschmer T, et al. Brain tumour surgery in the vicinity of short-term memory representation–results of neuronavigation using fMRI images. Acta Neurochir (Wien). 2006;148:733–739

[59] Crossen JR, Garwood D, Glatstein E, Neuwelt EA. Neurobehavioral sequelae of cranial irradiation in adults: a review of radiation-induced encephalopathy. J Clin Oncol. 1994;12:627–642

[60] Tofilon PJ, Fike JR. The radioresponse of the central nervous system: a dynamic process. Radiat Res. 2000;153:357–370

[61] Gage FH, Kempermann G, Palmer TD, Peterson DA, Ray J. Multipotent progenitor cells in the adult dentate gyrus. J Neurobiol. 1998;36:249–266

[62] Bellinzona M, Gobbel GT, Shinohara C, Fike JR. Apoptosis is induced in the subependyma of young adult rats by ionizing irradiation. Neurosci Lett. 1996;208:163–166

[63] Mizumatsu S, Monje ML, Morhardt DR, Rola R, Palmer TD, Fike JR. Extreme sensitivity of adult neurogenesis to low doses of X-irradiation. Cancer Res. 2003;63:4021–4027

[64] Monje ML, Vogel H, Masek M, Ligon KL, Fisher PG, Palmer TD. Impaired human hippocampal neurogenesis after treatment for central nervous system malignancies. Ann Neurol. 2007;62:515–520

[65] Shi L, Linville MC, Iversen E, Molina DP, Yester J, Wheeler KT, Robbins ME, Brunso-Bechtold JK. Maintenance of white matter integrity in a rat model of radiation-induced cognitive impairment. J Neurol Sci. 2009;285(1–2):178–84

[66] Greene-Schloesser D, Robbins ME, Peiffer AM, Shaw EG, Wheeler KT, Chan MD. Radiation-induced brain injury: a review. Front Oncol. 2012;2:73

[67] Lee WH, Warrington JP, Sonntag WE, Lee YW. Irradiation altersMMP-2/TIMP-2system and collagen type iv degradation in brain. Int J Radiat Oncol Biol Phys. 2012;82:1559–1566

[68] Gebicke-Haerter PJ. Microglia in neurodegeneration: molecular aspects. Microsc Res Tech. 2001;54:47–58

[69] Gaber MW, Sabek OM, Fukatsu K, Wilcox HG, Kiani MF, Merchant TE. Differences in ICAM-1 and TNF-alpha expression between large single fraction and fractionated irradiation in mouse brain. Int J Radiat Biol. 2003;79(5):359–366

[70] Dent P, Yacoub A, Fisher PB, Hagan MP, Grant S. MAPK pathways in radiation responses. Oncogene. 2003;22:5885–5896

[71] Lee WH, Sonntag WE, Mitschelen M, Yan H, Lee YW. Irradiation induces regionally specific alterations in pro-inflammatory environments in rat brain. Int J Radiat Biol. 2010;86:132–144

[72] Zhou H, Liu Z, Liu J, Wang J, Zhou D, Zhao Z, Xiao S, Tao E, Suo WZ. Fractionated radiation-induced acute encephalopathy in a young rat model: cognitive dysfunction and histologic findings. AJNR Am J Neuroradiol. 2011;32:1795–1800

[73] Monje ML, Palmer T. Radiation injury and neurogenesis. Curr Opin Neurol. 2003;16:129–134

[74] Shors TJ, Miesegaes G, Beylin A, Zhao M, Rydel T, Gould E. Neurogenesis in the adult is involved in the formation of trace memories. Nature. 2001;410:372–376

[75] Klein M, Heimans JJ, Aaronson NK, et al. Effect of radiotherapy and other treatment-related factors on mid-term to long-term cognitive sequelae in low-grade gliomas: a comparative study. Lancet. 2002;360:1361–1368

[76] Swennen MH, Bromberg JE, Witkamp TD, et al. Delayed radiation toxicity after focal or whole brain radiotherapy for low-grade glioma. J Neurooncol. 2004;66:333–339

[77] Schultheiss TE, Kun LE, Ang KK, Stephens LC. Radiation response of the central nervous system. Int J Radiat Oncol Biol Phys. 1995;31:1093–1112

[78] Taphoorn, Martin JB, Bromberg, Jacoline EC. Neurological effect of therapeutic irradiation. Continuum. 2005;11:93–115

[79] Meyers CA, Wefel JS. The use of the mini-mental state examination to assess cognitive functioning in cancer trials: no ifs, ands, buts, or sensitivity. J Clin Oncol. 2003;21:3557–3558

[80] Meyers CA, Hess KR, Yung WK, Levin VA. Cognitive function as a predictor of survival in patients with recurrent malignant glioma. J Clin Oncol. 2000;18:646–650

[81] Wefel JS, Kayl AE, Meyers CA. Neuropsychological dysfunction associated with cancer and cancer therapies: a conceptual review of an emerging target. Br J Cancer. 2004;90:1691–1696

[82] Mahoney FI, Barthel DW. Functional evaluation: the Barthel index. Md State Med J. 1965;14:61–65

[83] Weitzner MA, Meyers CA, Gelke CK, Byrne KS, Cella DF, Levin VA. The Functional Assessment of Cancer Therapy (FACT) scale. Development of a brain subscale and revalidation of the general version (FACT-G) in patients with primary brain tumors. Cancer. 1995;75:1151–1161

[84] Armstrong CL, Hunter JV, Ledakis GE, Cohen B, Tallent EM, Goldstein BH, et al. Late cognitive and radiographic changes related to radiotherapy: initial prospective findings. Neurology. 2002;59:40–48

[85] Aarsen FK, Paquier PF, Arts WF, Van Veelen ML, Michiels E, Lequin M, Catsman-Berrevoets CE. Cognitive deficits and predictors 3 years after diagnosis of a pilocytic astrocytoma in childhood. J Clin Oncol. 2009;27(21):3526–3532

[86] Reeves CB, Palmer SL, Reddick WE, Merchant TE, Buchanan GM, Gajjar A, Mulhern RK. Attention and memory functioning among pediatric patients with medulloblastoma. J Pediatr Psychol. 2006;31(3):272–280

[87] Hoppe-Hirsch E, Brunet L, Laroussinie F, Cinalli G, Pierre-Kahn A, Rénier D, Sainte-Rose C, Hirsch JF. Intellectual outcome in children with malignant tumors of the posterior fossa: influence of the field of irradiation and quality of surgery. Childs Nerv Syst. 1995;11(6):340–345

[88] Shortman RI, Lowis SP, Penn A, McCarter RJ, Hunt LP, Brown CC, Stevens MC, Curran AL, Sharples PM. Cognitive function in children with brain tumors in the first year after

diagnosis compared to healthy matched controls. Pediatr Blood Cancer. 2014;61(3):464–72

[89] Douw L, Klein M, Fagel SS, van den Heuvel J, Taphoorn MJ, Aaronson NK, et al. Cognitive and radiological effects of radiotherapy in patients with low-grade glioma: long-term follow-up. Lancet Neurol. 2009;8:810–818

[90] Surma-aho O, Niemela M, Vilkki J, Kouri M, Brander A, Salonen O, et al. Adverse long-term effects of brain radiotherapy in adult low-grade glioma patients. Neurology. 2001;56:1285–1290

[91] Jalali R, Mallick I, Dutta D, Goswami S, Gupta T, Munshi A, et al. Factors influencing neurocognitive outcomes in young patients with benign and low-grade brain tumors treated with stereotactic conformal radiotherapy. Int J Radiat Oncol Biol Phys. 2010;77:974–979

[92] Chang EL, Wefel JS, Hess KR, Allen PK, Lang FF, Kornguth DG, Arbuckle RB, Swint JM, Shiu AS, Maor MH, Meyers CA. Neurocognition in patients with brain metastases treated with radiosurgery or radiosurgery plus whole-brain irradiation: a randomised controlled trial. Lancet Oncol. 2009;10(11):1037–1044

[93] Gondi V, Tolakanahalli R, Mehta MP, Tewatia D, Rowley H, Kuo JS, Khuntia D, Tomé WA. Hippocampal-sparing whole-brain radiotherapy: a "how-to" technique using helical tomotherapy and linear accelerator-based intensity-modulated radiotherapy. Int J Radiat Oncol Biol Phys. 2010;78(4):1244–1252

[94] Weber DC, Ares C, Lomax AJ, et al. Radiation therapy planning with photons and protons for early and advanced breast cancer: an overview. Radiat Oncol. 2006;1:22–57

[95] Blomstrand M, Brodin NP, Munck Af Rosenschöld P, Vogelius IR, Sánchez Merino G, Kiil-Berthlesen A, Blomgren K, Lannering B, Bentzen SM, Björk-Eriksson T. Estimated clinical benefit of protecting neurogenesis in the developing brain during radiation therapy for pediatric medulloblastoma. Neuro-oncology. 2012;14(7):882–889

[96] Mitchell T, Turton P. 'Chemobrain': concentration and memory effects in people receiving chemotherapy—a descriptive phenomenological study. Eur J Cancer Care. 2011;20:539–548

[97] Gong X, Schwartz PH, Linskey ME, Bota DA. Neural stem/progenitors and glioma stem-like cells have differential sensitivity to chemotherapy. Neurology. 2011;76:1126–1134

[98] Dietrich J, Han R, Yang Y, Mayer-Proschel M, Noble M. CNS progenitor cells and oligodendrocytes are targets of chemotherapeutic agents in vitro and in vivo. J Biol. 2006;5(7):22

[99] Saykin AJ, Ahles TA, McDonald BC. Mechanisms of chemotherapy-induced cognitive disorders: neuropsychological, pathophysiological, and neuroimaging perspectives. Semin Clin Neuropsychiatry. 2003;8:201–216

[100] Han R, Yang YM, Dietrich J, Luebke A, Mayer-Proschel M, Noble M. Systemic 5-fluorouracil treatment causes a syndrome of delayed myelin destruction in the central nervous system. J Biol. 2008;7(4):12

[101] Seigers R, Schagen SB, Beerling W, et al. Long-lasting suppression of hippocampal cell proliferation and impaired cognitive performance by methotrexate in the rat. Behav Brain Res. 2008;186(2):168–175

[102] Ahles TA, Saykin AJ, Noll WW, et al. The relationship of APOE genotype to neuropsychological performance in long-term cancer survivors treated with standard dose chemotherapy. Psychooncology. 2003;12:612–619

[103] Keime-Guibert F, Napolitano M, Delattre JY. Neurological complications of radiotherapy and chemotherapy. J Neurol. 1998;245:695–708

[104] der Weid N, Mosimann I, Hirt A, et al. Intellectual outcome in children and adolescents with acute lymphoblastic leukaemia treated with chemotherapy alone: age- and sex-related differences. Eur J Cancer. 2003;39:359–365

[105] Wen PY. Central nervous system complications of cancer therapy. In: Schiff D, Wen PY, editors. Cancer neurology in clinical practice. Chichester: Totowa: Humana Press; 2003. pp. 215–231

[106] Herrlinger U, Kuker W, Uhl M, Blaicher HP, Karnath HO, Kanz L, et al. NOA-03 trial of high-dose methotrexate in primary central nervous system lymphoma: final report. Ann Neurol. 2005;57:843–847

[107] Fliessbach K, Helmstaedter C, Urbach H, Althaus A, Pels H, Linnebank M, et al. Neuropsychological outcome after chemotherapy for primary CNS lymphoma: a prospective study. Neurology. 2005;64:1184–1188

[108] Nolan CP, DeAngelis LM. Neurologic complications of chemotherapy and radiation therapy. Continuum. 2015;2:429–451

[109] Copeland DR, Moore BD, Francis DJ, et al. Neuropsychologic effects of chemotherapy on children with cancer: a longitudinal study. J Clin Oncol. 1996;14:2826–2835

[110] Dietrich J, Han R, Yang Y, Mayer-Proschel M, Noble M. CNS progenitor cells and oligodendrocytes are targets of chemotherapeutic agents in vitro and in vivo. J Biol. 2006;5(7):22

[111] Prabhu RS, Won M, Shaw EG, Hu C, Brachman DG, Buckner JC, Mehta MP. Effect of the addition of chemotherapy to radiotherapy on cognitive function in patients with low-grade glioma: secondary analysis of RTOG 98–02. J Clin Oncol. 2014;32:535–541. doi:10.1200/JCO.2013.53.1830)

[112] Taphoorn MJ1, Sizoo EM, Bottomley A. Review on quality of life issues in patients with primary brain tumors. Oncologist. 2010;15(6):618–626. doi:10.1634/theoncologist.2009–0291. Epub 2010 May 27

[113] Levin VA, Yung WK, Bruner J, et al. Phase II study of accelerated fractionation radiation therapy with carboplatin followed by PCV chemotherapy for the treatment of anaplastic gliomas. Int J Radiat Oncol Biol Phys. 2002;53:58–66

[114] Hilverda K, Bosma I, Heimans JJ, Postma TJ, Peter Vandertop W, Slotman BJ, et al. Cognitive functioning in glioblastoma patients during radiotherapy and temozolomide treatment: initial findings. J Neurooncol. 2010;97:89–94

[115] Liu R, Solheim K, Polley MY, et al. Quality of life in low-grade glioma patients receiving temozolomide. Neuro-oncology. 2009;11:59–68

[116] Osoba D, Brada M, YungWK, et al. Health-related quality of life in patients with anaplastic astrocytoma during treatment with temozolomide. Eur J Cancer. 2000;36:1788–1795

[117] Yang ES, Wang H, Jiang G, et al. Lithium-mediated protection of hippocampal cells involves enhance-ment of DNA-PK-dependent repair in mice. J Clin Investig. 2009;119:1124–1135

[118] Ramanan S, Kooshki M, Zhao W et al. The PPARa agonist fenofibrate preserves hippocampal neurogenesis and inhibits microglial activation after whole-brain irradiation. Int J Radiat Oncol Biol Phys. 2009;75:870–877

[119] Kuhnt D, Ganslandt O, Schlaffer SM, et al. Quantification of glioma removal by intraoperative high-field magnetic resonance imaging: an update. Neurosurgery. 2011;69:852–862

[120] Ahn ES, Goumnerova L. Endoscopic biopsy of brain tumors in children: diagnostic success and utility in guiding treatment strategies. J Neurosurg Pediatr. 2010;5:255–262

[121] St Clair WH, Adams JA, Bues M, et. Al. Advantage of protons compared to conventional X-ray or IMRT in the treatment of a pediatric patient with medulloblastoma. . Int J Radiat Oncol Biol Phys. 2004;58:727–734

[122] Lin SY, Yang CC, Wu YM, Tseng CK, Wei KC, Chu YC, Hsieh HY, Wu TH, Pai PC, Hsu PW, Chuang CC. Evaluating the impact of hippocampal sparing during whole brain radiotherapy on neurocognitive functions: a preliminary report of a prospective phase II study. Biomed J. 2015;38(5):439–449. doi:10.4103/2319-4170.157440

[123] Wahba HA, Abu-Hegazy M, Wasel Y, Ismail EI, Zidan AS. Adjuvant chemotherapy after reduced craniospinal irradiation dose in children with average-risk medulloblastoma: a 5-year follow-up study. JBUON. 2013;18(2):425–429

[124] Merchant TE, Hua CH, Shukla H, et al. Proton versus photon radiotherapy for common pediatric brain tumors: comparison of models of dose characteristics and their relationship to cognitive function. Pediatr Blood Cancer. 2008;51:110–117

[125] Kim YJ, Park HJ, Lee G, et al. Neuroprotective effects of human mesenchymal stem cells on dopami-nergic neurons through anti-inflammatory action. Glia. 2009;57:13–23

[126] Acharya MM, Christie LA, Lan ML, et al. Human neural stem cell transplantation ameliorates radiation-induced cognitive dysfunction. Cancer Res. 2011;71:4834–4845

[127] Berridge CW, Shumsky JS, Andrzejewski ME, et al. Differential sensitivity to psychostimulants across prefrontal cognitive tasks: differential involvement of noradrenergic a1- and a2-receptors. Biol Psychiatry. 2012;71:467–473

[128] DeLong R, Friedman H, Friedman N, Gustafson K, Oakes J, Methylphenidate in neuropsychological sequelae of radiotherapy and chemotherapy of childhood brain tumors and leukemia. J Child Neurol. 1992;7(4):462–463

[129] Meyers CA, Weitzner MA, Valentine AD, Levin VA. Methylphenidate therapy improves cognition, mood, and function of brain tumor patients. J Clin Oncol. 1998;16(7):2522–2527

[130] Shaw EG, Rosdhal R, D'Agostino RB Jr, et al. Phase II study of donepezil in irradiated brain tumor patients: effect on cognitive function, mood, and quality of life. J Clin Oncol. 2006;24:1415–1420

[131] Nazemi KI, Butler RW. Neuropsychological rehabilitation for survivors of childhood and adolescent brain tumors: a view of the past and a vision for a promising future: an interdisciplinary approach. J Pediatr Rehabil Med. 2011;4:37–46

[132] Butler RW, Copeland DR, Fairclough DL, et al. A multicenter, randomized clinical trial of a cognitive remediation program for childhood survivors of a pediatric malignancy. J Consult Clin Psychol. 2008;76(3):367–378

[133] Butler RW, Copeland RR. Interventions for cancer late effects and survivorship, In: Brown R. editor. Comprehensive Handbook of Childhood Cancer and Sickle Cell Disease. Chichester: New York, NY: Oxford University Press, Inc.; 2006. p. 297

[134] Gehring K, Aaronson N, Taphoorn M, Sitskoorn M. A description of a cognitive rehabilitation programme evaluated in brain tumour patients with mild to moderate cognitive deficits. Clin Rehabil. 2011;25(8):675–692. doi:10.1177/0269215510395791

[135] Richard NM, Bernstein LJ, Mason WP, Laperriere N, Chung C, Millar BA, Maurice C, 25 Edelstein K. Cognitive rehabilitation for brain tumor survivors: a pilot study. 2016 Cancer Survivorship Symposium.http://meetinglibrary.asco.org/content/119165?media=vm&poster=1

8

Medulloblastoma

Asifur Rahman

Abstract

Among the pediatric brain tumors, medulloblastoma (MB) is the most common solid variety and entirely occur in the posterior fossa with tendency to seed into CSF spaces. Despite innovations in technological developments and understanding of tumor biology, modern imaging facilities, advances in surgical practices, and newer chemotherapeutic and radiation techniques, this malignant type of tumor continues to be a formidable entity. Even though, the outcome in terms of survival rate is better than any time before, the overall result is still disappointing. With advances in management strategy, chances of survival with good quality of life have been amplified, where newer targeted therapies and rehabilitation plays an immense role. While the adverse effects of surgery and adjuvant therapies are still on play, researchers are trying ceaselessly to minimize those to give maximum wellbeing to these unfortunate children.

Keywords: medulloblastoma, surgery, radiotherapy, chemotherapy, molecular subgroup

1. Introduction

Medulloblastomas are a group of highly undifferentiated, rapidly growing, extremely malignant formidable solid tumor of childhood with worst estimated prognosis. Maximal safe resection, craniospinal irradiation (CSI) and chemotherapy remain the mainstays of first-line treatment of these aggressive embryonal tumors which are the most frequent primary malignant brain cancer in children.

The name "medulloblastoma" was first adapted by Harvey Cushing in 1930. Initially these tumors were termed as spongioblastoma indifferentiale, spongioblastoma multiforme, spongioblastoma cerebelli or simply spongioblastoma by different authors. Cushing presumed this subset of tumors to be originating from one of the five pluripotent stem cells, the medulloblast, thought to populate the primitive neural tube [1–5]. It has meanwhile been established that the concept of embryonal cell identified as medulloblast does not exist [6, 7]. Hence the term medulloblastoma that Cushing erroneously coined, which is so strongly concreted to the nomenclature, is actually a misnomer [7].

Medulloblastomas were considered as one of the most disappointing maladies in neurosurgery until the 1960s as survival was still equally poor as was in the early periods of neurosurgery when posterior fossa tumors were most daunting. Overall, improved diagnostic, surgical, and radiation technologies, newer and more effective chemotherapy regimens have led to dramatically improved patient outcomes with advanced research [8]. Multidisciplinary approach being the keystone of success for this formidable disease, significant clinical challenge still remains because of acute onset, rapid growth, rapid clinical course and early fatal termination leading to great number of morbidity and mortality despite aggressive therapeutic strategies [2, 3, 9, 10].

Survival of medulloblastoma patients have become better over the last few decades nonetheless in patients with relapse, the outcome is still miserable. Long-term survival rates have progressively improved from 22% by 1950s to 85% in 2015 with current approaches [11–14]. This significant development has resulted from combination of systemic chemotherapy and improvement in supportive care measures in addition to the regular treatment with surgery and radiotherapy [15–19]. Advances in genetic profiling with emergence of newer agents and development of newer strategies targeting the key molecular alterations have improved the outcomes further [20]. Efforts to improve survival results, dose reduction or elimination of radiation or trial with less offensive chemotherapeutic agents are going on to standardize the treatment of medulloblastoma.

2. Epidemiology

2.1. Incidence

Generally it is recognized that medulloblastoma is the most common malignant brain tumor in children. However, recent data shows that as a group, high-grade gliomas are marginally more prevalent. Approximately 350 new pediatric cases of medulloblastoma are diagnosed in the United States every year and that represents about 30% of pediatric brain tumors and 7–10% of all brain tumors [2, 6, 8, 9, 21–23].

2.2. Age

There are characteristic bimodal peaks, having a higher incidence in children between 3 and 4 years of age and between 8 and 10 years of age. About 70% of childhood medulloblastomas occur in this age range of the first decade. However, medulloblastoma has been reported in a 2-week-old infant and a 55-year-old adult [6, 9]. About 1–3% of cases are reported in adults, mostly before the age of 40 years [8, 24, 25].

2.3. Sex

Curiously enough, Cushing found medulloblastomas to be three times more common in males than females and since then most published reports indicate a continuing male predominance. On an average the male to female ratio is 2:1 [2, 8, 9].

2.4. Location

The typical medulloblastoma develops in the midline of the posterior fossa [9, 25]. Some 70–80% of medulloblastomas have been found in the midcerebellum with or without extension into the lateral cerebellar hemispheres. Medulloblastomas typically arise from the medullary velum and fill the cavity of the fourth ventricle and has the propensity to spread throughout the brain and spine via the cerebrospinal fluid (CSF) and about one third of the cases infiltrate the dorsal brainstem [8, 26].

3. Etiology

The etiologies of medulloblastoma are still obscure for most patients. Though Parental pesticide use and parental occupational contact with hydrocarbons, exposure to N-nitroso compounds and metals have been associated with higher incidence in some studies [25].

For development of medulloblastoma, the most ventured postulation in the earlier literatures was cell misplacements during early embryonic development where genetic factors play vital role [9]. This has been proven true with time with the advancement of genetic studies. Association between several familial cancer syndromes in children with medulloblastomas like TP53 germline mutation syndromes, Gorlin syndrome, and Turcot syndrome also supports predisposition of hereditary factors [8].

Studies have identified Human Cytomegalovirus (HCMV) protein pp65 immunoreactivity in medulloblastomas, but the oncogenic role of HCMV is still debated. Yet HCMV is believed to play role as a significant oncomodulator and based on that researchers are on the quest to utilize the potential of HCMV as a novel immunotherapeutic agent [25, 27–29].

4. Pathology

4.1. General

The World Health Organization (WHO) defines medulloblastoma as "a malignant, invasive embryonal tumor of the cerebellum with preferential manifestation in children, predominantly neuronal differentiation and an inherent tendency to metastasize via cerebrospinal (CSF) pathways" [30]. Although it is generally agreed that cerebellar medulloblastoma is an embryonic tumor, its origin is still a matter of speculation [9].

4.2. Macroscopic pathology

Macroscopically these midline globular, soft tumors are fairly well demarcated, and are apparently encapsulated. The marked vascularity gives them a dark, dirty brownish-red hue and occasionally they have extensive areas of necrosis. Consistency may vary from suckable to rubbery or to even firm sometimes. Calcifications are seen occasionally while hemorrhage in medulloblastoma is an extremely rare occurrence. Often marked edema of a wide zone of the neighboring tissue is also seen. They overlie the fourth ventricle as they develop in the midline in the roof of the fourth ventricle to occupy it, but most of the floors of the fourth ventricle in the great majority of cases are typically free. They usually block the aqueduct of Sylvius, with significant dilatation. These have a tendency to invade the meninges. Commonly they grow downward through the foramen magnum from the primary location between the tonsils of the cerebellum [1–3, 9]. CSF dissemination into the subarachnoid spaces often lead to local or widespread leptomeningeal metastases in the spinal axis or over the surface of the cerebral hemispheres or cerebellum and this also may cause characteristic pearly gray sheets of tumor in the meninges. Furthermore, widespread implantation of tumor can be found throughout the ventricles [9, 31].

4.3. Microscopic pathology

Generally medulloblastomas are categorized as small blue-cell tumors, based on presence of their deeply basophilic nuclei [25]. Histologically, these tumors comprise of densely packed rounded or pear-shaped or sometimes spindle-shaped cells having large ovoid nuclei containing plentiful network of chromatin with scanty cytoplasm and for the most part consisting of numerous embryonic glia fibrillae [1, 3, 8]. These are highly cellular tumors forming uniform sheets of cells, interposed with occasional thin-walled blood vessels. Low magnification reveals that the cells appear as a loose structureless mass, but the nuclei sometimes may form pseudo-rosettes or may show a palisade arrangement. Extensive areas of necrosis, numerous hemorrhagic foci and great vascularity often come across too [1, 3, 9]. Thin-walled blood vessels with delicate connective tissue confined to their walls can be demonstrated by special staining with Perdrau's stain [9].

4.4. Electron microscopic examination

The electron microscopic picture is a mosaic of cells, processes, and fibers. The tumor cells are arranged in a tightly packed mass as also seen in light microscopy. Both the glial and neuronal cells can be recognized on electron microscopic analysis [9].

4.5. Immunohistochemistry

Immunohistochemistry can help in diagnosis of medulloblastoma and can provide information augmenting the plan for further management. Mitosis is seen in up to 80% of tumors, as assessed by positive staining with the Ki-67/MIB1 antibody. Medulloblastomas are frequently positive for vimentin and synaptophysin staining [32].

4.6. Genetic aspects

With the advent of genetic profiling and molecular analysis, evolving evidences point to the fact that the different precursor cell populations that form the cerebellum are vulnerable to mutations in signal pathways that regulate their functions; these mutations modify normal development pathways and may result in the development of distinct variants of medulloblastoma [33].

5. Classification

From the very beginning of history of this special type of tumor, these has been tried to be classified in different ways. With the advent and development of molecular biology and incorporation of that with genetic profiling has taken the classification beyond the level of mere histological classification. The molecular subgroupings are helpful in prediction of course of the disease and outcome as well as choosing therapeutic options. Recently the treatment plan is devised in accordance with the classification that integrates both histological and the molecular subgroupings to have the best possible outcome on the basis of a personalized treatment for individual patients.

5.1. Histological classification

Histopathological classification of medulloblastoma has evolved with time. Rubinstein and Northfield [34] initially identified three variants of medulloblastoma: pigmented papillary medulloblastoma, medullomyoblastoma, and desmoplastic medulloblastoma. With newer technologies, newer histological types were being introduced. To alleviate the confusions, the World Health Organization (WHO) in 1976 developed a common classification of brain tumors in an effort to combine the various systems in use till then and the WHO publication "Histological Typing of Tumours of the Central Nervous System" in 1979 outlined and illustrated the new classification system [30, 35, 36]. Since then modifications, additions and characterization of classification of medulloblastoma has evolved a lot throughout the newer classifications of medulloblastoma of the WHO editions of classifications gradually in 1993 [35], 2000 [37, 38] and 2007 [30]. The present histological classification that is in practice has the following types:

1. **Classic medulloblastoma:** Most common histologic subtype (66%). Composed of sheets of densely packed, small to medium-sized, round to oval-shaped, blue cells (basophilic) with a high nuclear to cytoplasmic ratio and high mitotic and apoptotic activity. Reticulin staining shows a lack of nodular desmoplasia.

2. **Large cell/anaplastic medulloblastoma**: Large cell medulloblastomas have monomorphic cells with large, round, prominent nuclei, high mitotic activity, and frequent apoptosis, while the anaplastic medulloblastoma are characterized by hallmarks of anaplasia. Large cell and anaplastic medulloblastomas have a significant degree of cytologic overlap and are differentiated only by the degree of anaplasia.

3. **Desmoplastic/nodular medulloblastoma**: Widespread desmoplasia, characterized by presence of nodular, reticulin-poor "pale islands" of neurocytic differentiation surrounded by densely packed, mitotically active cells having pleomorphic and hyperchromatic nuclei. Reticulin staining highlights internodular desmoplasia.

4. **Medulloblastoma with extensive nodularity (MBEN)**: Similar to nodular type but has an expanded lobular architecture with more prominent reticulin-free zones that are more elongated and rich in neutrophil-like tissue. Reticulin staining highlights internodular desmoplasia. Advanced neurocytic differentiation in islands with strong nuclear NeuN expression is also seen.

Two other histologic types of medulloblastomas are also recognized but are not considered to be distinct variants. They are the Myogenic differentiation type and the Melanotic medulloblastoma. All the histopathological types have significant predictability of prognoses in accordance with the clinico-pathological characteristics of each tumor type as outlined in the WHO classification [6, 8, 30, 34].

5.2. Genetic classification and subgroups

Research in the molecular study has led to understanding of embryonal tumors of the CNS. This reflection has basically been driven by genomic studies characterizing prevalent genetic profiles and biological features. These have led to tumor reclassification, sub-typing and detection of novel entities [10, 39, 40]. Over the last two decades, individual molecular subgroups have been identified for medulloblastoma based on cytogenetic profiles. Each group is named for the cellular pathway activation or genomic alterations it exhibits and each subgroup is associated with distinct prognostic character and survival outcomes [8]. In 2010, in Boston, an international group of medulloblastoma authorities, came to a consensus to categorize medulloblastomas into four distinct subgroups: Wingless (Wnt), Sonic hedgehog (Shh), Group 3, and Group 4 based on their unique set of demographic and clinical features, genetics, gene expression, genome-wide transcriptomic and DNA methylomic profiles [41, 42]. Prediction of outcome and clinical behavior is more precise with the known molecular subgroups than the histopathology or clinical staging. [6, 43–45]. These molecular subgroups are distinct from the histologic subtypes, albeit there are certain areas of considerable overlap (**Figure 1**).

5.2.1. Wingless pathway tumors (Wnt pathway/Wnt-MB)

The Wingless pathway (also termed as the β-catenin pathway) comprises of secreted glycoproteins which are secreted to act through signal transduction to regulate various parts of embryonic development. Uncontrolled activation of Wnt pathway signaling results in accumulation of β-catenin, encoded by the CTNNB1 gene, leading to aberrant up regulation of transcription and ensues oncogenesis [46]. Wnt pathway tumors are the least common of the four molecular subgroups that represents merely about 10% of sporadic medulloblastomas [47]. Genetic features of this subgroup are characterized by the aberrations like monosomy 6, CTNNB1 mutations, and nuclear β-catenin positivity by immunohistochemistry [47]. This subgroup of medulloblastomas is more common in children and in adults than in infants. The outcomes of these medulloblastomas are outstanding and 5-year overall survival rate is 95% in children and 100% in adults [6, 10, 42]. TP53 mutations are invariably present in both the Wnt and Shh subgroup medulloblastomas [6, 42, 48]. As Wnt-MB has uniformly good prognosis, treatment regimen can be de-escalated with reduced dose of craniospinal radiation, reduced-intensity of chemotherapy, or a combination of both in patients without metastatic disease [49].

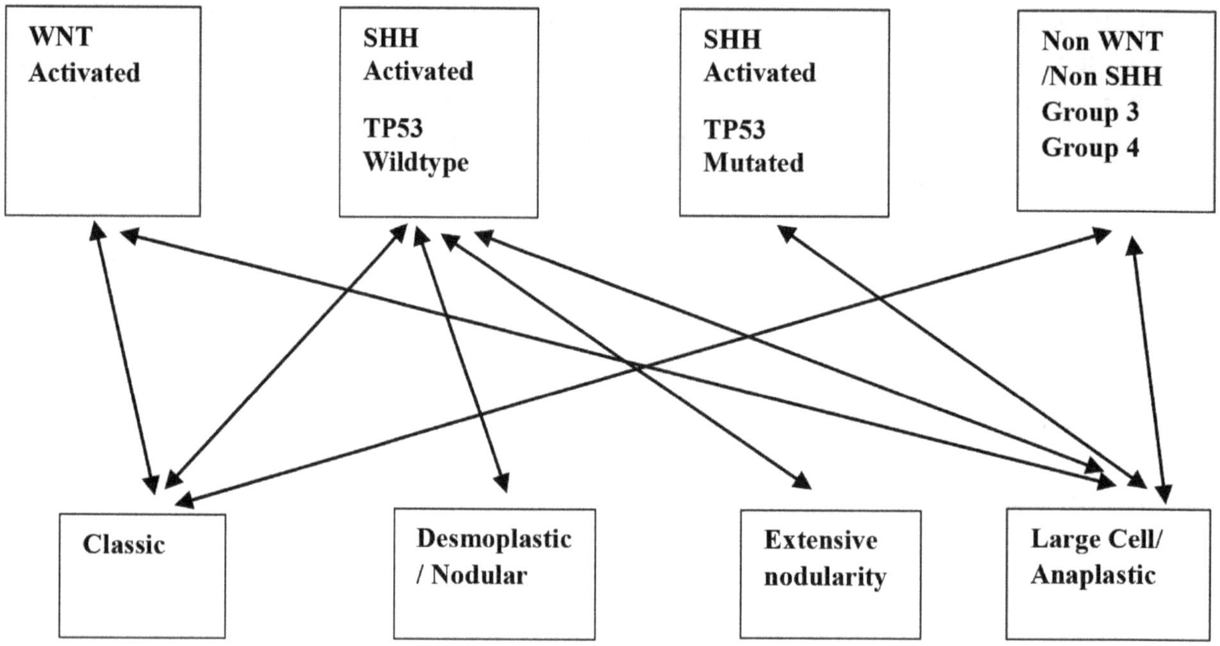

Figure 1. WHO 2016 classification of medulloblastoma subtypes, characterized by genetic and histological features.

5.2.2. Sonic hedgehog pathway tumors (Shh pathway/Shh-MB)

The Shh group of medulloblastomas is named after the Sonic Hedgehog signaling pathway, which is thought to drive this type of tumor initiation [42]. Medulloblastomas categorized by activation of Shh signaling are heterogeneous and are linked with a variety of genetic aberrations and outcomes, unlike the Wnt-MB [50]. As a whole, Shh subgroup tumors comprises nearly 30% of medulloblastomas overall [42, 48, 50].

Medulloblatomas of the Shh subgroup results from genetic predisposition of alteration of the sonic hedgehog pathway in the form of germline mutations in the patched-1 gene (PTCH1) or the suppressor of fused gene (SUFU). Loss of function PTCH1 and SUFU mutations lead to truncation of their associated protein products, leading to failure of their tumor suppressor effects and activation of Shh signaling with resultant tumorigenesis. Somatic mutations in PTCH1 and SUFU are also associated with sporadic medulloblastomas characterized by activation of the Shh pathway, along with PTCH2, MYC, SMO, GLI1 and GLI2 mutations [6, 42, 51, 52]. Deletion of chromosome 9q seems to be restricted to Shh medulloblastomas, which is fitting as the PTCH gene is located at chromosome 9q22 [42].

Clinical outcomes of individuals with Shh-MB can be divided into favorable and poor survival groups depending on TP53 mutation status which is particularly critical [48]. Patients with Shh/TP53 mutant variety medulloblastomas have extremely poor outcome than those with Shh/TP53 wild-type tumors as mutant TP53 has been associated with high rate of anaplasia and MYCN amplification, which are equally disastrous cellular events [48, 53]. Because of its clinical impact, TP53 mutation status has been incorporated into the 2016 WHO classification for CNS tumors and is part of routine assessment in all Shh-activated medulloblastomas [40].

Survival for Shh subgroup medulloblastomas is similar to Group 4 medulloblastomas and intermediate between that of Wnt and Group 3 medulloblastomas and varies significantly based on age and histologic subtype [10, 42, 48].

5.2.3. Non-Wnt/Shh tumors

The non-Wnt/Shh tumor subgroup encompasses Group 3 and Group 4, in which the underlying genetic predisposition of mutations have yet not been recognized [49]. These types are associated with a higher incidence of tumor dissemination and approximately 30% of patients have metastasis at the time of diagnosis [6]. Despite these similarities, features of Group 3 and Group 4 subgroup medulloblastomas vary regarding the demographic, clinical, transcriptional, and genetic differences between them and these advocate that they are actually distinct entities with molecular diversity [42, 54].

5.2.3.1. Group 3 MB

Nearly 30% of medulloblastomas are of the Group 3 subgroup and histologically mostly are of the "classic" variety of medulloblastomas [6, 55–57]. These tumors genetically are more likely to have high-level expression and amplification of MYC, MYCN and OTX2 with imbalance of chromosome 17 [42, 49, 51, 58]. Group 3 tumors show gain of chromosome 1q, and/or loss of chromosome 5q and chromosome 10q more than Group 4 tumors [42]. They occur more frequently in infants and children, and has the worst outcome among all molecular subgroups, with 10-year overall survival of 39% in infants and 50% in children [6, 42, 49, 51, 59].

5.2.3.2. Group 4 MB

About 35% of medulloblastomas overall are of Group 4 subgroup and the peak incidence for this subgroup is in late childhood and early adolescents [6, 42]. The prognosis of Group 4 tumors is similar to Shh subgroups tumors and is intermediate between those of Wnt and Group 3 subgroup tumors. Patients with metastatic disease or MYC amplifications in this Group have significantly poorer outcomes [49, 50]. Though isochromosome 17q is also seen in Group 3 tumors, it is more common in Group 4 tumors. Another prominent cytogenetic alteration among Group 4 tumors is loss of the X chromosome, which is found in 80% of females with Group 4 medulloblastoma [42].

Recently, the discovery of seven novel molecular subgroups has permitted to categorize patients further to envisage better disease subclassification and outcome predictions. These subgroup dependent grouping stratified patients into four clinical risk groups for 5-year progression-free survival: favorable risk (91% survival); standard risk (81% survival); highrisk (42% survival); and very high-risk (28% survival) [41]. Another study recommended total of 12 subgroups based on the integration of transcriptomic and methylation data. In that analysis medulloblastoma encompasses 12 subtypes; 2 Wnt, 4 Shh, 3 Group 3, and 3 Group 4 groups. These subtypes of each subgroup are clinically and biologically pertinent [54].

5.3. Integrated classification

In 2016, for the first time, the molecular characteristics was incorporated into the WHO classification for the diagnosis of CNS tumors. This integration of histological features with genetic information has considerably transformed the diagnostic work-up and reporting of tumors of the CNS. Nonetheless, this remains perplexing in embryonal tumors due to their de novo tumor heterogeneity that is being faced [10]. This integrated diagnosis is presented in a layered format; that includes the histological diagnosis, WHO grade, molecular genetic information and ultimately the integrated diagnosis. The value of this approach is clearly illustrated in embryonal tumors, in particular medulloblastoma, where the combination of molecular and histological data provides discrete diagnostic information [40]. In this new concept of a "layered diagnosis" brain tumors that are diagnosed purely morphologically are incorporated with molecular characteristics for an "integrated diagnosis" at the peak diagnostic level [60]. In the layered integrated classification, a patient would be labeled as having medulloblastoma of a definite histological subtype, the WHO grade and the molecular subgroup [61].

6. Staging

There is no well-established staging system for medulloblastoma for prediction from which treatment plan and outcome prediction can be made. In 1969, Chang et al. suggested an operative staging system for medulloblastomas adapting the TNM classification for other tumors [62]. According to the size and extent of primary tumor, T category was divided into four main groups with subdivisions of T3 (T1, T2, T3a, T3b or T4) and the M category had five groups (M0, M1, M2, M3 and M4) based on the degree of tumor spread in the CSF pathway or extra-CNS metastases [9]. Overall, M staging has remained more useful in prognostic evaluation, while the T staging is less valuable as a prognostic indicator [63]. Several studies have stratified the patients into "high-risk" and "average" or "standard-risk" groups depending on age of the patient, residual disease after surgery, pathologic variant, and M staging [8, 64]. This risk stratification is a good predictor of outcome. Standard-risk and high-risk categories have long term survival rates of approximately 85% and 70%, respectively [6].

7. Presentation

Because of its origin in the posterior fossa, the presenting symptoms of medulloblastoma are often vague complaints and understandably the diagnosis may be delayed. Presentation depends on various elements of the tumor subject to location, size, duration, compression on the surrounding structures. As these arise from the vicinity of cerebellum and brainstem, often the first feature to appear is instability of gait. Being a midline posterior fossa lesion, trunkal ataxia appears first and appendicular ataxia gradually ensues as the tumor grows bigger to compress the cerebellar hemispheres, and other common cerebellar signs follow with time. When the tumor is big enough to compress the brainstem, long tract signs begin to appear and add more difficulty in movement of the patients. As the tumor grows further, especially downwards, the lower cranial nerves start to get involved and lower cranial nerve palsies manifest. If the tumor grows bigger to occupy and block the Aqueduct of Sylvius, hydrocephalus ensues. Hydrocephalus may also result from blockage of the fourth ventricular outlets, by compression, by the growing tumor, individually or in combination. Hydrocephalus in turn may lead to features of raised Intracranial Pressure (ICP) resulting in headache, nausea, vomiting, irritability, lethargy, behavior alteration, personality change and impaired memory or attention, etc. Raised ICP occasionally gives rise to possibility of having seizure and 6th nerve palsy. Respiratory and cardiac manifestations may be evident, resulting from compromise of the respiratory and cardiac centers in the brainstem. Alteration of level of consciousness, starting from disorientation to deep coma, may result either from raised ICP or from compression on the brainstem. Papilledema or even visual impairment from raised ICP is not very uncommon, especially when presented in late stage.

Medulloblastoma is a very rapidly growing tumor and tends to follow a rapid progression in a very short period of time. The median time between onset of symptom until diagnosis (symptom interval) is 3.3 months (65 days) [65]. Rarely, patients may have symptoms for up to 6 months before diagnosis and younger patients have significantly longer interval to diagnosis while more aggressive subgroups of medulloblastoma have a shorter pre-diagnostic interval [66].

8. Diagnosis and differentials

The Accurate diagnosis of pediatric tumors is essential to ensure balance between achieving a long-term cure and avoiding treatment related disability in survivors. The tentative diagnosis of medulloblastoma is relatively straight cut one from the age of the patient, history and neurological examination findings. Nonetheless, there are other maladies that are to be kept in mind. The two commonest differential diagnosis of a posterior fossa mass in children are pilocytic astrocytoma and ependymoma. Other lesions to be considered are atypical teratoid/rhabdoid tumors, exophytic brainstem glioma and choroid plexus papilloma as well as teratoma in infants and hemangioblastoma in patients with Von Hippel-Lindau syndrome. Metastasis is the first to be thought in adults as that is the most frequently encountered posterior fossa lesion [6, 10].

9. Investigation work ups

A variety of diagnostic studies are used to confirm the clinical diagnosis of medulloblastoma and to localize the tumor exactly. The first-line diagnostic test for medulloblastoma is brain imaging.

Up until introduction of CT scan in 1971, air studies (pneumoencephalography and ventriculography) were most reliable and almost accurate in the diagnosis of medulloblastoma in all age groups. Angiography also yielded useful results regardless of age. With advent of MRI, CT scan has become an adjunct to that. Skull x-ray studies, once useful for the detection of brain tumors, is now rarely of value. Nucleotide brain scans and bone scans, myelographic examination, CSF cytology were also helpful in diagnosing a moderate number of cases [6, 8, 9, 67, 68].

9.1. Computerized tomography (CT)

CT is often used as the first-line diagnostic imaging because of its readily availability, fastness in imaging and comparatively cheaper price [8]. This is a good tool for early diagnosis with state of hydrocephalus, serial evaluation of tumor, postoperative assessment of extent of tumor removal, detection of residual and recurrent tumor, and tumor deposits in the CSF pathways as well as convenient follow-up studies [4, 15, 42]. Medulloblastomas appear typically hyperdense and sharply demarcated lesion near the fourth ventricle in the plain CT scan with a surrounding hypodense zone of edema which show better delineation with contrast enhancement showing moderate to marked increase in density (**Figure 2**). Cystic components may also be seen. Leptomeningeal tumor deposits appear as areas of increased density in the subarachnoid space. Calcification may be seen in about 10–20% of medulloblastomas [5, 62].

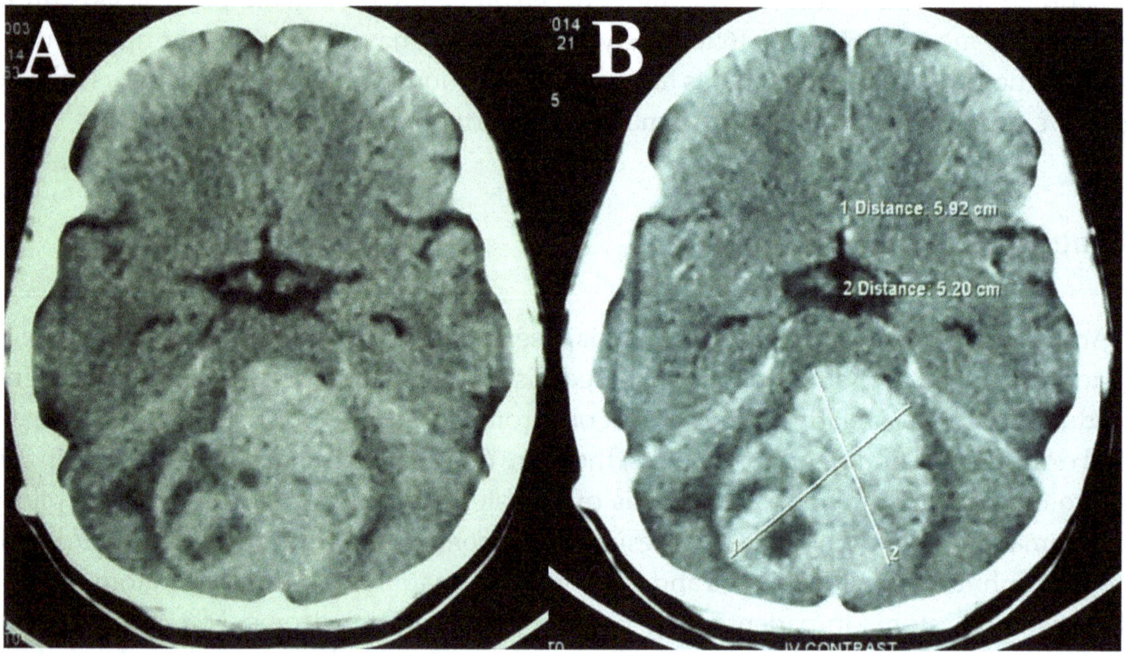

Figure 2. Plain axial CT scan (A) showing hyperdense and sharply demarcated lesion near the fourth ventricle with surrounding hypodense area of edema which with contrast enhancement (B) is well demarcated by increased density.

9.2. Magnetic resonance imaging (MRI)

The relationship between the tumor and the surrounding brain structures can be vividly demonstrated in MRI with and without gadolinium. Screening MRI of the whole spinal axis is capable of displaying and evaluating tumor dissemination, when present and pre-operative whole spine MRI is preferred [20, 21].

Different sequences of MRI can provide different information to help in diagnosis and treatment planning. Medulloblastomas are hypointense to gray matter on T1-weighted imaging (T1WI) with heterogeneous gadolinium enhancement in 90% of cases, while they are generally iso to hyperintense to gray matter on T2-weighted imaging (T2WI). The heterogeneity in T1WI and T2WI results from cyst formation, calcification or necrosis. Diffusion-weighted imaging (DWI) shows restricted diffusion and in fluid-attenuated inversion recovery (FLAIR) imaging, medulloblastomas are generally hyperintense to surrounding brain (**Figure 3**). MR spectroscopy (MRS) shows elevated choline peaks and decreased creatine and N-acetyl acetate peaks, with occasional elevation in lactic acid and lipid peaks [62].

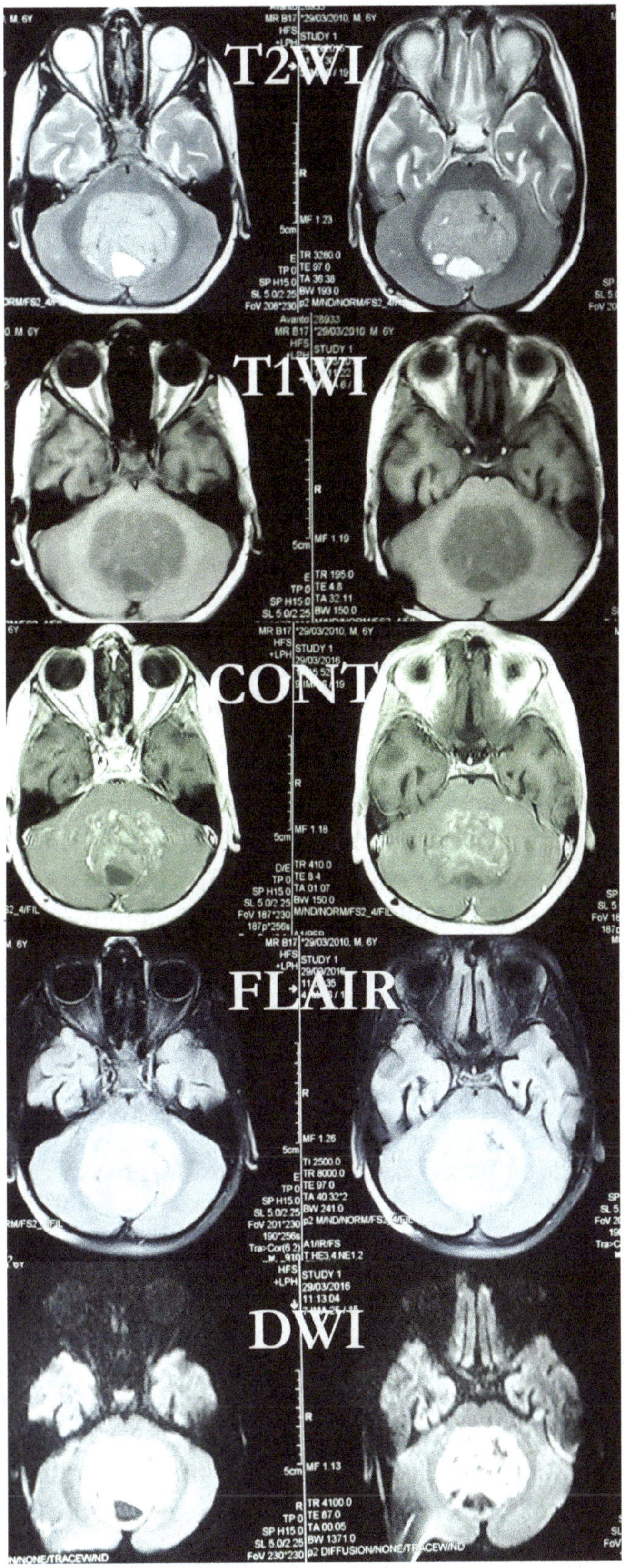

Figure 3. Medulloblastomas in T2-weighted imaging (T2WI), T1-weighted imaging (T1WI), with gadolinium enhancement (CONT), fluid-attenuated inversion recovery (FLAIR) (D) and diffusion-weighted imaging (DWI) in axial planes.

9.3. Molecular diagnosis

Molecular diagnosis is of immense importance and an integral part of the management protocol as it is invaluable in prediction of outcome and in formulation of dose of therapy, especially in cases of selection of agents for targeted therapy. As these state of the art assays are accessible merely in few laboratories of the first-world neuropathological institutions, it is often very difficult to come to an integrated diagnosis for most of the centers in the world. Nonetheless, molecular antibodies specifically targeting mutated proteins should be available in nearly all neuropathological laboratories.

10. Treatment

10.1. General

Treatment strategies for medulloblastomas have advanced slowly over the past 5 decades. Generally based on the histology and clinical factors, especially, disease dissemination at presentation and residual tumor after surgical resection, management of medulloblastoma has evolved to maximal safe surgical resection followed by radiation therapy and adjuvant chemotherapy [20, 22–24, 26, 69].

Adjuvant chemotherapy is recommended for all patients as this improves outcomes significantly. Following surgery, risks of recurrence and of neurocognitive effects of radiation therapy, doses of radiation and the type of chemotherapy protocol vary depending on extent of disease and age of the patient as well as institutional preferences [20, 29].

Though the medulloblastoma subgroups (Wnt, Shh, Groups 3 and 4) have distinct molecular and clinical profile, current adjuvant chemotherapy that are in practice are for the nontargated ones. However, significant improvements, approximately 70% 5-year survival rate with these combined therapies are achieved at the high cost of the quality of life, resulting mostly from the effects of radiotherapy and nonspecific, antimitotic agents on the developing brains of young medulloblastoma patients [27–31]. A general approach carries significant risk of over or under-treatment. [30, 34].

10.2. Surgery and surgical techniques

In March 1925, Cushing first succeeded in gross total removal of a medulloblastoma [1, 2]. Since then, the first-line treatment for medulloblastoma is surgery with the aim of maximal safe resection, along with treatment of any concomitant hydrocephalus [8]. But Cushing also cautioned that "the temptation will always be present for the surgeon to attempt an enucleation, a conservative attitude in this respect is the course of wisdom" [1, 8].

The basic principles of surgery for medulloblastoma have changed little in the modern era, but technological revolutions in surgical technique and supportive care have made surgery safer. Development of surgical skill and other facilities has dramatically reduced the perioperative mortality from 25.2% during the period of Cushing to less than 1% in expert hands at the present time [70]. With recent technological advancements the goal of surgery is always a complete excision, but practically it can safely be accomplished only in about one fourth of cases [71].

Most surgeons prefer the prone position than to the sitting position to minimize the risk of air embolism, frontal pneumocephalus, and systemic hypotension. The straight vertical skin incision employed by almost all neurosurgeons today was described first by Naffziger in 1928 [70]. A wide craniectomy or craniotomy extending from the transverse sinuses to the foramen magnum is performed with or without removal of the posterior arch of C1. The dura is usually opened in a Y-shaped manner extending down to the level of C1 when the posterior arch is removed. The tumor may be readily evident as a red, semi circumscribed mass peeping into the vallecula when the tumor is large. The dorsal surface of the tumor is exposed and even though not truly encapsulated, medulloblastomas often have a clear interface between the tumor and surrounding brain where a dissection plane can be created. The tumor is excised in piece meal fashion either through the telovaler approach or by splitting the vermis (**Figure 4**). With the goal

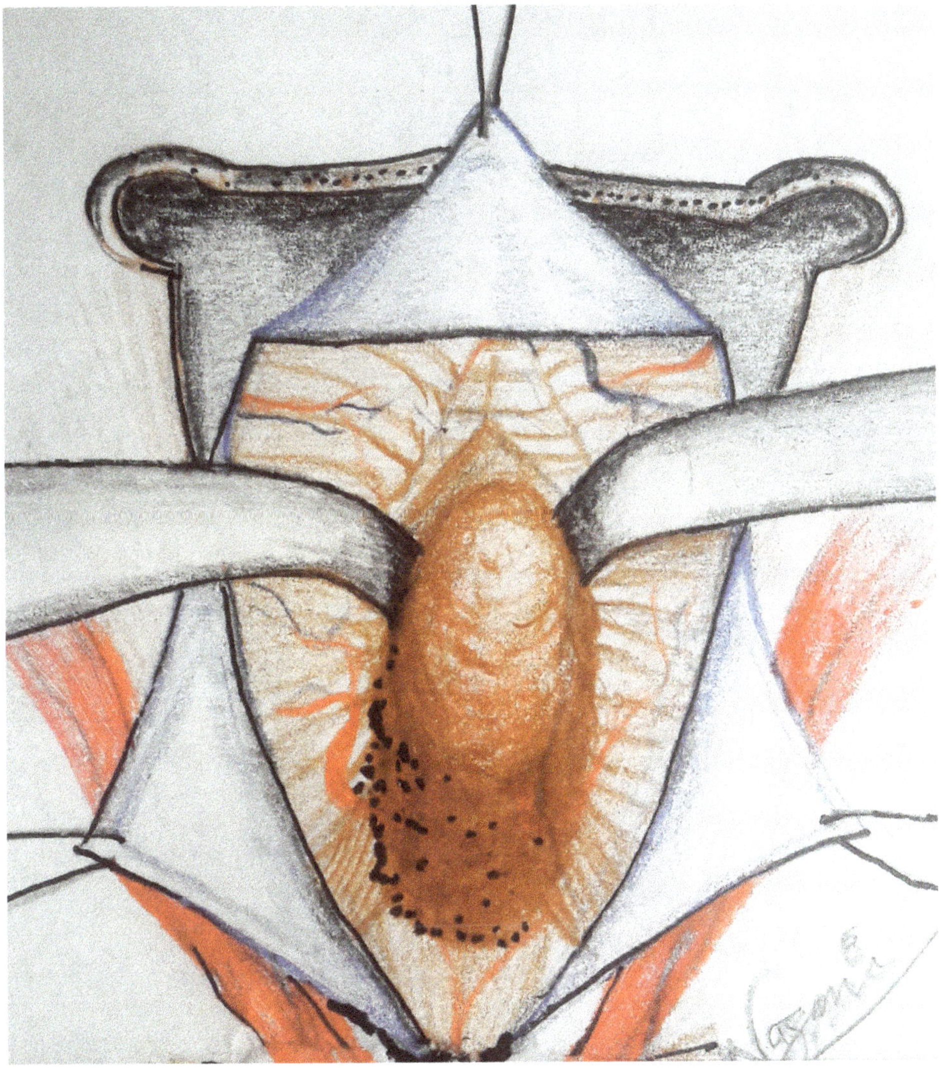

Figure 4. Schematic diagram showing the exposure of medulloblastoma after splitting the vermis in the midline.

of maximal safe resection, gross total resection can often be accomplished. Superiorly, the tumor is often projected into the aqueduct, filling it and obstructing the CSF pathway. The part projecting into the aqueduct can be meticulously removed with gentle suction, reestablishing the CSF flow (**Figure 5**). The part of the tumor that is attached to the brain stem or peduncles, is carefully removed, keeping a thin mantle leaving behind to ensure not to injure any vital structure. To alleviate the post-operative morbidity or mortality, immediate postoperative care of the patient is of immense importance. This is a factor that can make enormous difference in outcome.

Whether preoperative shunting should be done to relieve hydrocephalus prior to tumor surgery remains controversial. A ventriculoperitoneal (VP) shunt permanently or an external ventricular drain (EVD) as a temporary measure can be employed to treat hydrocephalus, if present at the time of diagnosis [8, 26, 71]. An EVD can be placed in the operating room, just prior to posterior fossa craniotomy, if the hydrocephalus is not treated preoperatively. About 20% of patients require long-term treatment of hydrocephalus with a VP shunt insertion or an endoscopic third ventriculostomy (ETV), when the hydrocephalus persists even after tumor removal [8, 71]. There is high possibility that a preoperative shunt

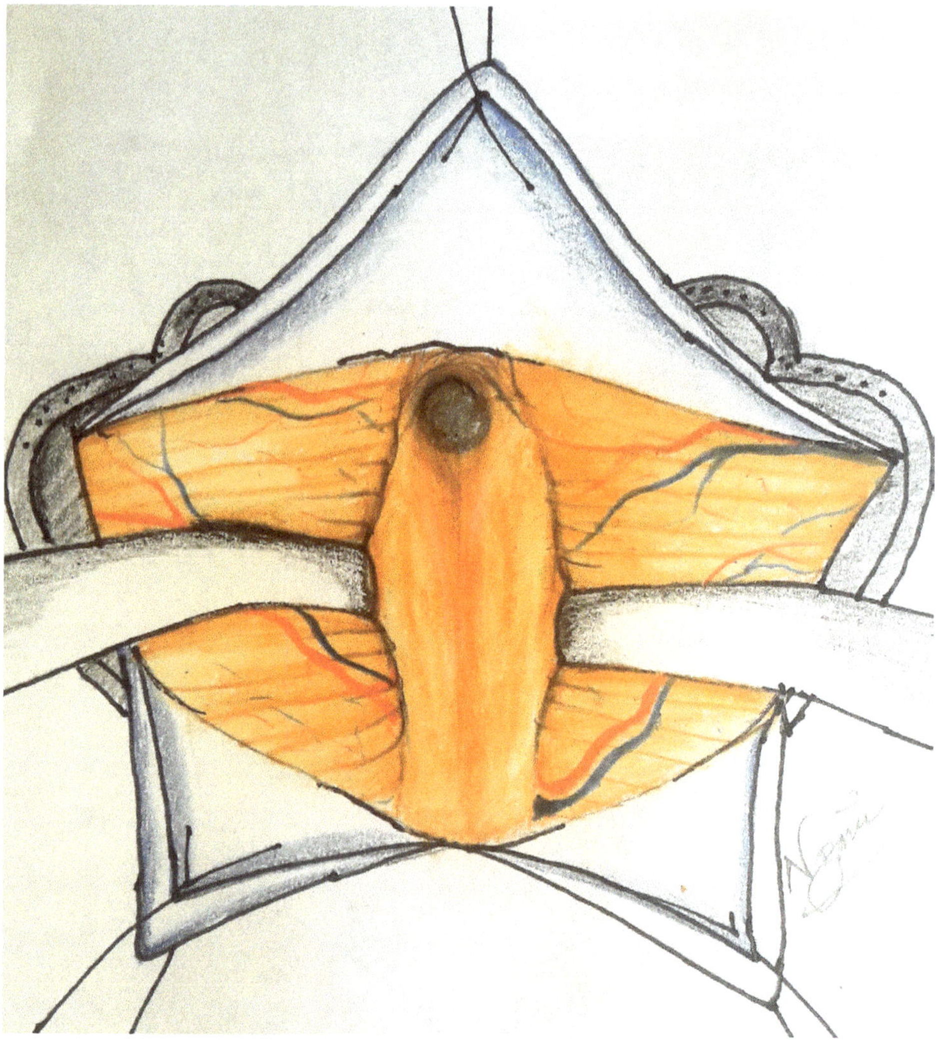

Figure 5. Schematic diagram of expanded aqueduct after removal of the medulloblastoma extending into the aqueduct.

may serve as a pathway of dissemination of the medulloblastoma, which has a tendency to spread by the CSF pathways. The use of millipore filters has been described to prevent dissemination [26, 70].

10.2.1. Complications of surgery

Clinical or subclinical venous air embolism, which is more common in sitting position, can happen in the prone position as well. With the goal of complete resection, major complications during tumor removal are usually caused by damage to the brain stem and injury to the lower cranial nerves. Aspiration pneumonia and respiratory failure often follows if the post-operative lower cranial nerve injuries are not handled meticulously. Though described frequently, cerebellar mutism, a commonly described complication of posterior fossa surgery, is less likely to occur now a days with microsurgical techniques. Meningitis, pseudomeningocele, postoperative tumor bed hematoma, epidural hematoma, subdural hematoma are among the other less often encountered complications.

10.3. Radiotherapy

Radiotherapy has been an adjunct of the treatment modality for medulloblastomas since the early twentieth century as these tumors are very responsive to radiotherapy. The survival rate has improved dramatically after the introduction of radiotherapy. Post-operative craniospinal irradiation (CSI) with or without boost to the posterior fossa are the customary protocol, as chosen by different centers [8, 72].

10.3.1. Treatment for average-risk patients ≥3 years of age

Post-operative radiotherapy dose for average risk medulloblastoma patients aged ≥3 years initially was set as 36 Gy CSI and 54 Gy boost for the posterior fossa (PF) because of high risk of local recurrence. Dose adjustment to 23.4–24 Gy CSI with the addition of adjuvant chemotherapy has been made with successful result [66, 73, 74]. Reduction in the posterior fossa radiation volume, in the form of 3-Dimensional conformal radiotherapy (3D CRT) has enabled to restrict the boost volume to the tumor bed plus a margin without compromising local control that minimizes morbidity associated with full PF irradiation by shielding normal vital structures [74–76]. Intensity-modulated radiotherapy (IMRT) or proton beam therapy similarly can reduce exposure to the heart and liver during CSI [72, 77–79].

10.3.2. Treatment for high-risk patients ≥3 years of age

The usual radiotherapy schedule for high-risk medulloblastoma patients of 3 years or more consists of standard dose regimen of 36 Gy CSI with a boost to both the posterior fossa and focal sites of metastasis of 55.8 Gy. Adjuvant chemotherapy, consisting of concurrent vincristine followed by maintenance chemotherapy with Lomustine, Vincristine, and Cisplatin has shown progression-free survival of 67% in M1, M2 and M3 stage [66, 80]. Outcomes for high-risk patients are equally poor even with inclusion of some neoadjuvant agents in addition to conventional chemotherapeutic agents [81–83].

10.3.3. Treatment of infants and children <3 years of age

As patients younger than 3 years are in risk of poor outcome of neurocognitive function following CSI, delay or omission of radiotherapy is recommended for this group of patients. M0 patients following gross total resection have commendable outcome with only chemotherapy after surgery [84].

10.3.4. Radiation hazards

The long-term sequelae of radiation therapy are well described, among which the most common ones are endocrinopathies, neurocognitive and neurosensory impairment following craniospinal irradiation depending on age of patient and radiation dose [85, 86]. Cancer survivors with a history of cranial irradiation have more tendency to have cerebrovascular disease and an increased risk of second malignancies in the radiation field [6]. Skin reactions, hair loss, growth problems, nausea and vomiting, chronic otitis media and/or otitis externa, myelosuppression are other commonly encountered side effects [71].

10.4. Chemotherapy and combined radio-chemo therapy

As medulloblastoma is a highly radiosensitive tumor, chemotherapy for this formidable tumor has been an adjunct in the treatment strategy for years. Various combinations of chemotherapeutic agents are used in conjunction with radiotherapy. The toxic effect of different chemotherapeutic agents have forced their use to be restricted in different circumstances. Now a days, the newer drugs are more soothing to the patients with better acceptability, tolerance and efficacy.

Penetrability of the blood-brain barrier of a drug is the most important feature for a chemotherapeutic agent to be a worthy regimen for brain tumors. Vincristine, Cisplatin, Cyclophosphamide, Lomustine, Etoposide, Methotrexate, Temozolomide, and Carboplatin are the commonly used effective chemotherapeutic agents for medulloblastomas [8, 87].

For average-risk medulloblastoma patients two common chemotherapy regimens are practiced. One is with a combination of Cisplatin, Lomustine, and Vincristine, while the second one comprises of a combination of Cisplatin, Cyclophosphamide, and Vincristine. These two regimens do not have significant difference in outcome regarding event-free survival (EFS) and overall survival (OS) [68]. Among conventional chemotherapeutics, Temozolomide-containing regimens have shown most promising activity. Two studies, one in monotherapy [88] and another in combination with Irinotecan [89], have shown the best results in a relatively large population, although follow up for disease-free survival is short. Its tolerable toxicity profile and synergies with other chemotherapeutics and targeted agents make it an attractive compound to serve as backbone for new strategies [20].

As children under the age of 3 years has worse long term cognitive effects, they are not commonly treated with the radiotherapy. To compensate this more intense chemotherapy is initiated instead [87]. In the last few decades, with the intension to avoid radiation and to have an equally better outcome in younger patients, protocols have been developed consisting of intense systemic chemotherapy, followed by a consolidation cycle with myeloablative chemotherapy along with autologous stem cell rescue (AuHCR) as an alternative management in these patients under the age of 3 years [90]. The 5 year EFS and OS varies between patients with localized disease, and patients with disseminated disease as well as between patients with desmoplastic, classical and anaplastic MB [91].

10.4.1. Side effects of chemotherapy

Adverse effects of adjuvant chemotherapy have been significant and needs to be modified in a good number of patients because of adverse reactions [92, 93]. The commonnest side effect of chemotherapy is hematologic toxicity in the form of leukothrombocytopenia. Other common adverse effects being anemia, somnolence, peripheral neuropathy, headaches, constipation, paresthesias, mucositis, nausea and vomiting, immune compromise and bone marrow suppression, renal toxicities with electrolyte abnormalities, hepatotoxicity, infertility [8, 71]. Some drugs carry the risk of development of treatment-related cancers which is 4.2% at 10 years [94]. Vincristine and cisplatin is known to cause various types of neurotoxicity particularly peripheral neuropathy and ototoxicity [95].

11. Recurrence

The majority of treatment failures develop within the first 2–3 years, and then the failure rate tends to decrease. Tumor recurrence occurs most frequently in the posterior fossa and that may or may not be associated with subarachnoid dissemination in the craniospinal axis [8, 9]. Inadequate post-operative dose of the radiotherapy and large volume of residual tumor are the major causes of recurrence. Commonly the outcomes in patients with relapsed disease are grave, with five-year survival rate of only about 25% and which has not improved much, even with development in treatment strategies [96–98]. Repeat surgical resection, re-irradiation, stereotactic radiosurgery, high-dose chemotherapy with AuHCR, low-dose oral Etoposide, the use of biologically targeted agents, singly or in combination, have been tried and success in control was more for localized recurrence than for disseminated recurrence [97–107]. At recurrence medulloblastomas often change towards a more anaplastic pathological variant. Interestingly Shh tumors tend to recur locally while Groups 3 and 4 recur almost entirely with metastases [10, 20, 44].

12. Metastasis

Medulloblastomas exhibit a strong propensity to metastasize through CSF pathways and tend to form tumors of variable size along ventricular surfaces, in subarachnoid space, or along nerve roots or may grow en plaque on surface of brain or spinal cord or may deposit in the ventricles [25]. Dissemination through the CSF route may be augmented by ventricular or spinal punctures or by manipulations of the lesion during operation. VP shunting has frequently been reported to cause extraneural metastases to the peritonium. Invasion of the meninges is not very uncommon [2, 9]. Extra CNS metastases have been reported to be in the bone marrow, lymph nodes, and viscera. Though very rare, metastasis to skin, liver, lung, mediastinum and retroperitoneal structures has also been reported [8, 9].

13. Surveillance

Surveillance is important as relapses encountered on surveillance imaging can be better dealt with and show improved survival as paralleled to those identified by reemergence of the clinical symptoms [108]. Though consensus about the schedule is debated, generally clinical and radiographic follow-up is recommended at three-month intervals during the first year after completion of scheduled therapy, at three to four-month intervals in the second year, every 6 months during the third year, and annually thereafter [109–112] (**Figure 6**). It is generally

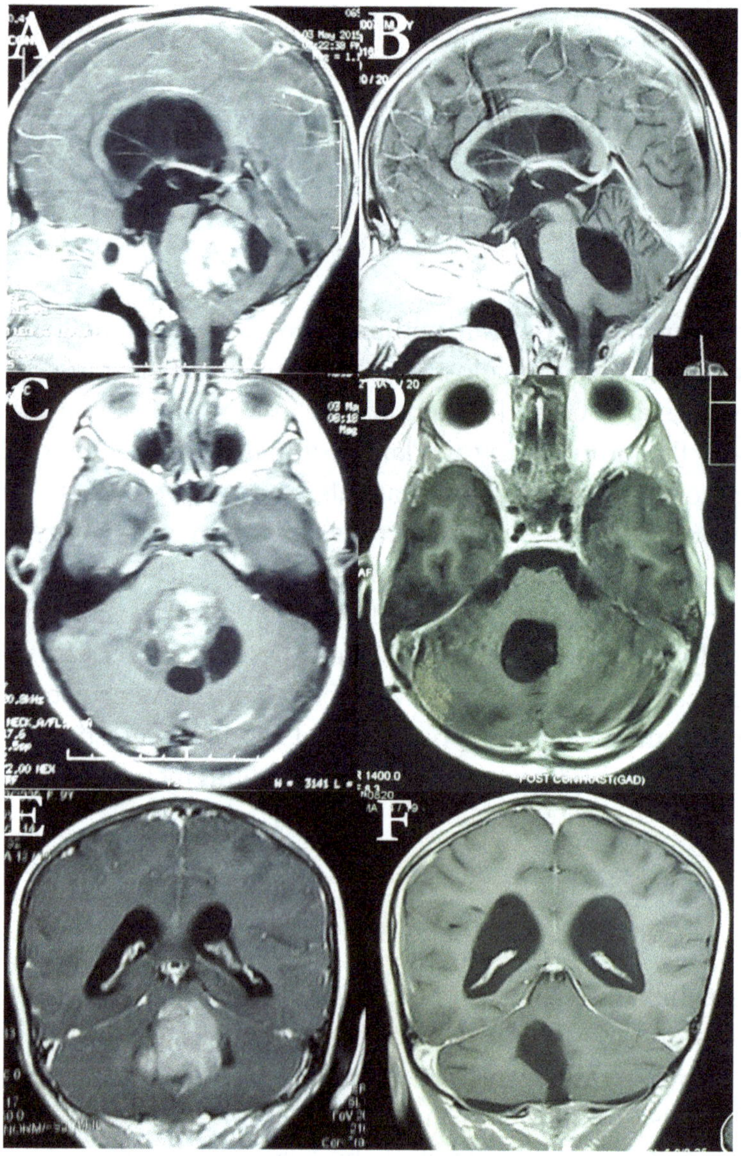

Figure 6. Preoperative contrast enhanced MRI in sagittal (A), axial (C) and coronal (E) planes and 1 year post-operative contrast enhanced MRI following radiotherapy in sagittal (B), axial (D) and coronal (F) planes of a 9 years old boy.

agreed that surveillance imaging of the brain should be complemented with full spinal MRI as it often might prove to be crucial and beneficial for the patient [110]. It is also recommended that, endocrine screening and neuropsychological testing be performed in those who were treated with craniospinal irradiation [6].

14. Medulloblastoma in adults

Medulloblastoma is much less common in adults, accounting for less than 1% - 3% of primary CNS tumors [24, 113, 114]. The annual incidence of medulloblastoma is 1–1.5 cases per million in the general adult population and 80% occur before the end of the fourth decade [24, 113–115]. Treatment protocols are limited for adults and they are treated by heterogeneous ways using various chemo-radiotherapy regimens with surgery with post-operative CSI being the mainstay of treatment [115]. As late relapse is common among adult medulloblastoma patients, long-term follow-up is warranted. Spinal seeding at presentation is a poor prognostic factor for recurrence [114, 115]. Adult medulloblastomas are clinically similar to that in the pediatric population, but lateral location and desmoplastic type is more frequent in adults as opposed to the pediatric age group. Adult medulloblastomas are thus, more amenable to complete resection and better outcome is expected because of their locations and histopathological variants respectively [24, 113–116]. Relapse following complete treatment is relatively late in adults as compared to children and they have a relatively prolonged time from relapse to death [116]. As most treatment recommendations for adults are extrapolated from the experience in pediatric patients, a protocol from the time of diagnosis includes: increasing the intensity to identify metastasis; increasing the radiotherapy dose to the primary site; adding chemotherapy following radiotherapy in medically fit patients; and following-up the patients with PET or bone scan every 6 months for at least 3 years [117, 118].

15. Outcome

Though the outcomes need to be judged cautiously because of the marked heterogeneity between studies, overall outcome of medulloblastoma patients has improved tremendously over the last decades. Still, outcome in a good number of patients with metastatic disease, adverse molecular or cytogenetic features, infants and relapsed or refractory patients remains depressing.

Many factors play role in outcome of medulloblastoma patients and outcomes have been variable in different series. The outcome has gradually improved from survival from onset to death of 8–9 months in 1930s to 54% 3-year survival in 1950s, about 75% 5-year survival in 1980s [71]. Till the last decade the five-year EFS and OS has raised to 81 ± 2.1 and 86 ± 9%, respectively [68]. Among the factors that play role in poor outcome, the noteworthy are younger age, larger residual tumor volume after surgery, inadequate dose of radiotherapy, presence of metastatic disease at diagnosis, presence of hydrocephalus, anaplastic or large cell histology, insufficient chemotherapy, MYC amplification or expression, 17p loss or 1q gain, and tumors of

Group 3 or Shh subgroup with TP53 mutations. On the contrary, patients having monosomy 6, mutation of CTNNB1, and trkC expression demonstrate a favorable outcome [6, 9, 33, 41, 49, 59]. Generally, OS for children with medulloblastoma are reported as 50–60%, whereas for average-risk and high-risk patients OS is 70–80 and 30–40% respectively [8, 119].

16. Newer therapies/future

The future of medulloblastoma treatment lies on the basis of its genetic coding and molecular subgroupings. A few drugs have been tested preliminarily and that made the researchers as well as the patients optimistic. Endeavor is going on to determine whether the intensity of treatment can be reduced safely, keeping the optimum efficacy, to mitigate the treatment-related long term developmental and cognitive morbidity without affecting survival rates, thus improving the quality of life for medulloblastoma survivors [6, 10]. The molecular biology of the subgroups have emerged to be the key elements of success in future and, with the early success and the potential utility of molecular biomarkers in prognostication and prediction, researchers are in search of more personalized and tailored therapies for the patients [8, 42, 49].

Of the different pathways of tumor origin and progression, the sonic hedgehog (Shh) pathway is a front-runner in research in this perspective. Smoothened (SMO), is an intriguing protein in developmental processes involving the hedgehog signaling pathway [120]. Assuming the role of SMO in the Shh pathway in tumorogenesis, molecules that target SMO are under intensive research and preliminary success have been achieved in some clinical trials [42, 121]. Of these, smoothened inhibitor Vismodegib showed promising result in studies with varying outcomes, having both short-term and long-lasting response, especially in standard-risk Shh medulloblastoma patients [122–125]. Trial with another SMO inhibitor Sonidegib, in cases of patients with relapsed disease also reveals promise for future [123]. Blocking GLI1 with Arsenic trioxide [126], combining SMO inhibitors with PI3K inhibitors [124], or inhibition of PIN1 by either Juglone or the flavonoids Epigallocatechin gallate and Quercetin [127], have attained certain levels of success as these aberrations are frequently encountered in this subset of patients [20]. Quercetin has been found to be a probable worthy radio-sensitizer [127]. Saridegib and Erismodegib are other potent SMO inhibitors under trial that seem to have potential in regression of tumor and inhibition of tumor progression [128].

For Non-WNT/Non-SHH medulloblastomas comprising molecular subgroups 3 and 4, Gemcitabine, a nucleoside analog, and Pemetrexed, a folate antimetabolite are currently being investigated in combination to evaluate their role in prognosis [20, 49]. Combination of these two drugs have been found to be active, particularly against Group 3 medulloblastomas [129]. These were tried separately previously in medulloblastoma patients but only combination of Gemcitabine with Oxaliplatin was found to have promising results with a disease control rate (DCR) of 50% [130]. On the other hand, the combination of Vorinostat and Retinoic acid was found to have a 5-month disease stabilization in patients with Group 4 medulloblastomas [131].

Temozolomide-containing regimens are well tolerable and have good antitumor activity against relapsed/refractory medulloblastomas [20]. Evaluation of temozolomide and

Irinotecan in a study with short follow-up has shown to have good prospect with a DCR of 73% [89]. Trials with multiagent oral antiangiogenic regimen like Bevacizumab, Cilengitide, Lenalidomide and Thalidomide either in monotherapy or in combination with Vincristine, Irinotecan, Temozolomide or Temsirolimus in patients with medulloblastoma yielded only short-lasting disease stabilizations with a tolerable toxicity profile [132–137].

Tyrosine kinase inhibitors (TKIs) like imatinib, sorafenib, lapatinib, nilotinib, dasatinib, ponatinib and bafetinib have shown to block the migration and invasion properties of MB cells which may prove to be effective alternative agents in the treatment of medulloblastomas [128].

In order to reduce treatment related side effects, newer radiotherapy techniques are being evaluated. IMRT and helical tomotherapy have been evaluated, but results were not very pleasing [24].

Immunotherapy is another novel therapeutic approach that is being evaluated for the treatment of medulloblastoma. The target antigens that have been identified are cancer testis antigens (CTAs), MAGE and GAGE proteins. MAGE-4, MAGE-A and GAGE expression have been found in 50, 62 and 84% of medulloblastomas respectively [138, 139]. MAGE antigens, are a promising targets for immunotherapy in patients with medulloblastoma as it has paved the way of immunotherapy already by targeting successfully in some other tumors [140, 141]. Vaccinations against EGFRvIII in combination with GM-CSF, is another potential immunotherapeutic approach, which have already been tested in other brain tumors [142].

In the post-surgery treatment process, delivery of anticancer drugs across the BBB remains a challenge. A number of methods have been tried to facilitate effective drug delivery across the BBB to the brain. Of those, a very promising technique is Nanoparticles (NP) encapsulating magnetic materials such as iron oxide. Upon entering the systemic circulation, through NPs a drug can be directed remotely to the disease site. The addition of receptor-specific ligands to magnetic NPs for active targeting can significantly increase their efficacy [128].

17. Rehabilitation

Quality of life and psychosocial outcomes following treatment of medulloblastoma are progressively recognized as crucial issues in decision-making regarding therapy. Long-term outcome was less emphasized than survival previously as survival was nominal in the earlier period of history of medulloblastoma, though the thought of prolongation of life and making it worth living was always there with the encouragement to persist in efforts [2]. Over the past decades, survival has improved significantly, and expectantly will continue to improve with the development of molecularly targeted agents and other modalities of treatment. With time, thoughts regarding quality of life is becoming increasingly vital both in decision-making concerning therapy and in the design of future treatment protocols where quality of life is the prime target next to survival [6]. Treatment-related endocrinologic, cognitive, and psychological sequelae, especially in Infants and very young children with medulloblastoma remain a difficult therapeutic challenge which can be tackled prudently with rehabilitation programs. For that it is an obvious need to develop active rehabilitative programs and special educational assistance for the children who survive the multi-modality therapy [71]. Optimum therapy has led to long-term survival in patients of medulloblastoma and it is expected to be increased with time with the anticipated need of more intense and dedicated rehabilitation regime for this group of patients. Thus the long-term survivors of medulloblastoma badly require multifaceted medical rehabilitation care involving team of subspecialists including oncologist, neurologist, endocrinologist, psychologist, psychiatrist and physiotherapist to overcome the challenges that they have to face in the longer run [8, 64].

18. Conclusion

Medulloblastomas have been neurosurgeons' nightmare for years. MB, a highly aggressive tumor of the cerebellum, treated with a combination of surgery, craniospinal irradiation and chemotherapy, still remains a challenge. Enriched knowledge of histological and molecular subgroups with their aberrant signaling pathways has provided novel therapeutic targets for MB to regress their growth and has enhanced both the prognostic and therapeutic implications. Efforts to modify and refine the MB treatment strategy are ongoing as toxicity and off-target effects of various newer drugs are yet not under total control. Regardless of marked advancements in overall survival for medulloblastoma patients over the past decades, substantial successes remain to be achieved, especially concerning improvement in survival, mitigating treatment-related morbidities as well as improving quality of life for survivors. These have led to modifications of therapies and research, with the emphasis on novel, less toxic and more targeted agents for the best possible survival with least long-term adverse consequences for a worthwhile post-therapy quality of life. The combination of molecular pharmacology, neurogenetics, cell biology, and biophysics will ultimately drive the utmost hope of a cure for medulloblastoma. With the advancement of modern research, medulloblastoma, once a dreaded and hopeless entity, is looming to be a potentially curable disease.

Acknowledgements

I am very grateful to my colleagues Dr. Abu Saleh Mohammad Abu Obaida and Dr. Muhtamim Chowdhury for their critical advices in preparing this chapter. I am immensely indebted to my colleague Dr. Nazmin Ahmed for her beautiful schematic diagrams that have made this chapter colorful.

Author details

Asifur Rahman

Address all correspondence to: bijoun14@yahoo.com

Department of Neurosurgery, Bangabandhu Sheikh Mujib Medical University, Shahbag, Dhaka, Bangladesh

References

[1] Bailey P, Cushing H. Medulloblastoma cerebelli: A common type of midcerebellar glioma of childhood. Archives of Neurology and Psychiatry. 1925;**14**(2):192-224

[2] Cushing H. Experiences with the cerebellar medulloblastomas. Acta Pathologica, Microbiologica, et Immunologica Scandinavica. 1930;**7**(1-2):1-86

[3] Globus JH, Strauss I. Spongioblastoma multiforme: A primary malignant form of brain neoplasm: Its clinical and anatomic features. Archives of Neurology and Psychiatry. 1925;**14**(2):139-191

[4] Ribbert H. Über das Spongioblastom und das Gliom. Virchows Archiv. 1918;**225**(2):195-213

[5] Strauss I, Globus J. Spongioblastoma with unusually rapid growth following decompression. Neurological Bulletin. 1918;**1**:273

[6] Millard NE, De Braganca KC. Medulloblastoma. Journal of Child Neurology. 2016;**31**(12):1341-1353

[7] Rorke LB. Presidential address: The cerebellar medulloblastoma and its relationship to primitive neuroectodermal tumors. Journal of Neuropathology & Experimental Neurology. 1983;**42**(1):1-15

[8] Quinlan A, Rizzolo D. Understanding medulloblastoma. Journal of the American Academy of PAs. 2017;**30**(10):30-36

[9] Chin HW, Maruyama Y, Young AB. Medulloblastoma: Recent advances and directions in diagnosis and management—Part I. Current Problems in Cancer. 1984;**8**(11):1-54

[10] Pickles JC, Hawkins C, Pietsch T, Jacques TS. CNS embryonal tumours: WHO 2016 and beyond. Neuropathology and Applied Neurobiology. 2018;**44**(2):151-162

[11] Farwell JR, Dohrmann GJ, Flannery JT. Medulloblastoma in childhood: An epidemiological study. Journal of Neurosurgery. 1984;**61**(4):657-664

[12] Packer RJ, Sutton LN, Goldwein JW, Perilongo G, Bunin G, Ryan J, et al. Improved survival with the use of adjuvant chemotherapy in the treatment of medulloblastoma. Journal of Neurosurgery. 1991;**74**(3):433-440

[13] Paterson E, Farr R. Cerebellar medulloblastoma: Treatment by irradiation of the whole central nervous system. Acta Radiologica. 1953;**39**(4):323-336

[14] Ramaswamy V, Remke M, Adamski J, Bartels U, Tabori U, Wang X, et al. Medulloblastoma subgroup-specific outcomes in irradiated children: Who are the true high-risk patients? Neuro-Oncology. 2015;**18**(2):291-297

[15] Allen J, Donahue B, Mehta M, Miller DC, Rorke LB, Jakacki R, et al. A phase II study of preradiotherapy chemotherapy followed by hyperfractionated radiotherapy for newly diagnosed high-risk medulloblastoma/primitive neuroectodermal tumor: A report from

the Children's oncology group (CCG 9931). International Journal of Radiation Oncology, Biology, Physics. 2009;**74**(4):1006-1011

[16] Jakacki RI, Burger PC, Zhou T, Holmes EJ, Kocak M, Onar A, et al. Outcome of children with metastatic medulloblastoma treated with carboplatin during craniospinal radiotherapy: A Children's oncology group phase I/II study. Journal of Clinical Oncology. 2012;**30**(21):2648-2653

[17] Lannering B, Rutkowski S, Doz F, Pizer B, Gustafsson G, Navajas A, et al. Hyperfractionated versus conventional radiotherapy followed by chemotherapy in standard-risk medulloblastoma: Results from the randomized multicenter HIT-SIOP PNET 4 trial. Journal of Clinical Oncology. 2012;**30**(26):3187-3193

[18] Taylor RE, Bailey CC, Robinson K, Weston CL, Ellison D, Ironside J, et al. Results of a randomized study of preradiation chemotherapy versus radiotherapy alone for non-metastatic medulloblastoma: The International Society of Paediatric Oncology/United Kingdom Children's Cancer study group PNET-3 study. Journal of Clinical Oncology. 2003;**21**(8):1581-1591

[19] von Hoff K, Hinkes B, Gerber NU, Deinlein F, Mittler U, Urban C, et al. Long-term outcome and clinical prognostic factors in children with medulloblastoma treated in the prospective randomised multicentre trial HIT '91. European Journal of Cancer. 2009;**45**(7):1209-1217

[20] Bautista F, Fioravantti V, Carceller F, Madero L, Lassaletta A, Moreno L. Medulloblastoma in children and adolescents: a systematic review of contemporary phase I and II clinical trials and biology update. Cancer medicine. 2017;**6**(11):2606-2624

[21] McNeil DE, Coté TR, Clegg L, Rorke LB. Incidence and trends in pediatric malignancies medulloblastoma/primitive neuroectodermal tumor: A SEER update. Pediatric Blood & Cancer. 2002;**39**(3):190-194

[22] Ostrom QT, De Blank PM, Kruchko C, Petersen CM, Liao P, Finlay JL, et al. Alex's lemonade stand foundation infant and childhood primary brain and central nervous system tumors diagnosed in the United States in 2007-2011. Neuro-Oncology. 2014;**16**(suppl_10):x1-x36

[23] Ostrom QT, Gittleman H, Fulop J, Liu M, Blanda R, Kromer C, et al. CBTRUS statistical report: Primary brain and central nervous system tumors diagnosed in the United States in 2008-2012. Neuro-Oncology. 2015;**17**(Suppl 4):iv1

[24] Brandes AA, Bartolotti M, Marucci G, Ghimenton C, Agati R, Fioravanti A, et al. New perspectives in the treatment of adult medulloblastoma in the era of molecular oncology. Critical Reviews in Oncology/Hematology. 2015;**94**(3):348-359

[25] Packer RJ, Cogen P, Vezina G, Rorke LB. Medulloblastoma: Clinical and biologic aspects. Neuro-Oncology. 1999;**1**(3):232-250

[26] Park TS, Hoffman HJ, Hendrick EB, Humphreys RP, Becker LE. Medulloblastoma: Clinical presentation and management: Experience at the hospital for sick children, Toronto, 1950-1980. Journal of Neurosurgery. 1983;**58**(4):543-552

[27] Baryawno N, Rahbar A, Wolmer-Solberg N, Taher C, Odeberg J, Darabi A, et al. Detection of human cytomegalovirus in medulloblastomas reveals a potential therapeutic target. The Journal of Clinical Investigation. 2011;**121**(10):4043

[28] Hortal AM, Vermeulen JF, Van Hecke W, Bovenschen N. Oncogenic role of cytomegalovirus in medulloblastoma? Cancer Letters. 2017;**408**:55-59

[29] Libard S, Popova SN, Amini R-M, Kärjä V, Pietiläinen T, Hämäläinen KM, et al. Human cytomegalovirus tegument protein pp65 is detected in all intra-and extra-axial brain tumours independent of the tumour type or grade. PLoS One. 2014;**9**(9):e108861

[30] Louis DN, Ohgaki H, Wiestler OD, Cavenee WK, Burger PC, Jouvet A, et al. The 2007 WHO classification of tumours of the central nervous system. Acta Neuropathologica. 2007;**114**(2):97-109

[31] Bailey P. Further notes on the cerebellar medulloblastomas: The effect of roentgen radiation. The American Journal of Pathology. 1930;**6**(2):125

[32] Crawford JR, MacDonald TJ, Packer RJ. Medulloblastoma in childhood: New biological advances. The Lancet Neurology. 2007;**6**(12):1073-1085

[33] Gulino A, Arcella A, Giangaspero F. Pathological and molecular heterogeneity of medulloblastoma. Current Opinion in Oncology. 2008;**20**(6):668-675

[34] Rubinstein L, Northfield D. The medulloblastoma and the so-called "arachnoidal cerebellar sarcoma" a critical re-examination of a nosological problem. Brain. 1964;**87**(2):379-412

[35] Kleihues P, Burger PC, Scheithauer BW. The new WHO classification of brain tumours. Brain Pathology. 1993;**3**(3):255-268

[36] Rorke LB, Gilles FH, Davis RL, Becker LE. Revision of the World Health Organization classification of brain tumors for childhood brain tumors. Cancer. 1985;**56**(S7):1869-1886

[37] Eberhart CG, Kepner JL, Goldthwaite PT, Kun LE, Duffner PK, Friedman HS, et al. Histopathologic grading of medulloblastomas. Cancer. 2002;**94**(2):552-560

[38] Kleihues P, Louis DN, Scheithauer BW, Rorke LB, Reifenberger G, Burger PC, et al. The WHO classification of tumors of the nervous system. Journal of Neuropathology & Experimental Neurology. 2002;**61**(3):215-225

[39] Gajjar A, Pfister SM, Taylor MD, Gilbertson RJ. Molecular insights into pediatric brain tumors have the potential to transform therapy. Clinical Cancer Research. 2014;**20**(22):5630-5640

[40] Louis DN, Perry A, Reifenberger G, Von Deimling A, Figarella-Branger D, Cavenee WK, et al. The 2016 World Health Organization classification of tumors of the central nervous system: A summary. Acta Neuropathologica. 2016;**131**(6):803-820

[41] Schwalbe EC, Lindsey JC, Nakjang S, Crosier S, Smith AJ, Hicks D, et al. Novel molecular subgroups for clinical classification and outcome prediction in childhood medulloblastoma: A cohort study. The Lancet Oncology. 2017;**18**(7):958-971

[42] Taylor MD, Northcott PA, Korshunov A, Remke M, Cho Y-J, Clifford SC, et al. Molecular subgroups of medulloblastoma: The current consensus. Acta Neuropathologica. 2012; **123**(4):465-472

[43] Gibson P, Tong Y, Robinson G, Thompson MC, Currle DS, Eden C, et al. Subtypes of medulloblastoma have distinct developmental origins. Nature. 2010;**468**(7327):1095-1099

[44] Ramaswamy V, Remke M, Bouffet E, Faria CC, Perreault S, Cho Y-J, et al. Recurrence patterns across medulloblastoma subgroups: An integrated clinical and molecular analysis. The Lancet Oncology. 2013;**14**(12):1200-1207

[45] Wang X, Dubuc AM, Ramaswamy V, Mack S, Gendoo DM, Remke M, et al. Medulloblastoma subgroups remain stable across primary and metastatic compartments. Acta Neuropathologica. 2015;**129**(3):449-457

[46] Northcott PA, Korshunov A, Pfister SM, Taylor MD. The clinical implications of medulloblastoma subgroups. Nature Reviews Neurology. 2012;**8**(6):340-351

[47] Ellison DW, Kocak M, Dalton J, Megahed H, Lusher ME, Ryan SL, et al. Definition of disease-risk stratification groups in childhood medulloblastoma using combined clinical, pathologic, and molecular variables. Journal of Clinical Oncology. 2010;**29**(11):1400-1407

[48] Zhukova N, Ramaswamy V, Remke M, Pfaff E, Shih DJ, Martin DC, et al. Subgroup-specific prognostic implications of TP53 mutation in medulloblastoma. Journal of Clinical Oncology. 2013;**31**(23):2927-2935

[49] Staedtke V, Dzaye OD, Holdhoff M. Actionable molecular biomarkers in primary brain tumors. Trends in Cancer. 2016;**2**(7):338-349

[50] Kool M, Korshunov A, Remke M, Jones DT, Schlanstein M, Northcott PA, et al. Molecular subgroups of medulloblastoma: An international meta-analysis of transcriptome, genetic aberrations, and clinical data of WNT, SHH, Group 3, and Group 4 medulloblastomas. Acta Neuropathologica. 2012;**123**(4):473-484

[51] Shih DJ, Northcott PA, Remke M, Korshunov A, Ramaswamy V, Kool M, et al. Cytogenetic prognostication within medulloblastoma subgroups. Journal of Clinical Oncology. 2014;**32**(9):886-896

[52] Smith MJ, Beetz C, Williams SG, Bhaskar SS, O'Sullivan J, Anderson B, et al. Germline mutations in SUFU cause Gorlin syndrome-associated childhood medulloblastoma and redefine the risk associated with PTCH1 mutations. Journal of Clinical Oncology. 2014;**32**(36):4155-4161

[53] Rausch T, Jones DT, Zapatka M, Stütz AM, Zichner T, Weischenfeldt J, et al. Genome sequencing of pediatric medulloblastoma links catastrophic DNA rearrangements with TP53 mutations. Cell. 2012;**148**(1):59-71

[54] Cavalli FM, Remke M, Rampasek L, Peacock J, Shih DJ, Luu B, et al. Intertumoral heterogeneity within medulloblastoma subgroups. Cancer Cell. 2017;**31**(6):737-754 (e6)

[55] Cho Y-J, Tsherniak A, Tamayo P, Santagata S, Ligon A, Greulich H, et al. Integrative genomic analysis of medulloblastoma identifies a molecular subgroup that drives poor clinical outcome. Journal of Clinical Oncology. 2010;**29**(11):1424-1430

[56] Kool M, Koster J, Bunt J, Hasselt NE, Lakeman A, Van Sluis P, et al. Integrated genomics identifies five medulloblastoma subtypes with distinct genetic profiles, pathway signatures and clinicopathological features. PLoS One. 2008;**3**(8):e3088

[57] Northcott PA, Korshunov A, Witt H, Hielscher T, Eberhart CG, Mack S, et al. Medulloblastoma comprises four distinct molecular variants. Journal of Clinical Oncology. 2010;**29**(11):1408-1414

[58] Hatten ME, Roussel MF. Development and cancer of the cerebellum. Trends in Neurosciences. 2011;**34**(3):134-142

[59] Pfister S, Remke M, Benner A, Mendrzyk F, Toedt G, Felsberg J, et al. Outcome prediction in pediatric medulloblastoma based on DNA copy-number aberrations of chromosomes 6q and 17q and the MYC and MYCN loci. Journal of Clinical Oncology. 2009;**27**(10):1627-1636

[60] Banan R, Hartmann C. The new WHO 2016 classification of brain tumors—What neurosurgeons need to know. Acta Neurochirurgica. 2017;**159**(3):403-418

[61] Louis DN, Perry A, Burger P, Ellison DW, Reifenberger G, Deimling A, et al. International Society of Neuropathology-Haarlem consensus guidelines for nervous system tumor classification and grading. Brain Pathology. 2014;**24**(5):429-435

[62] Chang CH, Housepian EM, Herbert C. An operative staging system and a megavoltage radiotherapeutic technic for cerebellar medulloblastomas. Radiology. 1969;**93**(6): 1351-1359

[63] Dufour C, Beaugrand A, Pizer B, Micheli J, Aubelle M-S, Fourcade A, et al. Metastatic medulloblastoma in childhood: Chang's classification revisited. International Journal of Surgical Oncology. 2012;**2012**:1-6

[64] Packer RJ, Vezina G. Management of and prognosis with medulloblastoma: Therapy at a crossroads. Archives of Neurology. 2008;**65**(11):1419-1424

[65] Wilne S, Collier J, Kennedy C, Jenkins A, Grout J, Mackie S, et al. Progression from first symptom to diagnosis in childhood brain tumours. European Journal of Pediatrics. 2012;**171**(1):87-93

[66] Ramaswamy V, Remke M, Shih D, Wang X, Northcott PA, Faria CC, et al. Duration of the pre-diagnostic interval in medulloblastoma is subgroup dependent. Pediatric Blood & Cancer. 2014;**61**(7):1190-1194

[67] Fouladi M, Gajjar A, Boyett JM, Walter AW, Thompson SJ, Merchant TE, et al. Comparison of CSF cytology and spinal magnetic resonance imaging in the detection of leptomeningeal disease in pediatric medulloblastoma or primitive neuroectodermal tumor. Journal of Clinical Oncology. 1999;**17**(10):3234-3237

[68] Packer RJ, Gajjar A, Vezina G, Rorke-Adams L, Burger PC, Robertson PL, et al. Phase III study of craniospinal radiation therapy followed by adjuvant chemotherapy for newly diagnosed average-risk medulloblastoma. Journal of Clinical Oncology. 2006;**24**(25):4202-4208

[69] Müller W, Afra D, Schröder R, Slowik F, Wilcke O, Klug N. Medulloblastoma: Survey of factors possibly influencing the prognosis. Acta Neurochirurgica. 1982;**64**(3):215-224

[70] Sutton LN, Phillips PC, Molloy PT. Surgical management of medulloblastoma. Journal of Neuro-Oncology. 1996;**29**(1):9-21

[71] Chin HW, Maruyama Y, Young AB. Medulloblastoma: Recent advances and directions in diagnosis and management—Part II. Current Problems in Cancer. 1984;**8**(12):1-51

[72] Yuh GE, Loredo LN, Yonemoto LT, Bush DA, Shahnazi K, Preston W, et al. Reducing toxicity from craniospinal irradiation: Using proton beams to treat medulloblastoma in young children. The Cancer Journal. 2004;**10**(6):386-390

[73] Gajjar A, Chintagumpala M, Ashley D, Kellie S, Kun LE, Merchant TE, et al. Risk-adapted craniospinal radiotherapy followed by high-dose chemotherapy and stem-cell rescue in children with newly diagnosed medulloblastoma (St Jude Medulloblastoma-96): Long-term results from a prospective, multicentre trial. The Lancet Oncology. 2006; **7**(10):813-820

[74] Merchant TE, Kun LE, Krasin MJ, Wallace D, Chintagumpala MM, Woo SY, et al. Multi-institution prospective trial of reduced-dose craniospinal irradiation (23.4 Gy) followed by conformal posterior fossa (36 Gy) and primary site irradiation (55.8 Gy) and dose-intensive chemotherapy for average-risk medulloblastoma. International Journal of Radiation Oncology Biology Physics. 2008;**70**(3):782-787

[75] Fukunaga-Johnson N, Lee JH, Sandler HM, Robertson P, McNeil E, Goldwein JW. Patterns of failure following treatment for medulloblastoma: Is it necessary to treat the entire posterior fossa? International Journal of Radiation Oncology Biology Physics. 1998;**42**(1):143-146

[76] Wolden SL, Dunkel IJ, Souweidane MM, Happersett L, Khakoo Y, Schupak K, et al. Patterns of failure using a conformal radiation therapy tumor bed boost for medulloblastoma. Journal of Clinical Oncology. 2003;**21**(16):3079-3083

[77] Clair WS, Adams J, Bues M, Fullerton B, La Shell S, Kooy H, et al. Advantage of protons compared to conventional X-ray or IMRT in the treatment of a pediatric patient with medulloblastoma. International Journal of Radiation Oncology Biology Physics. 2004;**58**(3):727-734

[78] Panandiker AP, Ning H, Likhacheva A, Ullman K, Arora B, Ondos J, et al. Craniospinal irradiation with spinal IMRT to improve target homogeneity. International Journal of Radiation Oncology Biology Physics. 2007;**68**(5):1402-1409

[79] Parker W, Filion E, Roberge D, Freeman CR. Intensity-modulated radiotherapy for craniospinal irradiation: Target volume considerations, dose constraints, and competing risks. International Journal of Radiation Oncology Biology Physics. 2007;**69**(1):251-257

[80] Packer RJ, Sutton LN, Elterman R, Lange B, Goldwein J, Nicholson HS, et al. Outcome for children with medulloblastoma treated with radiation and cisplatin, CCNU, and vincristine chemotherapy. Journal of Neurosurgery. 1994;**81**(5):690-698

[81] Kortmann R-D, Kühl J, Timmermann B, Mittler U, Urban C, Budach V, et al. Postoperative neoadjuvant chemotherapy before radiotherapy as compared to immediate radiotherapy followed by maintenance chemotherapy in the treatment of medulloblastoma in childhood: Results of the German prospective randomized trial HIT'91. International Journal of Radiation Oncology Biology Physics. 2000;**46**(2):269-279

[82] Taylor RE, Bailey CC, Robinson KJ, Weston CL, Walker DA, Ellison D, et al. Outcome for patients with metastatic (M2-3) medulloblastoma treated with SIOP/UKCCSG PNET-3 chemotherapy. European Journal of Cancer. 2005;**41**(5):727-734

[83] Zeltzer PM, Boyett JM, Finlay JL, Albright AL, Rorke LB, Milstein JM, et al. Metastasis stage, adjuvant treatment, and residual tumor are prognostic factors for medulloblastoma in children: Conclusions from the Children's Cancer group 921 randomized phase III study. Journal of Clinical Oncology. 1999;**17**(3):832

[84] Grill J, Sainte-Rose C, Jouvet A, Gentet J-C, Lejars O, Frappaz D, et al. Treatment of medulloblastoma with postoperative chemotherapy alone: An SFOP prospective trial in young children. The Lancet Oncology. 2005;**6**(8):573-580

[85] Gurney JG, Kadan-Lottick NS, Packer RJ, Neglia JP, Sklar CA, Punyko JA, et al. Endocrine and cardiovascular late effects among adult survivors of childhood brain tumors. Cancer. 2003;**97**(3):663-673

[86] Packer RJ, Gurney JG, Punyko JA, Donaldson SS, Inskip PD, Stovall M, et al. Long-term neurologic and neurosensory sequelae in adult survivors of a childhood brain tumor: Childhood cancer survivor study. Journal of Clinical Oncology. 2003;**21**(17):3255-3261

[87] De Braganca KC, Packer RJ. Treatment options for medulloblastoma and CNS primitive neuroectodermal tumor (PNET). Current Treatment Options in Neurology. 2013;**15**(5): 593-606

[88] Cefalo G, Massimino M, Ruggiero A, Barone G, Ridola V, Spreafico F, et al. Temozolomide is an active agent in children with recurrent medulloblastoma/primitive neuroectodermal tumor: An Italian multi-institutional phase II trial. Neuro-Oncology. 2014;**16**(5):748-753

[89] Grill J, Geoerger B, Gesner L, Perek D, Leblond P, Cañete A, et al. Phase II study of irinotecan in combination with temozolomide (TEMIRI) in children with recurrent or refractory medulloblastoma: A joint ITCC and SIOPE brain tumor study. Neuro-Oncology. 2013; **15**(9):1236-1243

[90] Dhall G, Grodman H, Ji L, Sands S, Gardner S, Dunkel IJ, et al. Outcome of children less than three years old at diagnosis with non-metastatic medulloblastoma treated with chemotherapy on the "head start" I and II protocols. Pediatric Blood & Cancer. 2008;**50**(6):1169-1175

[91] Dhall G, Ji L, Haley K, Grimm JP, Gilles FH, Gardner SL, et al. Outcome of infants and young children with newly diagnosed medulloblastoma treated on head start III protocol. Journal of Clinical Oncology.. 2011;**29**(15_suppl):2011

[92] Van Eys J, Chen T, Moore T, Cheek W, Sexauer C, Starling K. Adjuvant chemotherapy for medulloblastoma and ependymoma using iv vincristine, intrathecal methotrexate, and intrathecal hydrocortisone: A southwest oncology group study. Cancer Treatment Reports. 1981;**65**(7-8):681

[93] Pezzotta S, Knerich R, Butti G. Chemotherapy for medulloblastoma in children current status and future prospects. Pediatric Neurosurgery. 1982;**9**(3-4):294-298

[94] Packer RJ, Zhou T, Holmes E, Vezina G, Gajjar A. Survival and secondary tumors in children with medulloblastoma receiving radiotherapy and adjuvant chemotherapy: Results of Children's oncology group trial A9961. Neuro-Oncology. 2012;**15**(1):97-103

[95] Trobaugh-Lotrario AD, Smith AA, Odom LF. Vincristine neurotoxicity in the presence of hereditary neuropathy. Pediatric Blood & Cancer. 2003;**40**(1):39-43

[96] Bowers DC, Gargan L, Weprin BE, Mulne AF, Elterman RD, Munoz L, Giller CA, Winick NJ. Impact of site of tumor recurrence upon survival for children with recurrent or progressive medulloblastoma. Journal of neurosurgery. 2007;**107**(1 Suppl):5-10

[97] Dunkel IJ, Boyett JM, Yates A, Rosenblum M, Garvin JH Jr, Bostrom BC, et al. High-dose carboplatin, thiotepa, and etoposide with autologous stem-cell rescue for patients with recurrent medulloblastoma. Children's Cancer group. Journal of Clinical Oncology. 1998;**16**(1):222-228

[98] Dunkel IJ, Gardner SL, Garvin JH, Goldman S, Shi W, Finlay JL. High-dose carboplatin, thiotepa, and etoposide with autologous stem cell rescue for patients with previously irradiated recurrent medulloblastoma. Neuro-Oncology. 2010;**12**(3):297-303

[99] Kadota RP, Mahoney DH, Doyle J, Duerst R, Friedman H, Holmes E, et al. Dose intensive melphalan and cyclophosphamide with autologous hematopoietic stem cells for recurrent medulloblastoma or germinoma. Pediatric Blood & Cancer. 2008;**51**(5):675-678

[100] Wetmore C, Herington D, Lin T, Onar-Thomas A, Gajjar A, Merchant TE. Reirradiation of recurrent medulloblastoma: Does clinical benefit outweigh risk for toxicity? Cancer. 2014;**120**(23):3731-3737

[101] Bakst RL, Dunkel IJ, Gilheeney S, Khakoo Y, Becher O, Souweidane MM, et al. Reirradiation for recurrent medulloblastoma. Cancer. 2011;**117**(21):4977-4982

[102] Yamada A, Moritake H, Kamimura S, Yamashita S, Takeshima H, Nunoi H. Proposed strategy for the use of high-dose chemotherapy with stem cell rescue and intrathecal topotecan without whole-brain irradiation for infantile classic medulloblastoma. Pediatric Blood & Cancer. 2014;**61**(12):2316-2318

[103] Aguilera D, Mazewski C, Fangusaro J, MacDonald TJ, McNall-Knapp RY, Hayes LL, et al. Response to bevacizumab, irinotecan, and temozolomide in children with relapsed medulloblastoma: A multi-institutional experience. Child's Nervous System. 2013;**29**(4):589-596

[104] Ashley DM, Meier L, Kerby T, Zalduondo FM, Friedman HS, Gajjar A, et al. Response of recurrent medulloblastoma to low-dose oral etoposide. Journal of Clinical Oncology. 1996;**14**(6):1922-1927

[105] Gururangan S, Krauser J, Watral MA, Driscoll T, Larrier N, Reardon DA, et al. Efficacy of high-dose chemotherapy or standard salvage therapy in patients with recurrent medulloblastoma. Neuro-Oncology. 2008;**10**(5):745-751

[106] Guruangan S, Dunkel IJ, Goldman S, Garvin JH, Rosenblum M, Boyett JM, et al. Myeloablative chemotherapy with autologous bone marrow rescue in young children with recurrent malignant brain tumors. Journal of Clinical Oncology. 1998;**16**(7): 2486-2493

[107] Milker-Zabel S, Zabel A, Thilmann C, Zuna I, Hoess A, Wannenmacher M, et al. Results of three-dimensional stereotactically-guided radiotherapy in recurrent medulloblastoma. Journal of Neuro-Oncology. 2002;**60**(3):227-233

[108] Saunders DE, Hayward RD, Phipps KP, Chong WK, Wade AM. Surveillance neuroimaging of intracranial medulloblastoma in children: How effective, how often, and for how long? Journal of Neurosurgery. 2003;**99**(2):280-286

[109] Bartels U, Shroff M, Sung L, Dag-Ellams U, Laperriere N, Rutka J, et al. Role of spinal MRI in the follow-up of children treated for medulloblastoma. Cancer. 2006;**107**(6):1340-1347

[110] Perreault S, Lober RM, Carret A-S, Zhang G, Hershon L, Décarie J-C, et al. Surveillance imaging in children with malignant CNS tumors: Low yield of spine MRI. Journal of Neuro-Oncology. 2014;**116**(3):617-623

[111] Perreault S, Lober RM, Carret A-S, Zhang G, Hershon L, Décarie J-C, et al. Relapse patterns in pediatric embryonal central nervous system tumors. Journal of Neuro-Oncology. 2013;**115**(2):209-215

[112] Sethi RV, Giantsoudi D, Raiford M, Malhi I, Niemierko A, Rapalino O, et al. Patterns of failure after proton therapy in medulloblastoma; linear energy transfer distributions and relative biological effectiveness associations for relapses. International Journal of Radiation Oncology Biology Physics. 2014;**88**(3):655-663

[113] Greenberg HS, Chamberlain MC, Glantz MJ, Wang S. Adult medulloblastoma: Multiagent chemotherapy. Neuro-Oncology. 2001;**3**(1):29-34

[114] Chan AW, Tarbell NJ, Black PM, Louis DN, Frosch MP, Ancukiewicz M, et al. Adult medulloblastoma: Prognostic factors and patterns of relapse. Neurosurgery. 2000;**47**(3): 623-632

[115] Abacioglu U, Uzel O, Sengoz M, Turkan S, Ober A. Medulloblastoma in adults: Treatment results and prognostic factors. International Journal of Radiation Oncology Biology Physics. 2002;**54**(3):855-860

[116] Menon G, Krishnakumar K, Nair S. Adult medulloblastoma: Clinical profile and treatment results of 18 patients. Journal of Clinical Neuroscience. 2008;**15**(2):122-126

[117] Mokhtech M, Morris CG, Indelicato DJ, Rutenberg MS, Amdur RJ. Patterns of failure in patients with adult medulloblastoma presenting without extraneural metastasis. American Journal of Clinical Oncology. 2017;**14**:50

[118] Riffaud L, Saikali S, Leray E, Hamlat A, Haegelen C, Vauleon E, et al. Survival and prognostic factors in a series of adults with medulloblastomas. Journal of Neurosurgery. 2009;**111**(3):478-487

[119] Rutkowski S, von Hoff K, Emser A, Zwiener I, Pietsch T, Figarella-Branger D, et al. Survival and prognostic factors of early childhood medulloblastoma: An international meta-analysis. Journal of Clinical Oncology. 2010;**28**(33):4961-4968

[120] Chidambaram A, Gerrard B, Hanson M, Dean M. Chromosomal localization of the human and murine orthologues of the Drosophila smoothened gene. Genomics. 1998;**53**(3):416-417

[121] Wang C, Wu H, Evron T, Vardy E, Han GW, Huang X-P, et al. Structural basis for smoothened receptor modulation and chemoresistance to anticancer drugs. Nature Communications. 2014;**5**:4355

[122] Gajjar A, Stewart CF, Ellison DW, Kaste S, Kun LE, Packer RJ, et al. Phase I study of vismodegib in children with recurrent or refractory medulloblastoma: A pediatric brain tumor consortium study. Clinical Cancer Research. 2013;**19**(22):6305-6312

[123] Geoerger B, Aerts I, Casanova M, Chisholm JC, Hargrave DR, Leary S, et al. A phase I/II study of LDE225, a smoothened (Smo) antagonist, in pediatric patients with recurrent medulloblastoma (MB) or other solid tumors. American Society of Clinical Oncology. 2012;**2012**:9519

[124] Robinson GW, Orr BA, Wu G, Gururangan S, Lin T, Qaddoumi I, et al. Vismodegib exerts targeted efficacy against recurrent sonic hedgehog-subgroup medulloblastoma: Results from phase II Pediatric brain tumor consortium studies PBTC-025B and PBTC-032. Journal of Clinical Oncology. 2015;**33**(24):2646-2654

[125] Rudin CM, Hann CL, Laterra J, Yauch RL, Callahan CA, Fu L, et al. Treatment of medulloblastoma with hedgehog pathway inhibitor GDC-0449. New England Journal of Medicine. 2009;**361**(12):1173-1178

[126] DeSouza R-M, Jones BR, Lowis SP, Kurian KM. Pediatric medulloblastoma – Update on molecular classification driving targeted therapies. Frontiers in Oncology. 2014;**4**:176

[127] Bomgaars L, Geyer J, Franklin J, Dahl G, Park J, Winick N, et al. Phase I trial of intrathecal liposomal cytarabine in children with neoplastic meningitis. Journal of Clinical Oncology. 2004;**22**(19):3916-3921

[128] Kumar V, McGuire T, Coulter DW, Sharp JG, Mahato RI. Challenges and recent advances in medulloblastoma therapy. Trends in Pharmacological Sciences. 2017;**38**(12):1061-1084

[129] Morfouace M, Shelat A, Jacus M, Freeman BB, Turner D, Robinson S, et al. Pemetrexed and gemcitabine as combination therapy for the treatment of Group 3 medulloblastoma. Cancer Cell. 2014;**25**(4):516-529

[130] Geoerger B, Chisholm J, Le Deley M-C, Gentet J-C, Zwaan CM, Dias N, et al. Phase II study of gemcitabine combined with oxaliplatin in relapsed or refractory paediatric solid malignancies: An innovative therapy for children with Cancer European consortium study. European Journal of Cancer. 2011;**47**(2):230-238

[131] Fouladi M, Park JR, Stewart CF, Gilbertson RJ, Schaiquevich P, Sun J, et al. Pediatric phase I trial and pharmacokinetic study of vorinostat: A Children's oncology group phase I consortium report. Journal of Clinical Oncology. 2010;**28**(22):3623-3629

[132] Chintagumpala M, Blaney SM, Bomgaars LR, Aleksic A, Kuttesch JF, Klenke RA, et al. Phase I and pharmacokinetic study of thalidomide with carboplatin in children with cancer. Journal of Clinical Oncology. 2004;**22**(21):4394-4400

[133] MacDonald TJ, Stewart CF, Kocak M, Goldman S, Ellenbogen RG, Phillips P, et al. Phase I clinical trial of cilengitide in children with refractory brain tumors: Pediatric brain tumor consortium study PBTC-012. Journal of Clinical Oncology. 2008;**26**(6):919-924

[134] Piha-Paul SA, Shin SJ, Vats T, Guha-Thakurta N, Aaron J, Rytting M, et al. Pediatric patients with refractory central nervous system tumors: Experiences of a clinical trial combining bevacizumab and temsirolimus. Anticancer Research. 2014;**34**(4):1939-1945

[135] Robison NJ, Campigotto F, Chi SN, Manley PE, Turner CD, Zimmerman MA, et al. A phase II trial of a multi-agent oral antiangiogenic (metronomic) regimen in children with recurrent or progressive cancer. Pediatric Blood & Cancer. 2014;**61**(4):636-642

[136] Venkatramani R, Malogolowkin M, Davidson TB, May W, Sposto R, Mascarenhas L. A phase I study of vincristine, irinotecan, temozolomide and bevacizumab (vitb) in pediatric patients with relapsed solid tumors. PLoS One. 2013;**8**(7):e68416

[137] Warren KE, Goldman S, Pollack IF, Fangusaro J, Schaiquevich P, Stewart CF, et al. Phase I trial of lenalidomide in pediatric patients with recurrent, refractory, or progressive primary CNS tumors: Pediatric brain tumor consortium study PBTC-018. Journal of Clinical Oncology. 2010;**29**(3):324-329

[138] Kasuga C, Nakahara Y, Ueda S, Hawkins C, Taylor MD, Smith CA, et al. Expression of MAGE and GAGE genes in medulloblastoma and modulation of resistance to chemotherapy. Pediatrics. 2008;**1**(4):305-313

[139] Oba-Shinjo SM, Caballero OL, Jungbluth AA, Rosemberg S, Old LJ, Simpson AJ, et al. Cancer-testis (CT) antigen expression in medulloblastoma. Cancer Immunity Archive. 2008;**8**(1):7

[140] Atanackovic D, Altorki NK, Stockert E, Williamson B, Jungbluth AA, Ritter E, et al. Vaccine-induced CD4+ T cell responses to MAGE-3 protein in lung cancer patients. The Journal of Immunology. 2004;**172**(5):3289-3296

[141] Kim S, Castro F, Gonzalez D, Maciag P, Paterson Y, Gravekamp C. Mage-b vaccine delivered by recombinant listeria monocytogenes is highly effective against breast cancer metastases. British Journal of Cancer. 2008;**99**(5):741

[142] Kim W, Liau LM. Dendritic cell vaccines for brain tumors. Neurosurgery Clinics. 2010;**21**(1):139-157

9

Modern Management of Craniopharyngioma

Anirudh Penumaka and Ekkehard Kasper

Abstract

Craniopharyngiomas (CPs) have had a prominent place in neurosurgery due to both the technical difficulty and controversy regarding the optimal treatment of these benign tumors. Harvey Cushing famously described craniopharyngiomas in 1936 as "the most forbidding of the intracranial tumors." Seventy years later, Rutka still wrote: "There is no other primary brain tumor that evokes more passion, emotion, and as a result, controversy than does the CP." Craniopharyngiomas comprise 1–2% of all brain tumors and occur in a bimodal distribution, with 40% of cases occurring between age 5–15 years and 60% occurring at ages >55 years. The differential diagnosis for craniopharyngioma can include a variety of entities, including pituitary macroadenoma, metastasis, Rathke's cleft cyst, colloid cyst, glioma, meningioma, germinoma, abscess, sarcoid, or aneurysm. Imaging characteristics usually include a solid cystic lesion, speckled with calcifications in 50–80% of craniopharyngiomas (especially pediatric patients), as well a presentation with hypopituitarism and diabetes insipidus, which influence clinical thinking toward establishing this diagnosis.

Keywords: craniopharyngioma, endoscopic, radiation, QOL, molecular

1. Clinical case vignette

A 42-year-old woman presented, as a transfer from an outside hospital, with increased forgetfulness, fatigue, as well as intermittent double vision leading to accidents. In addition, she complained of increased thirst and urination. She was concurrently taking lithium and lorazepam for psychiatric reasons. Imaging with CT revealed a large suprasellar mass extending into the third ventricle (**Figure 1**). The patient had laboratory studies performed (**Table 1**) and underwent a formal ophthalmology examination, which revealed red desaturation and a depressed visual field consistent with compressive optic neuropathy.

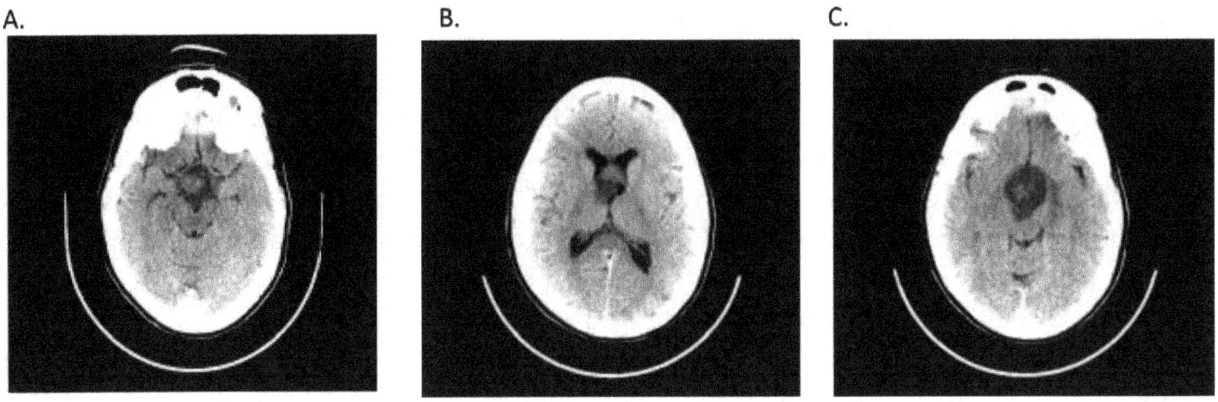

Figure 1. A–C. 4.0 × 3.3 × 4.0 cm, suprasellar mass with cystic and solid components extending into the third ventricle. No calcifications or hydrocephalus is seen.

Laboratory study	Result
Urine specific gravity	1.020
Prolactin	13
Thyroid function tests	TSH 0.17, T_4 4.9, T_3 71, Free T_4 0.8
Luteinizing hormone	< 0.1
Follicle stimulating hormone	< 0.1
IGF-1	201

Table 1. Patient's laboratory findings.

2. Overview

Craniopharyngiomas (CPs) have had a prominent place in neurosurgery due to both the technical difficulty and controversy regarding the optimal treatment of these benign tumors. Harvey Cushing famously described craniopharyngiomas in 1936 as "the most forbidding of the intracranial tumors." Seventy years later, Rutka still wrote: "There is no other primary brain tumor that evokes more passion, emotion, and as a result, controversy than does the CP" [1]. Craniopharyngiomas comprise 1–2% of all brain tumors and occur in a bimodal distribution, with 40% of cases occurring between age 5–15 years and 60% occurring at ages >55 years.

The differential diagnosis for craniopharyngioma can include a variety of entities, including pituitary macroadenoma, metastasis, Rathke's cleft cyst, colloid cyst, glioma, meningioma, germinoma, abscess, sarcoid, or aneurysm. Imaging characteristics usually include a solid cystic lesion, speckled with calcifications in 50–80% of craniopharyngiomas (especially pediatric patients), as well a presentation with hypopituitarism and diabetes insipidus, which influence clinical thinking toward establishing this diagnosis.

3. Subtypes of craniopharyngioma

Craniopharyngiomas are benign lesions which arise from the neuroepithelium in the sellar region. They are classically subdivided into two distinct entities based on both genetic and morphologic differences. Adamantinomatous CP (aCP), primarily seen in childhood, occurs more commonly than papillary CP (pCP), which is more often seen in adults [2]. In histologic sections, adamantinomatous CP is poorly circumscribed, often multi-cystic and calcified, and is associated with β-catenin and epidermal growth factor receptor (EGFR) overexpression. Papillary CP, on the other hand, is well-circumscribed, less calcified, characterized by solid components, and displays less adherence to surrounding structures [2]. Furthermore, pCP is made up of fibrovascular stroma lined by well-differentiated squamous epithelium [2, 3].

In terms of histologic appearance, aCP usually shows nests and trabeculae of epithelium in fibrocollagenous stroma, with peripheral cells showing nuclear palisading, loose central cells termed "stellate reticulum," and abundant keratin, cholesterol crystals, necrosis, and inflammation. Papillary CP is well circumscribed, composed of the cores of fibrovascular stroma lined by well-differentiated squamous epithelium that may separate to form pseudopapillae which resembles squamous papilloma and without xanthogranulomatous inflammation. In molecular staining of these tumors, the lack of expression of CK8 and CK20 keratin suggests a craniopharyngioma, which differentiates them from Rathke's cleft cyst or pituitary pars intermedia. More recently, VE1 staining has also been utilized to identify BRAF mutations which can help to differentiate between Rathke's cleft cyst and craniopharyngioma [4].

4. Origin of craniopharyngioma

Craniopharyngiomas were long thought to arise as an embryonic malformation from the anterior superior margin of the pituitary from residual Rathke's pouch. Due to their embryonic origin, they may even co-opt the blood supply of the wall and floor of the ventricle. More modern studies have demonstrated that aCP can arise due to paracrine actives of β-Catenin mutated cells, whereas pCP can arise via metaplastic transformation [2].

5. Clinical presentation

A triad of symptoms, involving visual impairment, neurological decline, and cognitive compromise, is generally seen in patients presenting with CP. The extent of morbidity associated with CP is closely related to both the specific tumor location and its size. Hypothalamic disease in patients can present as obesity (>50%), diabetes insipidus, thermoregulation disorder, somnolence, sleep apnea, and arrhythmia. Hypothalamic lesions, in particular, are associated with increased rates of neurocognitive decline, and the importance of these neuropsychological issues is evident in that fact that many of these patients continue to report cognitive issues at follow-up, preventing return to previous performance at work or school. Clinically significant hypopituitarism, usually involving several anterior pituitary hormones, occurs in the majority of patients presenting with CP. In nearly 90% of patients who are present with hypopituitarism in the long term, there is a significantly higher mortality risk related to both cardiovascular and cerebrovascular mortality, with an especially higher risk in females compared to males. The evidence from multiple cohorts of patients suggests that the increased exposure to sex hormones also manifests as cardiovascular risk greater in females compared to males [5].

6. Surgical treatment

Surgical resection of craniopharyngiomas is challenging due a number of different considerations, primary of which is the importance of the surrounding neurovascular structures. Risks of surgery include iatrogenic infarction, damage to the optic chiasm, cerebrospinal fluid (CSF) leak, anosmia, CN III–VI palsies, seizures, and a relatively high rate of incomplete resections and recurrences. Anatomic considerations play an especially important role when assessing the appropriate surgical approach. The location of CP can be described in relation to the optic chiasm, as either prechiasmatic (which displaces the chiasm posteriorly) or retrochiasmatic (which displaces the chiasm anteriorly) [6]. While prior classification schemes designed for transcranial surgery described CP in relation to the optic chiasm and the third ventricle, Kassam et al. developed a novel classification based on the infundibulum which was used for the expanded endoscopic approach. Craniopharyngiomas are grouped as pre-infundibular (Type I), trans-infundibular (Type II), or post-infundibular (Type III) locations and occasionally are located in the intraventricular region only (Type IV) [7]. Major variables that can also affect the outcome in these patients include the tumor configuration, patient's age, and medical comorbidities, as well as the surgeon and center experience and availability of essential facilities such as intra-operative imaging, ICU care, and multidisciplinary medical management under endocrinology and radiation oncology.

The risk of recurrence is significant in patients with CP, especially if gross total resection (GTR) is not achieved. Regardless of improved surgical techniques, post-mortem studies performed by Bartlett et al. demonstrated tumor remnants that can remain attached to vital structures such as the optic chiasm, hypothalamus, and/or critical vascular. These remnants can act as a nidus for tumor growth post-surgery, leading to the relatively high rates of recurrence (about 33% within 36 months of surgery) observed in CP patients [8] (**Figures 2** and **3**).

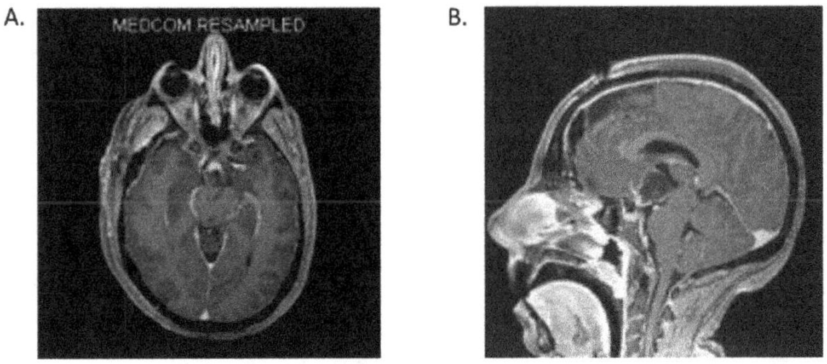

Figure 2. (A) Type IV supra-infundibular craniopharyngioma with intraventricular extension and (B) post-operative MRI demonstrates near-total resection of tumor with the opening of the lamina terminalis.

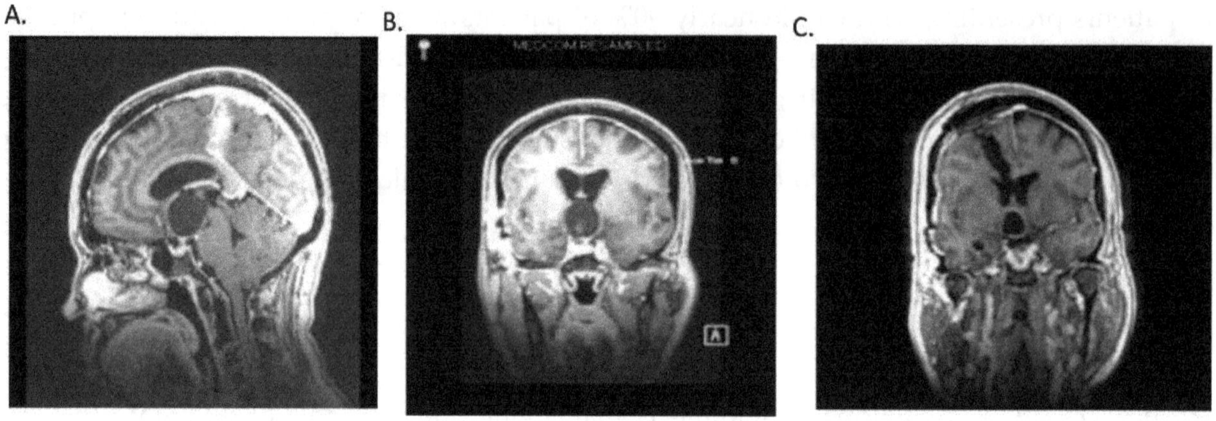

Figure 3. Recurrent cyst at 6 months follow-up. (A) Sagittal and coronal T1; (B) and (C) coronal T1 after transcortical approach involving septostomy with fenestration of the lateral ventricles and third ventriculostomy.

7. Modern case series

Surgical resection can involve an open craniotomy or—alternatively—an endoscopic transnasal approach. A series of open surgical resection employing the frontolateral approach for extensive craniopharyngiomas greater than 4 cm in size reported by Gerganov et al. demonstrated a gross total resection rate (GTR) of 87.5% by microscopic inspection and 62.5% when based on post-operative MRI. Visual improvement was achieved in a significant number of patients (37.5%) in this study. Side effects included new hormonal dysregulation (56.2%) and new diabetes insipidus (75%) [9]. The rate of GTR resection in adults employing this approach is comparable to rates achieved in pediatric patients and compares well with studies employing various other open techniques [10–13]. A complex transpetrosal approach was described by Al-Mefty et al. for CP located in the post-infundibular space [14].

A modern endoscopic series reported by Koutoursiou et al. of 47 adults and 17 children demonstrated comparable GTR, near-total, subtotal, and partial resection rates of 37.5, 34.4, 21.9, and 6.5%, respectively. Major complications reported in this series included CSF leak (23.4% initially and about 10% after the introduction of the modern endonasal flap) and again recurrence rates of 34.4% [15]. An analysis of the reported endoscopic series by Laws et al. found that endoscopic approaches for craniopharyngiomas are suitable especially if tumors are found to have a median intrasellar and subchiasmatic location, with no parasellar solid component and no growth along the pituitary stalk [16]. However, tumors that extend to the optic chiasm and the third ventricle may also be undertaken using the endoscopic approach if performed by experienced teams [17]. For patients requiring re-operation due to recurrence, the endoscopic approach was also shown to be effective, with no significant increase in the rates of complications according to some authors [18]. The endoscopic transsphenoidal approach offers a number of advantages including a surgical view in the axis of the tumor and the optic chiasm. Laws also suggest that while resection of craniopharyngioma is commonly associated with hypopituitarism, the transsphenoidal approach may offer the advantage of the reduced risk of permanent diabetes insipidus [19].

However, the endoscopic approach has certain disadvantages in that it is not well suited for masses that are postchiasmatic or for lesions with prominent lateral extensions [16]. In situations of a recurrent craniopharyngioma after craniotomy, the trans-nasal approach may offer the distinct advantage of a previously untouched approach to the lesion, and an endoscopy enables the surgeon to assess the anatomy of the subchiasmatic and retrochiasmatic regions more closely. If preservation or restoration of vision is the primary goal, this should be strongly considered. Endoscopic approaches also offer the advantage of reducing morbidity associated with brain retraction typically employed during transcranial approaches [16].

A comprehensive literature review performed by Komotar et al. claimed higher rates of GTR with endoscopic surgery compared to open resection (66 vs. 48%), higher likelihood of visual improvement (56 vs. 33%), although with a higher risk of CSF leak (18.4 vs. 2.6%). However, it is important to note that the paper suffers from systematic methodological flaws and selection bias since the mean follow-up time for the patients who underwent open resection in this study was 65 months, as opposed to 25.1 months for the endoscopically treated group [20]. More recent series comparing the two approaches were not able to establish similar significant differences in treatment outcomes.

In conclusion, the endoscopic approach may be most appropriate in certain patients who present with intrasellar and Type I lesions, whereas an open resection, employing a frontotemporal craniotomy, may be more suitable for intra-infundibular or post-infundibular lesions. In patients presenting with cystic CP, stereotactic management is appropriate to aspirate the cystic component of the mass before pursuing other avenues of treatment (e.g., radiation therapy).

8. Radiation therapy for craniopharyngioma

For much of the intervening decades since neurosurgery for CP was described, the debate largely revolved about the optimal treatment strategy, whether aggressive surgical resection or conservative surgery offered patients the best option. Among the two fundamental schools of thought regarding the optimal approach to treat craniopharyngioma, one advocated for GTR for all patients with radiation reserved for salvage therapy due to anticipated adverse effects of radiation [21]. The alternative management suggested was that of a subtotal resection or biopsy and cyst decompression in combination with adjuvant radiation therapy. Advantages of this approach include lower morbidity and improved quality of life [22]. Although the surgical goal remains maximal tumor resection with minimal morbidity, it is estimated that 33% of patients will present with some form of recurrence within the first few years. It is especially clear that radiation therapy is a key element of treatment for these patients with recurrent craniopharyngioma.

In a comprehensive review of a published series of CP patients, Yang et al. were able to demonstrate that subtotal surgery in conjunction with post-operative radiation results in improved survival in patients with CP [23]. This approach employing rather conservative surgery has the advantage of reducing the risks of hypopituitarism and hypothalamic injury. The results from various meta-analyses were corroborated and further expanded with evidence obtained from a large single-center series [24]. Conservative resection with adjuvant radiation was found to be a superior strategy in treating patients. Schoenfeld et al. reported a cohort of patients in which there was no significant difference between GTR and subtotal resection (STR) with radiation therapy (XRT) in terms of overall survival or progression-free survival at 2 years [25], with less endocrinological side effects observed in the STR group.

The key to progression-free survival appears to be conservative surgery with subsequent radiation therapy. Radiation therapy can include various regimens employing conventional external beam radiation therapy, stereotactic radiosurgery, or proton beam therapy. Although radiation offers patients the possibility of treatment with reduced morbidity and mortality, side effects of radiation include enlargement of a cystic tumor, fatigue, skin effects, increased intracranial pressure, and transient or permanent optic neuropathy. Moreover, radiation may have long-term effects such as hypopituitarism in 30–50% of patients, cranial nerve palsies, cerebrovascular diseases, and secondary malignancies. Fortunately, radiation therapy offers excellent outcomes with progressive-free survival between 5 and 10 years of 90% and 100%, respectively [26].

9. Future directions

As with many other cancers, targeted molecular therapies offer the promise of effective treatment without the need for extensive surgery or radiation. Genetic studies of aCP and pCP identified genetic characteristics of each subtype, that may eventually be targeted by specific molecular therapies for CP. Genomic analysis of aCP revealed mutations in CTNNB1 (β-catenin) in nearly all cases and BRAF mutations in most pCPs. These signaling pathways are currently being interrogated for targeted molecular therapies. Inhibitors of the BRAF proto-oncogene employing modern drugs such as Dabrafenib or Vemurafenib, or by prescribing MEK inhibitors, such as Trametinib, are already being studied as therapies for pCP. Inhibition of similar molecular pathways in melanoma, amelanoblastoma, hairy cell leukemia, and pleomorphic xanthoastrocytoma has already demonstrated the clinical promise of these therapies [27, 28]. Multicenter phase-2 clinical trials at the National Cancer Institute are currently underway evaluating BRAF/MEK inhibition in the treatment of craniopharyngioma [27].

Regardless of the therapeutic strategies that are utilized, it is evident that craniopharyngiomas continue to present a distinct oncologic challenge that still needs to be overcome. Quality of life is a key consideration in this disease, and long-term follow up, involving a multidisciplinary team, is a necessary element of care of these patients. The combination of minimally invasive surgery and radiosurgery will, in the near future, result in a minimally morbid approach to this disease to allow patients improved quality of life.

10. Conclusions

Since Cushing's early writings, describing surgery for craniopharyngioma, our strategies to treat this challenging disease have evolved with modern technology to include endoscopic and radiation therapy. The widespread availability and adoption of these techniques have led to endoscopic treatment and radiation therapy becoming indispensable facets of treatment of craniopharyngioma. As our molecular understanding of craniopharyngioma continues to grow, there is considerable hope for the development of effective targeted therapies.

Author details

Anirudh Penumaka and Ekkehard Kasper*

*Address all correspondence to: ekasper@bidmc.harvard.edu

Beth Israel Deaconess Medical Center, Boston, MA, USA

References

[1] Rutka JT. Craniopharyngioma. Journal of Neurosurgery. 2002;**97**(1):1-2. Discussion 2

[2] Larkin SJ, Ansorge O. Pathology and pathogenesis of craniopharyngiomas. Pituitary. 2013;**16**(1):9-17

[3] Hussain I et al. Molecular oncogenesis of craniopharyngioma: Current and future strategies for the development of targeted therapies. Journal of Neurosurgery. 2013;**119**(1):106-112

[4] Schweizer L et al. BRAF V600E analysis for the differentiation of papillary craniopharyngiomas and Rathke's cleft cysts. Neuropathology and Applied Neurobiology. 2015; **41**(6):733-742

[5] Erfurth EM, Holmer H, Fjalldal SB. Mortality and morbidity in adult craniopharyngioma. Pituitary. 2013;**16**(1):46-55

[6] Hoffman HJ. Surgical management of craniopharyngioma. Pediatric Neurosurgery. 1994; **21**(1 Suppl):44-49

[7] Kanaan HA et al. Expanded endoscopic endonasal resection of an olfactory schwannoma. Journal of Neurosurgery. Pediatrics. 2008;**2**(4):261-265

[8] Lober RM, GRt Harsh. A perspective on craniopharyngioma. World Neurosurgery. 2013; **79**(5-6):p. 645-646

[9] Gerganov V et al. Microsurgical resection of extensive craniopharyngiomas using a frontolateral approach: Operative technique and outcome. Journal of Neurosurgery. 2014; **120**(2):559-570

[10] Fahlbusch R et al. Surgical treatment of craniopharyngiomas: Experience with 168 patients. Journal of Neurosurgery. 1999;**90**(2):237-250

[11] Apuzzo ML, ML Levy, H Tung. Surgical strategies and technical methodologies in optimal management of craniopharyngioma and masses affecting the third ventricular chamber. Acta Neurochirurgica. Supplementum (Wien). 1991;**53**:77-88

[12] Karavitaki N et al. Craniopharyngiomas in children and adults: Systematic analysis of 121 cases with long-term follow-up. Clinical Endocrinology. 2005;**62**(4):397-409

[13] Elliott RE et al. Efficacy and safety of radical resection of primary and recurrent craniopharyngiomas in 86 children. Journal of Neurosurgery. Pediatrics. 2010;**5**(1):30-48

[14] Al-Mefty O, Ayoubi S, Kadri PA. The petrosal approach for the total removal of giant retrochiasmatic craniopharyngiomas in children. Journal of Neurosurgery. 2007;**106**(2 Suppl):87-92

[15] Koutourousiou M et al. Endoscopic endonasal surgery for giant pituitary adenomas: Advantages and limitations. Journal of Neurosurgery. 2013;**118**(3):621-631

[16] Cappabianca P, Cavallo LM. The evolving role of the transsphenoidal route in the management of craniopharyngiomas. World Neurosurgery 2012;**77**(2):273-274

[17] Cavallo LM et al. The endoscopic endonasal approach for the management of craniopharyngiomas involving the third ventricle. Neurosurgical Review. 2013;**36**(1):27-37. Discussion 38

[18] Dhandapani S et al. Endonasal endoscopic reoperation for residual or recurrent craniopharyngiomas. Journal of Neurosurgery. 2017;**126**(2):418-430

[19] Laws ER Jr. Surgical outcome in 90 patients with craniopharyngiomas: An evaluation of the transsphenoidal approach. World Neurosurgery 2010;**74**(2-3):254-255

[20] Komotar RJ et al. Endoscopic endonasal compared with microscopic transsphenoidal and open transcranial resection of craniopharyngiomas. World Neurosurgery. 2012;**77**(2):329-341

[21] Matson DD, Crigler JF Jr. Management of craniopharyngioma in childhood. Journal of Neurosurgery 1969;**30**(4):377-390

[22] Kramer S, Southard M, Mansfield CM. Radiotherapy in the management of craniopharyngiomas: Further experiences and late results. The American Journal of Roentgenology, Radium Therapy, and Nuclear Medicine. 1968;**103**(1):44-52

[23] Yang I et al. Craniopharyngioma: A comparison of tumor control with various treatment strategies. Neurosurgical Focus. 2010;**28**(4):E5

[24] Clark AJ et al. A systematic review of the results of surgery and radiotherapy on tumor control for pediatric craniopharyngioma. Child's Nervous System. 2013;**29**(2):231-238

[25] Schoenfeld A et al. The superiority of conservative resection and adjuvant radiation for craniopharyngiomas. Journal of Neuro-Oncology. 2012;**108**(1):133-139

[26] Aggarwal A, Fersht N, Brada M. Radiotherapy for craniopharyngioma. Pituitary. 2013; **16**(1):26-33

[27] Martinez-Gutierrez JC et al. Diagnosis and management of craniopharyngiomas in the era of genomics and targeted therapy. Neurosurgical Focus. 2016;**41**(6):E2

[28] Brastianos PK et al. Dramatic response of BRAF V600E mutant papillary Craniopharyngioma to targeted therapy. Journal of the National Cancer Institute. 2016;**108**(2):djv310

Permissions

All chapters in this book were first published in BTAU, by InTech Open; hereby published with permission under the Creative Commons Attribution License or equivalent. Every chapter published in this book has been scrutinized by our experts. Their significance has been extensively debated. The topics covered herein carry significant findings which will fuel the growth of the discipline. They may even be implemented as practical applications or may be referred to as a beginning point for another development.

The contributors of this book come from diverse backgrounds, making this book a truly international effort. This book will bring forth new frontiers with its revolutionizing research information and detailed analysis of the nascent developments around the world.

We would like to thank all the contributing authors for lending their expertise to make the book truly unique. They have played a crucial role in the development of this book. Without their invaluable contributions this book wouldn't have been possible. They have made vital efforts to compile up to date information on the varied aspects of this subject to make this book a valuable addition to the collection of many professionals and students.

This book was conceptualized with the vision of imparting up-to-date information and advanced data in this field. To ensure the same, a matchless editorial board was set up. Every individual on the board went through rigorous rounds of assessment to prove their worth. After which they invested a large part of their time researching and compiling the most relevant data for our readers.

The editorial board has been involved in producing this book since its inception. They have spent rigorous hours researching and exploring the diverse topics which have resulted in the successful publishing of this book. They have passed on their knowledge of decades through this book. To expedite this challenging task, the publisher supported the team at every step. A small team of assistant editors was also appointed to further simplify the editing procedure and attain best results for the readers.

Apart from the editorial board, the designing team has also invested a significant amount of their time in understanding the subject and creating the most relevant covers. They scrutinized every image to scout for the most suitable representation of the subject and create an appropriate cover for the book.

The publishing team has been an ardent support to the editorial, designing and production team. Their endless efforts to recruit the best for this project, has resulted in the accomplishment of this book. They are a veteran in the field of academics and their pool of knowledge is as vast as their experience in printing. Their expertise and guidance has proved useful at every step. Their uncompromising quality standards have made this book an exceptional effort. Their encouragement from time to time has been an inspiration for everyone.

The publisher and the editorial board hope that this book will prove to be a valuable piece of knowledge for researchers, students, practitioners and scholars across the globe.

List of Contributors

Ilhan Yaylim and Özlem Küçükhüseyin
Institute of Experimental Medicine, Department of Molecular Medicine, Istanbul University, Istanbul, Turkey

Sumeyya Azam
First Affiliated Hospital of Xinjiang Medical University, Xinjiang, Urumqi, PR China

Ammad Ahmad Farooqi and Muhammad Ismail
Institute of Biomedical and Genetic Engineering (IBGE), Islamabad, Pakistan

Ali Metin Kafadar
Department of Neurosurgery, Cerrahpaşa Medical Faculty, Istanbul University, Istanbul, Turkey

Santosh Valvi and Nicholas G. Gottardo
Perth Children's Hospital, Perth, Australia

Ahmed Rizk
Benha University Hospital, Benha, Egypt
Barmherzigen Brüder Hospital, Trier, Germany

Ligia Gabriela Tataranu
University of Medicine and Pharmacy "Carol Davila", Bucharest, Romania
Department of Neurosurgery,"Bagdasar-Arseni" Emergency Clinical Hospital, Bucharest, Romania

Vasile Ciubotaru and Tabita Larisa Cazac
Department of Neurosurgery,"Bagdasar-Arseni" Emergency Clinical Hospital, Bucharest, Romania

Oana Alexandru
Department of Neurology, University of Medicine and Pharmacy of Craiova, Romania

Oana Stefana Purcaru, Daniela Elise Tache, Stefan Alexandru Artene and Anica Dricu
Department of Biochemistry, University of Medicine and Pharmacy of Craiova, Romania

Romana Richterová and Branislav Kolarovszki
Clinic of Neurosurgery, Jessenius Faculty of Medicine of Commenius University in Bratislava, University Hospital in Martin, Martin, Slovak Republic

Alexander Hegarty and Yulia Furlong
Perth Children's Hospital, Perth, WA, Australia
University of Western Australia, Crawley, WA, Australia

Mohammad Abu-Hegazy
Neurology Department, Mansoura University, Mansoura, Egypt
Faculty of Medicine, Mansoura University, Mansoura, Egypt

Hend Ahmed El-Hadaad
Clinical Oncology and Nuclear Medicine Department, Mansoura University, Mansoura, Egypt

Asifur Rahman
Department of Neurosurgery, Bangabandhu Sheikh Mujib Medical University, Shahbag, Dhaka, Bangladesh

Anirudh Penumaka and Ekkehard Kasper
Beth Israel Deaconess Medical Center, Boston, MA, USA

Index

www.ingramcontent.com/pod-product-compliance
Lightning Source LLC
LaVergne TN
LVHW060517210926
848485LV00005B/1095